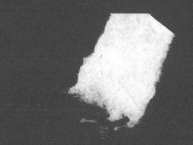

MEDICAL EDUCATION
PAST, PRESENT AND FUTURE
Handing on Learning

Commissioning Editor: Ellen Green
Development Editor: Barbara Simmons
Copy Editor: Jim Killgore
Project Manager: Gail Wright
Text Design: Keith Kail
Cover Design: Stewart Larking

MEDICAL EDUCATION
PAST, PRESENT AND FUTURE
Handing on Learning

SIR KENNETH C. CALMAN
KCB MD PhD FRCS FMedSci FRSE

Vice-Chancellor, University of Durham, UK

Foreword by BILL BRYSON

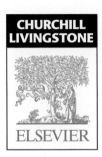

Edinburgh   London   New York   Oxford   Philadelphia   St Louis   Sydney   Toronto   2007

CHURCHILL
LIVINGSTONE
ELSEVIER

First published 2007

ISBN-13: 978-0-443-07473-8
ISBN-10: 0 443 07473 9

British Library Cataloguing in Publication Data
A catalogue record for this book is available from the British Library

Library of Congress Cataloging in Publication Data
A catalog record for this book is available from the Library of Congress

Working together to grow
libraries in developing countries

www.elsevier.com | www.bookaid.org | www.sabre.org

ELSEVIER | BOOK AID International | Sabre Foundation

ELSEVIER your source for books, journals and multimedia in the health sciences
www.elsevierhealth.com

The
publisher's
policy is to use
**paper manufactured
from sustainable forests**

Printed in China

Contents

Foreword

You could be excused for supposing that Sir Kenneth Calman is not one person but several. Doctor, surgeon, professor, author, vice-chancellor of one great British university, chancellor of another, this is a man with a world-class workload.

Even so, it is astonishing to reflect that amid all the challenges, distractions and commitments of his normal occupations he has found the time and energy to produce what would be, for almost anyone else, a lifetime's work—a history of medical education across multiple societies over some five thousand years.

It is an exhilarating journey, but one replete with surprises. Who would have thought, for instance, that the invention of movable type and quality paper was as central to the development of medicine as any technical or clinical breakthrough? Indeed, what comes radiantly through in these pages is that the history of medicine is the history of civilization.

It would be hard to think of a more important or vital job for any society than creating good doctors. Yet, like most people outside the medical profession, I had never really considered what this entails. Insofar as I had thought about it at all, I had always supposed that doctors were people with an aptitude for science, a tolerance for hard work and absurdly long hours, and (one would hope) a more than usual measure of compassion.

What had never occurred to me was how much thought and effort have been put into finding and training suitable physicians through the ages. I would never have dreamed that these are issues that worried and exercised the ancients just as profoundly as those working in medical education today.

As the pages that follow make clear, the history of medicine is not unrelievedly heroic—a point vividly underscored in the story of the Chamberlen family of England, who kept the development of obstetric forceps secret from the world for 150 years, producing generations of needless suffering for the sake of their own enrichment.

It is salutary, too, to be reminded just how rudimentary, and occasionally even primitive, medical treatment could be right up to comparatively modern times, as we are reminded when we read the confident boast of Dr. Benjamin Rush, one of the first doctors trained on American soil, that he could unlock the mystery of every ailment 'with the assistance of a single key—bloodletting', a sentiment that seems to owe more to the Middle Ages than the Enlightenment.

But I think perhaps the most startling fact I encountered in the whole of this astonishing and busy volume was that until well into the 16th century the medical library of the University of Paris consisted of a mere 26 volumes. The inundation of learning that we associate with medicine is, in the grander scheme of things, quite a recent development, it would seem.

Yet, despite the limitations and superstitions of past scholarship, and the occasional frailties and greed of human nature, the history of medical education is, as Sir Kenneth comprehensively documents, mostly a story of good, smart, compassionate people applying themselves in good, smart, compassionate ways to understanding and caring for that greatest of all machines, the human body.

It is a story that takes some telling. Here are all the familiar and important names of medicine—Hippocrates, Galen, Avicenna, Vesalius, Paracelsus—but also such unsung (at least unsung to me) worthies as Abu Bakr Muh al-Razi and the female scholar Trotula, the distaff star of the Salerno School, the first medical school in Europe. And on the chronicle continues through more modern figures such as Jean Fernal, Thomas Linacre, John Caius and Nicholas Tulp, the Dutch surgeon so deftly immortalised in Rembrandt's 'The Anatomy Lesson.' That the author also finds space for Bede, Molière, Shakespeare and countless others of unexpected relevance is both a delight for the reader and a testament to the ambition of the book's scope.

This is a thoroughly enthralling work by someone who knows more, and cares more, about medicine, society and the preparation of young minds than any other person I know. As with Sir Kenneth's earlier classic work, *A Study of Story Telling, Humour and Learning in Medicine*, this is a book to inspire and gladden the heart. It would be hard to imagine such an important subject in better hands.

Bill Bryson

Preface

Writing a book on any subject requires time, research and reflection. There were several times during the long, laborious and intermittent writing of this book that I asked myself why I was doing it. I was often reminded of the preface to Dr. Johnson's great 'Dictionary' where he notes in the bustle and noise of 18th-century London that his writing was pursued not in the 'soft obscurities of retirement, or under the shelter of academick bowers but amidst inconvenience and distraction, in sickness and sorrow.' I have been spared the latter two but being a modern vice-chancellor is not about sitting in academick bowers and thinking and reflecting quietly.

I continued because of my fascination with the subject—how do doctors learn?—and the implications for medical education, for doctors, patients and the public. It began as a history, not written by a historian but an educator, and during the writing it broadened in scope, incorporating a substantial final section on emerging themes and a discussion on how these might be taken forward. It is personal and eclectic and as such suffers from my own weaknesses and prejudices.

At the beginning of the text I refer to three journeys this book takes (the geographical, professional and personal), but the writing of it was an additional journey, and an even more exciting one. I read things, was told things, visited places and heard things during the writing which made me recognise what a fertile field this is for scholarship. In one sense it is a rather long, extended essay.

I was also aware, having myself written reports on medical education, that it is unfair to be too critical of those who have gone before. As I comment in the text, such reports have been written in a particular professional, social and political context. This requires therefore a broad interpretation of outcomes and of initiatives over the years and must make us conscious of the views expressed and how they have been derived. I have tried wherever possible to use the language in the original documents and reports to express the sentiments and context more clearly.

Writing this book has been great fun. I've really enjoyed it, squeezed as it has been between meetings and jotted down in planes and trains. If it has any value, it will be in opening the debate on medical education and encouraging others to challenge the views and pursue more effective and in-depth scholarship. Its basis (my hidden agenda) was to ensure that medical education serves the public, and the endpoint of the process is the improvement of health and healthcare for individuals and communities.

This book was conceived on a bus journey at a meeting of the Association for the Study of Medical Education when I met Ellen Green of Elsevier. She has nurtured this book and gently pressed me to complete it. I should also like to thank Barbara Simmons and her staff at Elsevier for their support.

I would like to thank many colleagues who have listened to my ramblings and commented at seminars and meetings. I would like to thank especially the Margaret Black Fellowship in New Zealand for providing me with an opportunity to present the findings in this book to a critical audience and gain from their experience. As always, libraries have been invaluable and it is a pleasure to acknowledge in particular the National Library of Scotland, the British Library, university libraries in Durham and Glasgow (especially the Special Collections), The Royal Society of Medicine, the British Medical Association, the General Medical Council and the magnificent Wellcome Library in London. The many Royal Colleges in the UK have also been very helpful, as have the staff of the General Medical Council. Sir William Reid, Professor Peter Rubin, Professor Ken Wood, Professor David Knight, Professor Philip Jones, Sir Andrew

Watt Kay and Richard Marshall gave invaluable help. I should also like to thank Julie Bryce and John Blyth from the journal *Medical Education* for their advice and prompting. I should also like to thank the cartoonists who contributed to the book and illuminated the finer points of medical education. A special thanks to Dr Bill Bryson, Chancellor of the University of Durham, for writing the Foreword.

As is expected in such a preface, I would like to thank my family for their tolerance and forbearance: to my wife for her insights into the health service and patient needs and to my daughter, Dr Lynn Calman, for commenting on the final sections of the book. I should especially like to thank my dog, Mungo, for taking me walks and encouraging me to reflect on the difficult parts of this book. My little notebook on such walks contains most of the ideas presented in this volume.

K. C. C.

2006

Durham

PART 1
The Past

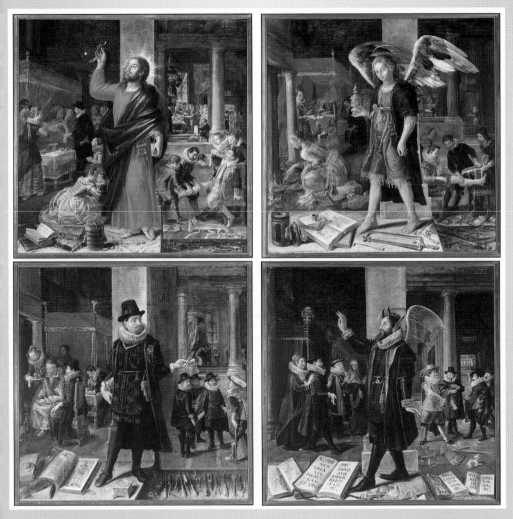

The four guises of the Physician. Anonymous, based on the drawings of Hendrik Goltzius, 1587

In the first a physician attends a critically ill man. The pulse is being taken while the family look on in anguish. To the right we see a surgeon with his assistants examining a man with a head wound, while another treats a patient with a broken leg. The three cases are in great need, and the doctor is represented as the person who can save them.

In the second the doctors are seen as hard at work and patients and the family see them as ministering angels.

The third scene shows the patients well on the way to recovery. They no longer regard the physician as a supernatural being but a mortal who has done his work as a healer satisfactorily.

The fourth scene carries the moral of the story. The patients are fully recovered and no longer remember how serious their illnesses were. The physicians now want to be paid but their bills are considered to be too high. The ungrateful patients now see their saviours as the devil incarnate.

1

Introduction

Properly planned and carefully conducted medical education is the foundation of a comprehensive health service.[1]

The Goodenough Report 1944

*I*t is always a difficult task to tell a story which has no beginning and no end. Medical education is such a story. It begins in prehistory as part of magic, mystery and religion, and it reaches the 21st century with an increasing role for technology and science. But it is not finished, and as a subject continues to evolve and grow. It has developed increasing links with the sciences and with related disciplines such as philosophy, anthropology, education and the arts. The knowledge base in medicine is expanding at an exponential rate, and opportunities to improve health, healthcare and quality of life increase by the day. In such circumstances how can we best educate our doctors and ensure that those working in hospitals or the community keep in touch with developments and put new findings into practice for the benefit of patients and society? Trying to answer this question is the substance of this book, based as it is on an historical analysis of medical education through the centuries.

Our story begins in a medical school, somewhere in the world on the first day of the first term. A small group of students sits nervously in a corner talking, and questions are raised. How did I get here? Do I really want to be a doctor? What will the course be like? What does being a doctor mean? What will the next 50 years of professional life be like? How will I cope? Should I leave now? How will I know where the heart is? How will I deal with my first death? How will I learn to break bad news? These questions, and many others, have been asked by medical students over the centuries.

Similarly, the newly qualified doctor embarking on a career as a specialist in any branch of medicine from family practice to surgery will have a similar series of questions. So too the established specialist, who has a separate set of questions including: How will I keep up to date? How will I maintain my competence?

Patients too ask a similar series of questions. How will my doctor know what's wrong with me? How do I know she is up to date? Will I be treated as person or the appendicitis in bed 6?

Three journeys

This book is about how medical education has tried to address these questions. It involves three related journeys. The first is both chronological and geographical, and moves from China to Egypt, to Greece, Rome and Arabia. It then moves to Salerno, Bologna, Paris Leiden, Edinburgh, Paris, Glasgow, Berlin, London and the USA. It finishes in Canada, Australia, Norway and Israel, and the many new medical schools around the world.

The second journey is that of the student (undergraduate, postgraduate and life-long learners) as they have, over the centuries, gone through a process of learning to care for patients and the public. This latter aspect, life-long learning or continuing professional development (CPD), has become increasingly important in the last few years and is associated with re-accreditation or validation.

Third is the personal journey undertaken by the author as he has read, observed, been a learner (and still is), and taught over a 40-year period. Much has been learned and the final section of the book is a summary of that experience, based on conclusions drawn from the review of the history.

Medical education: a broad view

This book is not a history of medicine, but a history of medical education. The scope is considerable (indeed too broad), and the book will concentrate on a series of case studies and selected writings from a wide range of sources. The history is divided into arbitrary periods, and the text cannot, and does not, claim to be exhaustive or comprehensive. Education is not just about the assimilation of knowledge and skills; it is also about attitudes, behaviour, values and beliefs and the purpose of medicine. This book aims to explore this broader view of medical education as well as its hidden agenda and the secret and tacit knowledge of the doctor.

The book begins in international and worldwide settings but gradually focuses on Great Britain for the more recent documentation. Reading papers by the great and the good of bygone years is humbling. They did their best with the best of intentions. People will read our reports (my reports) in years to come and wonder why we wrote what we did. We hope they will treat us kindly. The main objective is to draw out lessons and experience from different countries, settings and time periods. Themes emerge from the early sections and these form the basis of the conclusions and suggestions for a way forward. As always, the interpretation of data and ideas requires reflection upon the social and political context in which they were derived. This is well described by Hughes.[2] It is also clear that different countries have developed quite different systems of medical education though the outcome in terms of quality and patient care is essentially the same.

A word of interpretation on the use of language and, in particular, the gender used. Many of the documents quoted in this analysis assume that the doctor is male, and many references are to 'him'. At the present time over 50% of medical school entrants in Great Britain are female, and if the author uses the male term too often he is to be forgiven.

Values and beliefs, and the concept of a profession

In any historical review an author will present the information gleaned from original documents in a particular way. Quotations, points of interest and the document coverage will be selective and thus subject to bias. It is perhaps best that the author declare up front the values and beliefs (and prejudices) upon which this book is based.

Before doing so it is worth noting an important publication by Burnham.[3] In it he describes how writers on medical history changed the concept of a 'profession' by their writing and, indeed, created the concept. In one sense they idealised doctors and developed the professional image. Where before surgeons and apothecaries practiced in trades and guilds now they become professionals. So successful have such writers been that every member of the healthcare team is a professional! This historical context is of course interesting, and it is possible that the process could be reversed if medicine once again becomes a trade and subject to external pressures from government and others. The need to stick to the rules, prescribe and treat and be paid for particular forms of treatment could lead to de-professionalisation. The medical 'profession' itself needs to be clear what it wants and how it wishes to be regulated, and the history of regulation is a theme which runs through this book.

So what then are the author's values and beliefs? Many of them were set out in an article written in 1994 on the concept of a profession.[4] They include:

+ Serving patients and the public are at the heart of being a doctor.

✦ It is important to really like teaching and meeting new learners.

✦ Medicine is and has been the author's life, from laboratory to public health. The purpose of medicine for me has been about combining the science with the art.

✦ It is important to continue to learn (obvious but true).

✦ Medical education can and should be improved.

✦ Professional values are important.

✦ Teaching and research go hand in hand.

✦ There should be a continual review of practice, which should be evidence-based.

✦ The medial profession can and should be self regulating, with some important caveats and with the active involvement of the public.

There have been many other histories of medical education, many of which are listed in the bibliography. So what is different about this one? This book is written by someone who is not an historian, but a clinician with a special interest in learning. It is concerned with the interpretation of the historical data, gathered as described above. It is primarily about people and the way in which they have shaped the educational process and facilitated the process of learning. It is about the stories they tell.[5] An essential part of the study is the examination of the role of medicine, since without a clear understanding of this it is difficult to know how to develop a curriculum, how to assess the outcome and how to select doctors. We need to consider what we want to produce, before we decide what is to be learned.

The main audience for this book is medical teachers and all concerned with professional education in healthcare. It may also be of interest to those in other professions, as many of the lessons and possible solutions may be the same. The title of the book has been through various changes, culminating in 'Handing on learning', a phrase which comes from the Hippocratic oath. This makes clear that one of the responsibilities of a doctor is to hand on his or her learning to others. Other translations use the phrase 'impart my knowledge' but 'handing on' seems more active and suggests greater involvement of the learner, with the teacher being a facilitator of the learning process.

The phrase 'handing on learning' can be interpreted in at least three different ways. The first is in the transmission of knowledge, skills and attitudes—the traditional role of the teacher. The second is the transmission of the ability **to** learn, and to understand the need to learn and keep up to date. The need to continually challenge one's own practice and to record the outcome of the process of care is part of this. Finally, there is the handing on of the **love** of learning, of study and of scholarship—not for its own sake but for the benefit of others. This is the sharing part of learning, which is one interpretation from the original Greek (*mathesios, metadosin, poiesasthai*) which captures the real essence behind this book. Learning is something which is worthwhile, and sharing that learning, and handing on what you know for the benefit of patients and the public is a unique experience. Handing on what you know, and to learn from the experience of others, is part of being a doctor. The transmission of enthusiasm for the subject, of making it come alive, is a major part of this. This is the 'contagious' part of the learning process, being 'infected' with the excitement for a subject.

The problem of 'handing on learning' is perhaps best illustrated by a story from Sir James Mackenzie, a general practitioner who changed the face of cardiology while practising in the Northern English mill town of Burnley in the early years of the 20th century. He went to work with a Dr. Briggs in his surgery in Bank Parade and he admired the man enormously. Dr. Briggs seemed to know what to do, and whether patients were unwell or not. But on asking how the doctor did this, Mackenzie noted:

Unhappily Dr. Briggs was quite unable to impart or hand on his secret. He didn't know how he knew. His experience was entirely personal to himself.[6]

The art and the science of medicine

Over the centuries there have been debates about the distinction between the art and the science of medicine. The former emphasises the need for sensitivity, judgement and a concern for people. The latter highlights the need for data, the understanding of biological processes, and the importance of evidence and the testing of hypotheses. Both are, of course, essential if the patient and the public are to be given the best of care and advice. There will always be uncertainty and the need for judgement. The doctor will always have to consider the whole patient and the whole population. This uncertainty is where the art and the science of medicine meet, and throughout the book there will be repeated examples of this relationship.

This volume is also a history of books and libraries and their impact and influence, some having been used and quoted over centuries. These sources bring to us a glimpse of the required knowledge and the methods and mores of doctors in past times. Of course, it is an assumption that such writings reflect actual practice and ways of working, but a reasonable one. Most textbooks of today do the same though the pace of change in knowledge may be such that they become quickly out of date in details of diagnosis and treatment.

So what will be the future of textbooks? With the rapid expansion of knowledge will textbooks become obsolete and be replaced by e-learning on the world wide web? This is a question to which we will return at the end of this book.

Determinants of health

Medical education must relate to what it is that determines the health of an individual or the public. Five issues emerge as determinants of health:

1. Genetic and biological make-up.

2. Environment within which patients live. This includes the

climate and the condition of the air, soil and water. It also includes infection transmitted through any of these environmental routes.

3. Lifestyle: diet, exercise, addictions to alcohol, smoking, drugs, etc.

4. The impact of social and economic factors such as deprivation, employment, poverty, etc.

5. The delivery of a health service and effective therapies.

For most of the 4000 years covered by this book it is the first four determinants which have had the most impact on health. Indeed, at the present time, they are still arguably more important than therapy. Only in the last 200 years has there been sufficient knowledge to change in any effective way the outcome of an illness. Even now, at the start of the 21st century, there are many diseases in which we are unable to change the natural history of the illness. For example, our understanding of genetics has increased enormously but the impact of this knowledge is still limited, though the promise is there. Public health measures and the health implications of deprivation and poverty remain at the top of the agenda in most parts of the world.

Doctors over the centuries have had to learn about these five determinants in order to try to change the natural history of disease. Early on, the effects of climate, the environment, life style and social factors were recognised and, indeed, acted upon with advice on healthy living, diet, etc., although the knowledge base was limited. Study of these determinants set the curriculum for generations of students, the existing knowledge base and theories of disease determining the content. The balance of the curriculum has changed over the centuries as we shall describe, but the same determinants still operate.

The potential to change health is based on our knowledge of how best to maintain health and of the determinants of illness.[7] We already know a great deal, and the key is how to put this current knowledge into practice. This will be a further theme in this book, that of dealing with new knowledge and the diffusion of that knowledge into practice. We need more research to improve the health of the population. But we also need to act on what we already know. Hence the importance of the education of doctors and their need to keep up to date. The potential to change health is enormous.

Many of the efforts to improve health, to understand disease and to deliver an effective health service are carried out in conjunction with other professional groups: scientists, epidemiologists, nurses, dieticians, pharmacists, etc. The doctor cannot work alone but must be part of a team, delivering improved health and patient care. This ability to work effectively with other professionals is a key part of medical education, and this has also changed over the years and will be reflected in the book.

The scope of this book covers the period from 4000 BCE until the present day. Surprisingly perhaps, it is the most recent period which is most interesting and has shown the most change. This is not only in terms of the huge development in knowledge but also in relation to the considerable changes in medical education and our understanding of the learning process. Indeed the last 15–20 years have seen significant and important changes. It has been difficult to know how best to deal with these since time is needed to reflect on the outcome of the changes. Thus, only a brief summary is provided of the current initiatives, and it is left for others to comment on the long-term implications.

Emerging themes

Another function of this book is to identify themes which emerge from the historical background and consider them in a modern context. For some of these themes there are answers, for others research and debate must continue. This differs from other books on the history of medical education in that it tries to identify major questions and to provide some answers, and this analysis can be found in the second part of the book. A brief discussion of the themes is set out below to assist readers in the interpretation of each section and chapter. The themes are ones which the author has identified; others may be noted by different readers. If one of the purposes of the book is to stimulate discussion then the topics below are good starting points.

Note that there is considerable overlap between themes; this is both inevitable and necessary if the complexity of the role of the doctor is to be understood.

The role of medicine. What is medicine for? What are the roles of a doctor? What are the boundaries with other professional groups, and how have they changed? How should doctors interact with patients and the public? It is essential that roles are clear before the educational implications are developed. The doctor in society is a subset of this theme. The doctor has roles as educator, advocate and agent for change. He or she is a teacher, a mentor, advisor and friend.

The quest for competence. There is a long history of trying to identify the qualities of the 'good' doctor and how this might be measured. Again, it is necessary that this should be clear before learning programmes begin.

Who should be a doctor? Considerable resource has gone into identifying and selecting medical students over the generations. It is as active an issue at the start of the 21st century as it was in the time of Hippocrates.

Learning medicine. This covers the nature of the curriculum, the learning resources required, methods of assessment, preparation of the teacher, and the different aspects of under-graduate, postgraduate and continuing education.

Beyond learning, discovering new knowledge. One of the features of medicine which might therefore be reflected in medical education is the importance of research and development. Learning is the process of discovering what someone else already knows. Beyond learning is about finding out new ways of caring and of understanding disease. It also includes the challenge of change and the ways in which change is implemented. Numerous references will be made to the difficulties of diffusion of innovation and how new knowledge is assimilated into practice. 'Medical magnets' is a phrase which will be used repeatedly in this book and needs some explanation. It illustrates the journey to the best. One of the most interesting aspects of the history of medical education has been the way in which students from all parts of the world have been attracted and gravitated to various teachers and medical schools worldwide. These have varied from generation to generation but leadership has been a constant feature of the system, and continues to this day.

Structure and aim

The book is set out in three parts. The first (and largest) is a review of the history of medical education over the ages. This is followed by a development of the major themes which have emerged, with comments and some suggestions as to how the issues might be tackled. Finally, there is a short section with some conclusions and pointers for the future.

The aim of the book is to provide a forum for the discussion of issues in medical education, based on a review of the past and a look into the future. The book will be judged to be successful if that debate is stimulated.

REFERENCES

1. Report of the Inter-Departmental Committee on Medical Schools (The Goodenough Report) London: HMSO; 1944.
2. Hughes B. The many and conflicting histories of medical

education in Canada and the United States: An introduction to the paradigm wars. Medical Education 2005; 39: 613–21.

3. Burnham J C. How the idea of profession changed the writing of medical history. Med Hist Suppl 1998; (18): 1–95.

4. Calman K C. The Profession of Medicine. BMJ 1994; 309: 1140–3.

5. Calman K C. A study of storytelling humour and learning in medicine. London: The Stationery Office; 2000.

6. Wilson R M. The beloved physician: Sir James Mackenzie. London: John Murray; 1926.

7. Calman K C. The potential for health. Oxford: Oxford University Press; 1998.

2

Ancient medicine: the beginnings of the art

I think I have discussed this subject sufficiently, but there are some doctors and sophists who maintain that no one can understand the science of medicine unless he knows what man is; that anyone who proposes to treat men for their illnesses must first learn of such things…I do not believe that any clear knowledge of nature can be obtained from any source other than a study of medicine and then only through a mastery of this science.[1]

Hippocrates, *The Tradition in Medicine*

Where to begin? Where to start the story? The particular interest of this history is education, and as it will be based on the evidence available this must exclude those aspects which are only supposition.

The earliest records of medical people can be found on tablets of clay from Mesopotamia, that ancient land between the Tigris and the Euphrates rivers where the Sumerian civilisation began. In the Wellcome Museum there is the seal of a Sumerian physician who lived around 3000 BCE, and a similar Babylonian seal can be found in the Louvre Museum dating from 2300 BCE. The Code of Hammurabi, a law code drawn up by the sixth king of the first Babylonian dynasty (1948–1905 BCE) and also preserved in the Louvre, contains regulations relating to medical practice. It says, for example, that:

...if a doctor shall treat a gentleman and shall open an abscess with a bronze knife and shall preserve the eye of the patient he shall receive ten shekels of silver... If the doctor shall open an abscess with a bronze knife and shall kill the patient or shall destroy the sight of his eye, his hands shall be cut off.[2]

An example of early evidenced-based practice?

In India, the earliest Sanskrit document, the Rig-Veda, written about 1500 BCE, indicates that treatment of disease was mainly about spells and incantations. It was in surgery that Hindus excelled. Plastic surgery was pioneered in India with the technique of skin grafting to replace damaged noses. Operative procedures were taught using hollow plant stems, leaves and gourds as models for practice.[3,4] Perhaps the first recorded use of simulators in surgical practice.

However, there is insufficient detail to discuss these developments at length. Instead we will move first to China and record the details of medical education in that ancient land. But why begin here? Perhaps the best reason is *The Yellow Emperor's Canon of Internal Medicine*, a manuscript probably dating from 1000 BCE and still in use in modern China. Some 3500 years old and it remains a working document, still debated and discussed. Other medical texts may be older but none has this immediacy and relevance—a remarkable continuity of learning resources.

CHINESE MEDICINE

But to begin at the beginning. China has a rich and fascinating intellectual tradition. Its philosophy, found in the wisdom of sages such as Confucius, has captured the world's imagination and has had a major impact on developments in medicine and related areas. There are many Chinese legends surrounding the beginnings of medicine, and the most important feature Shen

Nung, the Divine Husbandman, and Huang Ti, the Yellow Emperor.

Shen Hung is said to have lived between 2838 and 2698 BCE and is considered the founder of Chinese medicine. He studied the effects of hundreds of herbs and established the art of medicine. He remains venerated as the father of medicine and there are shrines to him in many cities.

Huang Ti (2698–2598 BCE) is credited with writing *Nei Ching*, or the *The Yellow Emperor's Canon of Internal Medicine*, in conjunction with one of his chief ministers Ch'I Po. This book is one of the oldest and greatest medical classics and has formed the basis of much of Chinese medicine. It was probably first written down in the Chou dynasty (1000 BCE) and represents a tradition and method of learning practiced up to the present day. Based on a dialogue and question–and–answer format it is readily read and assimilated. It is a sort of catechism which is presented as a series of conversations between Huang Ti and Ch'I Po. It covers theory of disease, humoral pathology, pulse indications, anatomy, health conservation, principles of treatment, acupuncture, diet and other topics. While much of the anatomy is inaccurate, there are some fascinating insights. For example:

All the blood flow is under control from the heart.

The heart regulates all the blood in the body.

Blood flows continually in a circle and does not stop.[5]

These seem to predate Harvey though not with the physiological evidence.

In the Yellow Emperor's classic text, it is the dialogue which is of interest. For example:

The Emperor asks: "When people grow old they cannot give birth to children. Is this because they have exhausted their strength in depravity or is it because of natural fate?"

Ch'I Po answered "When a girl is seven years of age she begins to change, her teeth and her hair grows longer. When she reaches her 14th year she begins to menstruate and is able to become pregnant and the movement in the great thoroughfare pulse is strong. When the girl reaches 21 the emanations from the kidneys are regular, the last tooth has come out and she is fully grown. When the woman reaches 28 her muscles and bones are strong, her body is flourishing and fertile. When the woman reaches 35 the pulse indicating the "sunlight" deteriorates, her face begins to wrinkle and her hair begins to fall. When she reaches 42 the pulse in the three regions of Yang deteriorates, in the upper body her entire face is wrinkled, and her hair begins to turn white. When she reaches 49 she can no longer become pregnant. Her menstruation is exhausted, her body deteriorates and she is no longer able to bear children."

The Yellow Emperor asked, "When the physicians treat diseases, do they treat each differently from the others and can they all be healed?"

Ch'I Po answered "Yes they can all be healed according to the physical features of the place where one lives."

The Emperor said "I should like to be informed about the essential doctrines of healing."

Ch'I Po answered "The most important requirement of the art of healing is that no mistakes or neglect occur."

The Yellow Emperor asked "What constitutes a healthy person?"

Ch'I Po answered " Man has one exhalation to one pulse beat which is then repeated."

Such a small selection of the *Canon* (translated by Ilza Veith[6]) continues to provide a source and a way of learning which is still used in China today.

Philosophy has always played a great part in Chinese medicine and it has sometimes been difficult for the unversed to understand the background to the practice of the art. Students learning medicine would need to have been fully aware of the philosophical base. For example, an important principle is that of 'Tao' or 'the Way', which is concerned about how to lead one's life and achieve harmony. Another key concept is that of Yin and Yang, which are two primal opposing but complementary forces. Everything under the sun originates from them, and they are generally represented by a circle, the great or absolute void within which the two bodies are drawn. This circle is surrounded by eight symbols, each representing different objects. A third important principle or doctrine is that of the five elements—metal, wood, water, fire and earth. The human being is a balanced mixture of all these forces and elements. Ill health is the result of an imbalance.

The great philosopher Confucius (551–479 BCE) was very influential in the way that Chinese medicine developed, or rather why, from such exciting beginnings, it did not. He spent much of his life educating a small group of disciples, and Confucianism is seen as synonymous with learning. It is sometimes viewed as a system of philosophy, with such key concepts as Jen, the love of men, and the need for no material reward, virtue and righteousness, decorum, code of conduct, and the superior person is one who has arrived there through devotion. Learning is a key part of this.

However, the opposite is the consequence of such beliefs; that is the wish to remain the same: 'A man is worthy of being a teacher who gets to know what is new by keeping fresh in his mind what he is already familiar with'. And again: 'The master said, "I transmit, but do not innovate. I am truthful to what I say and devoted to antiquity"'.[7]

Perhaps this was the reason why such a promising beginning (with Shen Hung and Ch'I Po) slowed down. However, there were some other remarkable advances and developments.

In the Chou dynasty (1122–255 BCE) the medical department was well organised. There were two high-grade doctors, four lower grade doctors, two registrars, two clerks and twenty servants. There were also specialists in dietetics, and a surgical department, although surgeons were always of a lower grade.

Doctors were concerned with health and believed that prevention was better than cure. Confucius taught that: 'The sage does not treat those who are ill but those who are well.' Hygiene was encouraged, as was healthy living. Confucius said: 'If a man is irregular in his sleep, intemperate in his eating, and immoderate in his work, sickness will kill him'.[8] Hospitals were available for those who were unwell or disabled. Acupuncture was widely practised.*

The pulse was a key part of the examination of the patient, and formed the basis of medical practice. The nature, location, course and treatment of every disease depended on the pulse. Interestingly, *Nei Ching* states there are four standard methods of diagnosis: observation, auscultation, interrogation and palpation. Palpation is examination of the pulse. Wang Shu-ho in ACE 280 wrote *Mo Ching* (or *Pulse Classic*) in ten volumes, and it is considered the standard work on the subject.

Medical schools were set up and there were state examinations as early as the 10th century BCE. The Chou Rituals state that:

...at the end of the year work of the doctors is examined and the salary of each fixed according to the results shown. If the statistics show that out of ten cases treated all get well, every satisfaction may be felt. If, however, one out of ten dies, the results may be regarded as good, if two out of ten die, the results are only fair, if three out of ten die they are poor, if four out of ten they are bad.[9]

Formal medical education was first started in the T'ang dynasty (AD 618–906) and mostly confined to the Imperial Court. In the Sung dynasty (AD 960-1279), regular schools were organised, first in the capital and then in other parts of China. In CE 1076, an Imperial College was established, and

---

* Acupuncture was first introduced into Europe by a Dutch surgeon, Ten-Rhyne, who wrote an article on the practice which appeared in London in 1683.

300 students enrolled. They were taught medicine, surgery and acupuncture. Each candidate was examined in the theory of the subject, orally and clinically. In the first examination, the subject matter was *The Yellow Emperor's Canon of Internal Medicine*, including the structure of the body, functions of the organs, and methods of treatment. In the oral examination, there were questions on materia medica, typhoid fever, actions of drugs, modes of infection and causes of disease. In the clinical examination, the candidate had to demonstrate the results of his treatment and the reasons for adopting the methods employed. There were six examination questions, and the successful candidates were classified into two grades. The first-grade candidates were given official appointments and ordered to compile and write medical books, or engage as teachers. Those who obtained second grades were given a licence to practise. Those who failed were ordered to change profession. Officers, teachers and other medical staff were appointed by competitive examinations.

Medical education evolved little over this period and the schools gradually declined and ceased to exist. However, they were revived in 1262 CE. By this time the course covered ten subjects: diseases of adults and children; diseases due to wind; obstetrics and diseases of women; diseases of the eye, mouth and teeth, and throat; fractures and wounds; swellings and sores; acupuncture; charms and incantations. A wide range of textbooks was used.

Teachers were held responsible for the progress of their students. Those who did not compel students to attend lost a month's salary. Fines were imposed for more than one offence. If a teacher was found incompetent, lax in discipline and lazy in teaching, he was fined a half month's salary for the first offence and one month's salary for the second offence. For a third offence he was referred to a disciplinary board.

All candidates were to be above 30 years of age, of good medical knowledge, high moral character and esteemed by their friends. Out of all the candidates, 100 were chosen from each place, but in examinations held in the capital, only 30 candidates were chosen, an early example of norm referencing. Women doctors were also given recognition.

A fascinating book by Elizabeth Hsu, *The Transmission of Chinese Medicine*, written in 1999, is a contemporary study of medical education in China. She returned to China to learn traditional medicine as a Cambridge-based ethnographer and anthropologist. Learning is grounded in medical texts and practice, and *The Yellow Emperor's Canon* is still used as a major source. There are three modes in the transmission of learning:

1. **Secret.** This is intentionally secret and is crucial for the social relationship between the pupil and the teacher.

2. **Personal.** This depends on the mentor–follower relationship and is about the personal transmission of knowledge.

3. **Standardised.** This is the Western way of thinking and acquiring knowledge.[10]

The training of a disciple took nine years. Three years for the master to evaluate the disciple, three years for the disciple to consider his choice of master, and the last three years for the master to transmit essential knowledge. A disciple (as opposed to a student) was expected to know and accept all aspects of the master's personality—equivalent to the respect that a son has for a father. The study by Hsu provides an up-to-date reference on current methods of learning traditional Chinese medicine and shows how little has changed in both the knowledge base and learning methods over the last few thousand years.

MEDICAL EDUCATION IN ANCIENT EGYPT

Our knowledge of medical education and medicine in ancient Egypt is based on an astonishing range of material in the form of papyri, statues, inscriptions and buildings and monuments.

They provide a wide range of evidence upon which to reconstruct the past. Physicians in ancient Egypt were famed for their skill, and people and physicians travelled widely to gain and give medical care. Homer refers to them in the *Odyssey* when he notes: 'In Egypt the men are more skilled in medicine than any of human kind'.[11] Herodotus records that Egyptian specialist physicians attended Royal personages in distant lands. One of the key findings of this book is that there are medical 'magnets' which attract pupils and patients, and we will see it as a recurring theme in all ages and places.

Key resources exist in the form of papyri written between 3000 BCE (Edwin Smith Papyrus) and 1200 BCE (the Carlsberg Papyrus) and include the Berlin, Brooklyn Museum, Chester Beatty, Ebers, Kahoun, Hearst, and London papyri. The Ebers Papyrus is the longest and was written in 1550 BCE, in the 9th year of the reign of Amenophis I. It contains considerable medical knowledge, including physiology and pathology. In this papyrus there is a chapter entitled 'Beginnings of the secret physician; knowledge of the heart's movement and knowledge of the heart'.[12] Apart from the knowledge of the heart which existed at the time, it is also interesting to note the use of the term 'secret'. Once again this will be a recurring theme: that the physician has 'secret knowledge' and can use this for his own benefit, and can exclude others from the inner circle.

The Ebers Papyrus contains many accurate clinical descriptions and ethical precepts very like the Hippocratic Oath in sentiment and expression. As will be mentioned on several occasions, this link between Egyptian and Greek medicine is strong. The main difference was that whilst medicine in Egypt was in the hands of the priests, in Greece the practitioner was independent of a religious link.

The Edwin Smith Papyrus (sometimes called the 'Secret book of the physician') is probably the oldest surgical treatise in the world and has been attributed to Imhotep, the great physician and architect who built the first pyramid around 3000 BCE and was also a high priest of Heliopolis. Imhotep is worthy of further note. He was regarded by Osler as the first physician to emerge from the mists of antiquity, and should be regarded as the father of medicine.[13] He had a high reputation as a magician and physician. He was said to be the Grand Vizier to King Zoser, who lived between 2980 and 2900 BCE. He was worshiped as a god for many centuries, and numerous statues and temples were built in his honour at Memphis, Thebes, Philae and Sais. His statues show him as almost human, reading a scroll or thinking. He is buried near Memphis.

Imhotep is described as the god who looks after the sick; another testimony says that he visited the suffering 'to give them peaceful sleep and heal their pains and diseases'.[14] He is important in educational terms in the methods of transmission of learning. Breasted, in his *History of Egypt*, notes that people sang of Imhotep's proverbs centuries later—the power of the oral transmission of knowledge.[15] His influence is significant. J.B.Hurry has written:

> *Strange it is that the claims of Imhotep to be recognised as the tutelary deity of medicine have been so neglected. Many centuries before the exodus of the Israelites from Egypt, long before the recognition of Asklepios by the Greeks as their legendary God of Medicine, long before the days of Homer, long before the birth of Hippocrates, there lived in Egypt a magician–physician so famous for his skill in healing disease that he became recognised eventually as the Egyptian God of Medicine. To him surely belongs the highest place in our Hagiography; to him should all physicians look up as the patron spirit or the ars medendi, as the emblematic God of Medicine.*[16]

Indeed, the Greeks identified him with their own deity, Asklepios. He is a true role model and hero.

Egyptian medicine begins in magic and with the priest-hood, and there were different orders among practitioners. The priest–physician was the highest, and lay physicians the next rank. They all had the important ability to write, and physicians were often depicted with a writing instrument in statues and reliefs. Students of medicine were not drawn only from the ruling classes; industry and talent were said to be the only conditions imposed upon those who sought to study. They were an unruly mob as the following quotations show:

> *Let not idleness overtake thee else thou shalt be severely chastised. Hang not thy affection on pleasures and take care that the books fall not from thy hand. Exercise thyself in conversation and speak with thy superiors in learning.*[17]

> *It has been reported to me that thou neglectest thy studies and seekest only pleasure, wandering from tavern to tavern. But what profiteth the odour of beer? Avoid it; for it drives people away from thee, impoverishes thy wits, and likens thee to a broken oar upon the deck of a ship.*[18]

Such extracts from translations of papyri show that little has changed.

Students lived in houses attached to the school, under the inspection and discipline of their teachers. Instruction was founded on the sacred books, the last six of which related to medicine. These covered parts of the body, disease, surgical instruments and operations, materia medica, diseases of the eye and diseases of women. The assumption is that students also received practical instruction on the examination and treatment of the sick. In Egypt, patients were brought to the temple to await help from the priest, so there was always a source of patients for instruction and care. Such temple schools were associated with other scholars, such as judges, astronomers and mathematicians. The greatest schools were at Heliopolis, Memphis, Thebes, Sais and Chennu.

Subjects covered in medical training included a study of the pulse, history taking, general appearance, state of consciousness, smell, and examination of urine and faeces. Surgery included the treatment of wounds, and there was a huge range of medications, including decoctions, infusions, lozenges, pills, pessaries, suppositories, ointments and eye drops. The theory of humours, developed later by the Greeks, was the prevailing paradigm of health. Students were taught to be kind and deal gently with patients, and the sick were never seen to be untouchable. In the Ebers Papyrus, it is written: 'Go to him and do not abandon him'[19], and there are a number of maxims which set out ethical duties.

Books would have been difficult to get and keep. The ability to write would have allowed information to be transmitted and taken with the student upon leaving the school. Memory was another great asset, and the use of proverbs (referred to by Imhotep) may have been one way in which learning could be retained. This is another theme which runs for many centuries in medical learning—use of proverbs, questions and answers and catechismal-like statements.

Attached to the temples were the per-ankh or 'houses of life'. These were not formal medical schools but acted as centres for documentation, where books and manuscripts were collected and copied. They would thus act as resource centres for students or visitors. It is difficult to find any evidence of examination processes from the papyri. Large collections of books could be found in such places, and as late as the 3rd century CE Galen wrote that Greek physicians still visited the library of the school of Memphis. The creation of the great university and library at Alexandria was a natural outcome of this process.

As has been mentioned, the ability to write was crucial. The earliest recorded physician, Hesy-Re, had himself portrayed with a scribe's palette. Some ostraca (flakes of limestone or potsherds used for writing on as they were cheaper than papyrus) covered with medical recipes have been found and interpreted as student exercises.

Specialisation seems to have been common. A table of physicians has been found listing those who specialised in diseases of different organs. There were also medical aids, nurses, masseurs and specialists in bandaging. Herodotus notes:

The art of medicine is thus divided: each physician applies himself to only one disease and not more. Some are for the eyes, others for the head, others for the teeth, others for the intestines, and others for intestinal disorders.[20]

Not all agreed with this statement but some from of specialisation seems clear.

Egyptian medicine did not progress beyond this stage and its concepts and therapies were taken up by the Greeks, which is the subject of our next section. There is a huge debt owed to Egyptian medicine and its legacy lives on. The basic principles of learning medicine were established in this long period between 3000 and 500 BCE.

A co-incidence of symbolism: a quiver of arrows

It is traditional to use the symbol of the caduceus to represent medicine. This symbol derives from Hermes or Mercury, the winged messenger, and is a staff intertwined by two snakes. Greek mythology suggests that Hermes came across two fighting snakes and, throwing his wand at them, they became intertwined and stopped fighting. The head of the staff generally has two wings. It is important that this should be distinguished from the wand of Aesculapius, god of medicine, whose staff is rough hewn and intertwined with a single snake. The mythological background suggests that the Hermes story of the creation of the caduceus began around 600 BCE.

This symbol is, however, somewhat ambiguous. Hermes is also the patron of thieves, not a particularly good association for doctors. Snakes have often had a mystical connection to medicine, and they have an association with rebirth. Throughout history, the link between Hermes and medicine has always been disputed. Although the connection between medicine and the symbol of the caduceus goes back many centuries,[21] it essentially dates to 1902 when the US Army adopted it as the symbol of the Medical Corps.

When the symbol was used in the USA, there was considerable argument. Even Fielding Garrison, probably the most distinguished medical historian of his day, was challenged on this point when he described the caduceus as the symbol of the non-combatant in war.[22] Part of the problem was that the English and Prussian Armies had used the Aesculapian staff from the 1860s, and so its meaning may have been misinterpreted. Interestingly, the Royal College of Physicians and Surgeons of Glasgow and the Royal College of Surgeons of Edinburgh both use the staff of Aesculapius.

Readings in both Chinese and Egyptian medicine, however, suggest that another symbol may be more appropriate: that of the arrow, or quiver of arrows. The Chinese character for a doctor is a complex one that comprises three elements—a quiver of arrows, a hand grasping a weapon, and the symbol for a sorcerer or priest. The character denotes that the priest uses strong weapons to kill or drive away the demons of sickness.[23] Later, the lower part of the character was modified to be the symbol for wine. This may be seen as indicating a change in the role of medical practitioners, and reflects the use of alcohol, either as a constituent of medication or as a propitiatory offering.

In hieroglyphic writing, the word for doctor *swnw* (pronounced sewnew in English) also contains a quiver of arrows or a single arrow.[24] The reason for this symbol is not clear, but it has been suggested that it is because the doctor is one skilled in removing arrows. Whatever the derivation, it is striking that in two different cultures at about the same time (2500–1500 BCE) the symbol of the arrow is chosen (in combination with others) to signify the doctor. This predates the legend of the caduceus by several hundred years.

Perhaps, therefore, we should rethink the symbol of the doctor. Remove the caduceus and replace it with an arrow, a symbol of precision and of accuracy in attacking disease and illness. The quiver of arrows suggests that there are several ways of doing this, and the doctor is not limited to one therapeutic method. In any case, no ancient Greek would have thought of Hermes as a god of medicine. Apollo was the favourite, the archer god, whose arrows bring healing or disease, and whose hymn, the Paean, means the 'Healing song'. The arrows of Apollo are seen as smeared either with disease or cure. The sick Greek man always prayed to Apollo first and foremost (a woman might start with Artemis, Apollo's archer sister).

Thinking ahead it would also be easier to present the doctor with an arrow on graduation rather than a caduceus and the Chiron, one of the symbols of the Royal College of Physicians of Edinburgh (a centaur with a bow and arrow), would become immediately relevant. The Worshipful Company of Apothecaries already has Apollo as part of its crest. Is it too fanciful to suggest that 'arrow clubs' might spring up everywhere, where doctors could meet and discuss new and exciting methods of treatment? Hospitals and postgraduate centres would use arrows in their coat of arms. Fanciful perhaps, but possible.

MEDICAL EDUCATION IN ANCIENT GREECE

The great debt of Greek medicine to that of Egypt has already been noted. While much of the focus is on Hippocrates and his writing, the towering figure of Imhotep should not be forgotten. This section will concentrate on the educational implications of medicine in ancient Greece rather than on the treatment of disease or on its aetiology.

Hippocratic writings are a primary source of information on education and the process of learning in ancient Greece. As noted in previous sections, the lack of books meant that some other format had to be used for learning, and aphorisms provided the means. Remembering such short statements was at the heart of the learning process and allowed the trainee physician to move around the country armed with basic medical knowledge. Teaching was almost always oral and the vision of Hippocrates teaching under the plane tree on the Island of Cos is a very powerful one.

The writings of Hippocrates (brought together between 430 and 330 BCE) provide a glimpse of the difficulties of learning medicine. For example, in the translation of theory into practice, it is noted in *On Regimen in Acute Diseases*: 'Finally medical teaching is subject to the difficulty which besets all doctrine, that is indeed to say what should be done in a particular case when one is confronted by it, but that one cannot give general advice about what should be done without seeing the particular case'.[25]

Some of the writings are clearly for a medical audience but others are for the public at large. For example, in the introduction to *On The Nature of Man* Hippocrates states: 'This lecture is not intended for those who are accustomed to hear discourses which inquire more deeply into the human constitution than is profitable for medical study'.[26]

Learning communication skills is essential in medical training and there is a comment on this in *On The Nature of Man*: 'Thus the physician in his practical daily activity is in need of oratorical skill, and it is not astonishing that he should train as a speaker'.[27] This is an important statement in relation not only to individual patients but also the ability to communicate to a wider audience. It fits well with the derivation of the word 'doctor' which means teacher. Libraries were important and the great one at Alexandria, founded in 332 BCE nine years before Alexander's death, had 70,000 books.

Practising medicine in ancient Greece did not require an examination, and there was no set period of training. Nor were there any restrictions to practice. Reputation was key, a perspective which remains today (reputations matter to patients). Doctors were able to move around and set up shop wherever they wished, and practices were classified as trades or businesses. It was seen as a 'techne' or craft, whose learning was empirical in origin. Knowledge was passed on from family to family, and again the possible 'secret' nature of the knowledge was clear. Without books, this was the only way in which knowledge could be passed on. Therefore, the teacher was a key individual, as he had the knowledge and the secrets. A reference from the teacher (for example, 'I was a pupil of Hippocrates') was important, and such teachers acquired a reputation and attracted students. Such 'medical magnets' have already been mentioned as a common theme in this book. In ancient Greece, the Schools of Cos and Cnidos were the most famous. Epidaurus was another important centre, situated close to the theatre and with a special place for those dying. The status of doctors was mixed, although Eryximachus, the doctor in Plato's *Symposium*, gets a place at the table with poets and statesmen, even though he is pictured as rather pompous but liked.

The breadth and depth of knowledge required to be learned was also seen to be relevant, as this extract from Hippocrates' *Tradition in Medicine* shows:

> *I think I have discussed this subject sufficiently, but there are some doctors and sophists who maintain that no one can understand the science of medicine unless he knows what man is; that anyone who proposes to treat men for their illnesses must first learn of such things. Their discourse tends to philosophy as may be seen in the writings of Empedocles and all of the others who have ever written about nature; they discuss the origins of man and of what he was created....I do not believe that any clear knowledge of nature can be obtained from any source other than a study of medicine and then only through a thorough mastery of this science.*[28]

Selection of potential doctors is also covered in the Hippocratic writings. The sons of physicians were the obvious choices but this was not exclusive. Apart from slaves and women, anyone could become a student, and there was to be an agreement as set out in the *Oath* that the student would be looked after as if he was a son, and vice versa:

> *To hold my teacher in this art equal to my own parents; to make him partner in my livelihood; to consider his family as my own brothers, and to teach them this art, if they want to learn it, without fee or indenture; to impart precept, oral instruction, and all other instruction to my own sons, the*

sons of my teacher, and to pupils who have taken the Physician's oath and no other.[29]

The desirable characteristics of the medical student are listed in the *Canon*:

For a man to be truly suited to the practice of medicine he must be possessed of a natural disposition for it, the necessary instruction, favourable circumstances, education, industry and time. The first prerequisite is a natural disposition, for a reluctant student renders every effort vain. But instruction in the science is easy when the student follows a natural bent, so long as care is taken from childhood to keep him in circumstances favourable to learning and his early education has been suitable. Prolonged industry on the part of the student is necessary if instruction firmly planted in the mind is to bring forth good and luxuriant food.[30]

Such sentiments, and in particular 'prolonged industry', were to be reflected centuries later in Osler's *Masterword in Medicine*.[31]

There was no real curriculum in ancient Greek medicine. The theoretical basis was based on the four humours (blood, phlegm, yellow bile and black bile) and the four qualities (hot, cold, dry and moist). We will see throughout this history how such paradigms of health and illness determine the curriculum and the content of the learning. What we do know is that the knowledge base was wide and not solely related to therapeutics. In Hippocrates' *Of the Epidemics*, it is clear that diet, conditions of climate and locality, the patient's physical condition, mode of life, pursuits and age all mattered.[32] There has always been an aura of secrecy about medicine, and this was also true in ancient Greece. In the Hippocratic writings it is noted that: 'Holy things are revealed only to Holy men. Such things must not be made known to the profane until they are initiated into the mysteries of the science.'[33]

Hippocratic aphorisms presented a remarkable means of remembering key facts about disease and its treatment. They provided a way of retaining the knowledge and the skills learned at the feet of the master. Re-reading them today, some are quaint, inaccurate and unhelpful. However, most are easily remembered and recalled. For example:

Desperate cases need the most desperate remedies.

When the disease is at its height, then the lightest diets must be employed.

When a disease has attained its crisis, or when a crisis has just passed, do not disturb the patient with innovation in treatment either by the administration of drugs or by giving stimulants. Let them be.

Unprovoked fatigue means disease.

It is unwise to prophesy either death or recovery in acute diseases.

Every disease occurs at all seasons of the year, but some of them more frequently occur and are of greater severity at certain times.

It is a bad sign in acute illnesses when the extremities become cold.[34]

There are many others, full of commonsense and written in a form which can be recalled and put into practice. Such methods of learning, by rote, are currently frowned on and perhaps rightly so. But they had their uses.

Another document, 'Anonymus Londonensis', a papyrus written in Greek around the 2nd century CE, covers a range of medical and philosophical issues. It was probably compiled by a student or lecturer and includes sections on definitions, aetiology of disease, and the development of physiology. It refers to established medical names and comments on their views. For example, it refers to Herodicos of Cnidos and notes that, in terms of causes of disease, he is 'partly in agreement with Euryphon and partly in disagreement'.[35] There are numerous quotes from Hippocrates. This gives some insight into the way in which medical teaching was prepared, quoting as it does from various medical authorities as evidence of then current thought and debate.

There was no specialisation in ancient Greek medicine but practitioners were divided into three categories: the ordinary practitioner, the master craftsman, and the man educated in the art. The relevance of breadth of knowledge was clear. The methodology was also evident from the writings. There was a great emphasis on case studies, and the details remain fascinating even today. There is recording of the outcome and a belief that scientific method will assist in understanding of disease. Observation of individual cases was crucial to generate general rules as to treatment and outcome.

However, the doctor had to know his limitations. Noted in the lecture *The Science of Medicine* is 'the refusal to undertake to cure cases in which the disease has already won mastery, knowing that every thing is not possible in medicine'.[36] Prognosis was also critical.

It seems highly desirable that a physician should pay much attention to prognosis. If he is able to tell his patients when he visits them not only about their past and present symptoms, but also to tell them what is going to happen, as well as fill in the details they have omitted, he will increase his reputation as a medical practitioner and people will have no qualms in putting themselves under his care. Moreover, he will the better be able to effect a cure if he can foretell, from the present symptoms, the future course of the disease.[37]

The Hippocratic Oath,[38] while not the first statement of ethical principles, is by far the best known. It has served as a model for generations and is still relevant today. The importance in educational terms is not in the substance of the Oath (some aspects are not as relevant today) but the concept. The fact that a student or doctor had to agree on a series of values which would determine the way he practised is of great significance. It demonstrated to the outside world that the closed community of medicine had values and believed in certain things. Taking the 'oath' was the public demonstration of these beliefs, together with a recognition of the shame inherent in abusing the privilege of being a doctor. For a while it became unfashionable to take such an oath, but many medical schools now invite students to subscribe to some form of declaration, and the public acknowledgement of it is a powerful moment in the life of the student.

In summary, medical education in ancient Greece was based on personal contact with the teacher. Most learning was done through oral teaching and the use of aphorisms and case studies which allowed details to be memorised. Teaching was based on observation and an evaluation of the outcome. The whole process of learning centred on a series of values encapsulated in the Oath, which set out the principles of practice. Such a process was so powerful that it lasted for a thousand years and more, and still forms the basis of clinical practice.

The knowledge base was of course limited, but imagine today's knowledge being available to those Greek teachers. They would still have felt a responsibility for their pupils, for observation, and considering broad aspects of health and illness. They would still have had an Oath, and values would have remained relevant. The libraries would have been different and larger, but perhaps the greatest difference would have been in the public face of medicine. There were no examinations, and a reference from a great teacher would have sufficed to demonstrate competence. Nowadays, the examination and the question of competence are paramount, as is the demonstration to the public of the qualities of the individual doctor. This is again a theme which will develop over the next few chapters, and is a theme which will be picked up in the conclusions to this book.

MEDICINE IN ANCIENT ROME

Over the period of the Roman Empire, there was a gradual but limited increase in medical knowledge. Medical education also changed little. Most teaching was oral and by demonstration and, for this reason, the great libraries in Alexandria, Pergamon,

Athens, Rome and Ephesus were particularly important. An important part of Roman society was the apprenticeship system: not only was teaching transmitted but there was an extra pair of hands to do the work in a medical practice. Much of medicine was carried out by Greeks; the Romans had, at least initially, little use for medicine and did not like doctors. They thought of the family as the unit of healing and used their own drugs.

As in Greece, it was not difficult to become established as a doctor in Rome. There was no formal training or examinations, no legal requirements, and schools of medicine were loose associations. The key was to join a good and established physician and learn from him. In one of Martial's epigrams there is a note of how things were done: 'I was sickening; but at once you attended me Symmachus, with a train of a hundred apprentices. A hundred hands frosted by the North wind have pawed me; I had no fever before Symmachus; now I have'.[39]

Many doctors in Rome were of Greek descent, and Julius Caesar granted citizenship to foreign doctors. They were generally independent practitioners, but some were paid by civic authorities. For state appointments they were chosen by seven other doctors. They had tax immunity, but often had a bad press as shown in this epigram, again from Martial: 'Lately Diaulus was a doctor, now he is an undertaker. What the undertaker now does the doctor, too, did before'.[40] Pliny records in his *Natural History* that 'it is at the expense of our perils that they learn, and by conducting experiments they put us to death; a physician is the only man who can kill with sovereign impunity... I shall not even attempt to denounce their avarice, their rapacious haggling while their patients' fate hangs in the balance'.[41]

The army was an important employer of doctors, and all Roman legions had medical staff. The army offered great opportunities to learn, especially anatomy and the care of wounds. Roman army doctors were of importance in several respects. First, as the Empire spread over wide regions, so too did Roman medical knowledge. Second, knowledge of public health matters, such as clean water, sewage and the concept of a hospital, also spread widely, and there are numerous examples of the sophistication of this work. In the army, the medical service was one of the responsibilities of the camp prefect. The number of staff would depend on the size of the unit and the hospital was part of the fort (Valetudinarium). Plants were grown in a herbarium. Romans also learned remedies from local people and used them as appropriate.

The loose body of Roman medical knowledge comprised dietetics, exercise and bathing, pharmacology and surgery. Preventative medicine was also part of this general curriculum. Doctors could form their own guilds, and colleges were found across the Empire. They were regarded as learned men, and their tombstones are often decorated with a scroll. The guilds or colleges were mainly social, for dinners and for funerals. They held meetings to discuss practice and give advice and instruction. In one of the codes of practice it is noted that the doctor should:

> *Look healthy, and as plump as nature intended him to be; for the common crowd consider those who are not of this excellent bodily condition to be unable to care for others. Then he must be clean in person, well dressed and anointed with sweet smelling unguents…in appearance let he be serious but not of harsh countenance; for harshness is taken to mean arrogance and unkindness, while a man of un-controlled laughter and excessive gaiety is considered vulgar, and vulgarity must be avoided.*[42]

Such statements and how they are put into practice support the 'hidden agenda' in medical education, and the ways in which new doctors learn to behave. The same is true today. The relationship with patients is recorded, sometimes favourably and sometimes not. For example:

> *The intimacy also between physician and patient is close. Patients in fact put themselves into the hands of their*

physicians, and at every moment he meets maidens and possessions, very precious indeed.[43]

He spent more time than the average doctor on me; it was for my sake that he took precautions, not to preserve the reputations of his art; he sat beside those in distress; he was always present in time of crisis; no duty burdened him, none sickened him; he heard my groans with sympathy; amid a crowd of patients, my health was his first concern; he attended others only when my health permitted it; I was bound to him, not as to a doctor, but by ties of friendship.[44]

At a time when one learned as an apprentice by watching, such statements would have been very powerful, and part of the education of the doctor, part of the 'hidden agenda'.

Medical authorities frequently argued with each other and rival schools were set up. Pliny also comments on the fact that medicine was un-regulated:

Unfortunately there is no law which punishes doctors for ignorance and no one takes revenge on a doctor, if, through his fault, someone dies. It has permitted him by our danger to learn for the future, and our death to make experiments, and without having to fear punishment to set at nought the life of a human being.[45]

Instruction was by individual teachers who took on students. Doctors practised out of shops (tabernae medicae) where they treated patients and performed operations assisted by students. Galen notes that these were large buildings with high doors, letting in air and light, and with a range of surgical instruments and medical appliances. Many patients were also seen in their own homes; students accompanied the doctor on these visits and observed the treatment and the progress of the patient.

As Greek physicians arrived in Rome they changed the patterns of care. One of the first of the Roman physicians was Asclepiades, the 'Prince of Physicians'. Born in 124 BCE and educated in Athens and Alexandria, he taught that disease should be treated speedily, safely and agreeably (cito, tuto, and jucunde). He noted that health was a balance between tension and relaxation. His doctrines were modified by his pupils and the 'Methodist' sect was set up. This was not based on the Hippocratic humours, but on a corpuscular theory. Diagnosis was reduced to a series of common conditions, and treated by a limited range of methods. In this way it was possible to reduce the period of training to around six months, so saving time and money. Its advantage was that it was short, simple and easy to learn (a shortened medical course is not a new idea). Galen, who was educated for 11 years, was totally opposed to this short-term expedient. He was scathing about them: 'It is not the doctor who is most skilful in his profession but the one who knows best how to flatter who enjoys the regard of the multitude'.[46]

The Roman period of medical history, like all others, is dominated by major teachers, of whom Galen was pre-eminent. He was born in Pergamon, a great cultural centre in central Asia. His early studies were in Greek rhetoric and philosophy. He began the study of medicine when he was 16, first at Pergamon with the physician Satyros and then at Smyrna, Corinth and Alexandria. This latter centre was still one of the great places of study. Students from many countries learned there and one of the best recommendations to being a practitioner was to have studied at Alexandria.

Galen had undertaken around 11 years of study when he returned to Pergamon and became a surgeon to the school of gladiators. In CE 162 he went to Rome where he was already famous as a practitioner and anatomist. He was outspoken and was forced to return to Pergamon. Three years later at the request of Marcus Aurelius and Lucius Verus (co-emperors) he returned to Rome as court physician.

Galen had a huge literary output and there are 21 volumes of his writing in existence. Many of them have strong philosophical components. He claimed to have perfected the principles of ancient medicine, embracing the whole of medicine, and to have developed a systematic approach to medicine. He was known to be constantly revising his own conclusions by research and observation, though this concept is perhaps different from the modern one. One of his most interesting books is *The Pulse for Beginners.*

According the Galen, the physician should be skilled in the three branches of philosophy: **logic**, the science of how to think; **physics**, the science of nature; and **ethics** the science of what to do. He liked public display in teaching, and his dissections were attended by large numbers of people, not only those studying medicine. Galen emphasised the humours in the causation of disease. He was concerned that not all physicians, or those who would be physicians, had the motivation to learn. He said that doctors, like athletes, need to train and to have innate ability, and wondered:

> *Are today's doctors deficient on both counts? Do they lack potential and sufficient eagerness in their preparation for the art? Or do they have one but lack the other?…It would be easy, for example, to learn thoroughly in a few years what Hippocrates discovered over a long period of time, and then devote the rest of one's life to the discovery of what remains. But it is impossible for one who puts wealth before virtue, and studies the art for the sake of personal gain rather than public benefit, to have the art as a goal. It is impossible to pursue financial gain at the same time as training oneself in so great an art.* [47]

Galen died in CE 210 rich and successful, and spent most of his wealth on books and scribes, who copied works from other libraries. He wrote a whole treatise entitled 'On my own books' and says: 'During this time I collected and brought into a coherent shape all that I had learned from my teachers or discovered for myself. I was still engaged on research on some topics and wrote a lot in connection with this research, training myself in the solution of all sorts of medical and philosophical questions'.[48] He makes it clear that 'the best doctor is also a philosopher' and he issues an exhortation to study the arts.

Galen was interested in the question of health and wrote a substantial piece on whether healthiness should come under medicine or 'gymnastics' in 'To Thrasyboulos'.[49] He argues in a very philosophical way about this question and raises other issues on the way. For example: 'What is medicine?' One answer is 'the understanding of things healthy and morbid'. He concludes that health is part of medicine. In addition, he has a fascinating section on 'The thinning diet', an up-to-date account of a low-fat, low-calorie diet.

He also writes on teaching and notes:

There are three types of teaching in all, each with its place in the order. First is that which derives from the notion of an end, an analysis. Second is that from the putting together of the findings of analysis. Third is that from the dialysis (the separating out) of a definition; and this is now what we will embark on. This type of dialysis may also be referred to as unfolding, simplification or explication.[50]

His comments on anatomy teaching and on the recognition of drugs from plants show how important the practical aspects of learning medicine were to him.

A man cannot learn anatomy from books alone, neither can he from a superficial observation of the parts of the body.[51]

Young students must see specimens [of plants] not once or twice but often. For it is only by applying oneself with intelligence to these things and by examining them frequently that one gets a thorough knowledge of them.[52]

Galen comments on this need for practical training and condemns the learned theorists and sophists who 'from their high chairs shower down upon their pupils detailed explanations but if called to a patient have no idea of the complaint he is suffering from'.[53] He also recognises bad teachers.

Even in early youth I held many teachers in contempt—the sort who would give "proofs" of propositions which were in conflict with the demonstrable truths of geometry...remove the qualities of boastfulness, self regard, love of honour and respect, false pretence of wisdom, and acquisitiveness from the seeker after truth, and you will have a man who approaches that quest with a preparation not of months, but perhaps even of years, before making the enquiry into the doctrines which lead to happiness or unhappiness.[54]

He knew that to become a doctor would be a hard road.

Galen also recognised his own importance as he notes: 'I have done as much for medicine as Trajan did for the Roman Empire when he built bridges and roads through Italy. It is I, and I alone, who have revealed the true path of medicine. It must be admitted that Hippocrates already staked out this path...he prepared the way, but I have made it passable'.[55]

Celsus was another major figure and lived in the 1st century CE. His book *De Medicina* survives as an encyclopaedia and compendium of his writing. He was a member of the noble family of Cornelli, and as his works were written in Latin, and he a Roman, they were not noted by Greek physicians and overlooked even in the Middle Ages until Pope Nicholas V (1397–1455). He identified *De Medicina* in Florence and had it printed, one of the first medical books to be printed.

Celsus describes how to approach the patient:

A practitioner of experience does not seize the patient's forearm with his hand as soon as he comes. But first sits down and with a cheerful countenance asks how the patient finds himself; if the patient has any fear, he calms him with entertaining talk, and only after that moves his hands to touch the patient.[56]

His comments on the surgeon are equally apt:

Now a surgeon should be youthful or at any rate nearer youth than age; with a strong and steady hand which never trembles, and ready to use the left hand as the right; with vision sharp and clear, and spirit undaunted. Filled with pity so that he wishes to cure his patient yet is not moved by his cries, to go too fast, or cut less than is necessary. But does everything as if the cries of pain cause him no emotion.[57]

Here Celsus details the procedure in an eye operation:

The patient is to be seated opposite the surgeon in a light room, facing the light, while the surgeon sits on a slightly higher seat; the assistant from behind holds the head so that the patient does not move; for vision can be destroyed permanently by a slight movement. In order also that the eye to be treated may be held more still, wool is put over the opposite eye and bandaged on: further the left eye should be operated on with the right hand, and the right eye with the left hand.[58]

His books covered the preservation of health and diet, signs of disease, diseases of the whole body such as fevers, anatomy, drugs, diseases of specific parts of the body and several books on surgery. He described the cardinal signs of inflammation—rubor, dolor, calor and tumor (redness, pain, heat and swelling).

Dioscorides is the third major figure in Roman medical education, and his book *De Materia Medica*[59] was widely used and went into over 70 editions after the invention of printing in Europe. It contains very detailed information on the collection and preparation of plants and their effects on man. Drugs were collected from all over the world and the use of the herb garden developed.

These vignettes illustrate one further thing and that is the importance of books and libraries. These were places where information could be collected and shared, but the cost limited their availability. Only with the invention of printing did this change, though manual methods of book production could be rapid, as we shall see. It determined the mode of learning for many—knowledge had to be memorised. On the other hand, oral instruction meant that reading was not essential, though all real physicians saw the ability to read as one of the marks of the profession.

Roman medicine contributed little to the advance of knowledge by the time of Rome's 'fall', though it showed a great example in the inauguration of a public health system and of hygiene.

SOME CONCLUSIONS

The first few thousand years of the history of medical education have been compressed into a few thousand words. Even so, the major principles and practices have been established. These were to remain dominant for another thousand years until the knowledge base began to expand and extend the understanding of disease, and new and more effective treatments became available. So what was achieved in this early period?

First it was recognised that medicine is both a science (hypothesis-driven, evidence-based and testable by experiment) and an art. Judgement and wisdom are required to contend with uncertainties and specific individual patient problems. Medicine deals with human beings, and with feelings and values. These are important concepts, and the distinction remains even though the scientific nature of medicine has developed out of all recognition and would be inconceivable to the Greek physician of ancient times.

From the beginning, the selection of students and teachers has been recognised as key, and the characteristics of the 'good' student or teacher have been recorded from earliest times. Both require enthusiasm, commitment, knowledge and skills, and a special set of values and attitudes. Not much has changed, though the words used today may be different. The behaviour of the doctor and the ethical principles by which he or she should operate were also set out early on, and once again, though the knowledge base has changed, many such principles hold fast and need to be re-affirmed with every generation. Communication skills, for example, remain important. It is also clear that the 'hidden agenda' in medical education is of considerable importance. People learn from others; they watch and imitate behaviour. Habits and attitudes are passed on invisibly, for good or ill.

Teaching methods have changed little. Oral teaching in small or large groups, the use of books and libraries, methods of memorising the knowledge and putting it into practice were all present in early medical education. The importance of being an apprentice and of learning by watching and doing were clear. Perhaps less nowadays is learned by rote and catechism, or by the use of aphorisms, than in the past. Methods of assessment of competence were very limited, as was specialist education (though well recorded in Egypt). Formal assessment of the competence of doctors was to become a major issue in the next few stages in our journey and will be described later.

The paradigms of health and illness, on which much early learning was based, are now known to be false. The theory of humours is inadequate to explain changes in health. However, another thousand years was needed to change that. Crucially, the importance of health was recognised.

Of particular interest is the development of a major theme of this book, that of the 'medical magnet'. By this is meant the willingness of those wishing to become a doctor, or to take further training, to travel to the best teachers, no matter where they might be. Such individuals and schools dominate the development of medical education, and this concept persists into the present. These medical leaders set the standards and the tone for learning. As noted above they also set the 'hidden agenda' for behaviour and practice.

Perhaps the one aspect which was most missing in early medical education was that of research. While it is mentioned in sources, for example in relation to Galen, there was no real system for research, and the methodology was weak. This had the profound effect of limiting change in understanding disease and treatment, and much of what was then the knowledge base was not challenged for centuries. There was no real culture of curiosity and enquiry.

REFERENCES

1. Chadwick J, Mann W N. Hippocratic writings. London: Penguin Books; 1978; 83.
2. Comrie J D. Medicine among the Assyrians and the Egyptians in 1500 BC. Edin Med J 1909; New Series Vol II; 101.
3. Hammett F S. Anatomical knowledge of the ancient Hindus. Ann Med Hist 1929; I: 325–333.
4. Sharma P J. Hindu medicine and its antiquity. Ann Med Hist 1931; III: 318–324.
5. Wong K C, Wu, Lien-The. A history of Chinese medicine. Shanghai; 1932; 20.
6. Veith, I. The Yellow Emperor's Classic of Internal Medicine. 1972. Los Angles: University of California Press; 1972.
7. Confucius. The Analects. London: Penguin Classics. London; 1979 edition; 64, 86.
8. Wong, 26–27.
9. Ibid, 24.
10. Hsu E. The transmission of Chinese medicine. Cambridge: Cambridge University Press; 1999; 1–2.
11. Homer. Odyssey. Rieu E V (trans). London: Penguin Books; 1946; 227.
12. Ghalioungui P. The house of life: per ankh: magic and medical science in Ancient Egypt. Amsterdam: B M Israel; 1973; 35.
13. Osler W. The evolution of modern medicine. New Haven, Connecticut; 1921; 10.
14. Hurry J B. Imhotep: the vizier and physician of King Zoster and afterwards, the Egyptian god of medicine. Oxford: Oxford University Press; 1926; 55.
15. Breasted J H. History of Egypt from earliest times to the Persian conquest. London: Hodder and Stoughton; 1909; 117.
16. Hurry, 88.
17. Puschman T. A history of medical education. Facsimile of 1891 edition. New York: Hafner Publishing; 1966; 19.
18. Ibid.

19. Ebbell B. The papyrus Ebers. Copenhagen: Levin and Monksgaard; 1937.
20. Hurry, 78–79
21. Friedlander W J. The golden wand of medicine. A history of the Caduceus the symbol of medicine. New York: Greenwood Press; 1992.
22. Garrison F H. The prehistory of the caduceus. JAMA 1919; 72: 1843.
23. Wong, 7.
24. Nunn I F. Ancient Egyptian medicine. London: British Museum Press; 1996; 115–117.
25. Temkin O, Temkin C L, eds. Ancient medicine: selected paper of Ludwig Edelstein. Baltimore: John Hopkins Press; 1967; 109.
26. Chadwick J, Mann W N (trans). Hippocratic writings. London: Penguin Books; 1978; 260.
27. Temkin, 100.
28. Chadwick, 83.
29. Hippocrates.
30. Chadwick, 68.
31. Osler W. Aequanimitas and other addresses. 3rd edn. London: H K Lewis; 1906; 347–371.
32. Chadwick, 87–138.
33. Ibid, 69.
34. Ibid, 206–236.
35. Anonymus Londonensis. Translated by W.H.S.Jones. Cambridge: Cambridge University Press; 1947.
36. Chadwick, 140.
37. Ibid, 170.
38. Ibid, 67.
39. Ker W C A, trans. Martial Epigrams I. London: Heinman; xlvii.
40. Ibid.
41. Lewis N, Reinhold M, eds. Roman civilization: selected readings edited with an introduction and notes. New York: Harper and Row; 1966; vii: 18–21.
42. Jackson R. Doctors and diseases in the Roman Empire. London: British Museum Publications; 1988; 59.
43. Ibid.
44. French R, Greenaway F. Science in the early Roman Empire: Pliny the Elder, his sources and influence. London: Croom Helm; 1986, 32.
45. Puschman, 97.

46. Ibid,
47. Galen. Selected Works. Translated by Singer P N. Oxford: Oxford University Press; 1997; 47 [In: The best doctor is also a philosopher].
48. Galen. Selected Works. Translated by Singer P N. Oxford: Oxford University Press; 1997; 8 [In: My own books].
49. Galen. Selected Works. Translated by Singer P N. Oxford: Oxford University Press; 1997; 53–99 [In: To Thrasyboulos].
50. Galen. Selected Works. Translated by Singer P N. Oxford: Oxford University Press; 1997; 345 [In: The art of medicine].
51. Puschman, 109.
52. Ibid, 99.
53. Ibid, 113.
54. Ibid, 133.
55. Porter R. The greatest benefit to mankind. London: Fontana Press; 1999; 77.
56. Jackson R. Doctors and diseases in the Roman Empire. London: British Museum Publications; 1988; 69.
57. Ibid, 112.
58. Ibid, 121.
59. Dioscorides P. The Greek herbal of Dioscorides, 512 CE. Englished by John Goodyer 1655. Oxford: R T Gunther; 1933.

3

Arabian medicine and the rise of the universities

The sages said "Much wisdom I have learned from my masters, more from my friends, but most from my pupils." Even a small twig kindles a great fire so a little pupil stimulates the rabbi and there goes out from his questions marvellous wisdom.

Maimonides, *The Book of Knowledge*, quoting from the Babylonian Talmud[1]

INTRODUCTION

The period between the fall of Rome and the Renaissance is an interesting one for medical education. The earlier part, from CE 500–1000, was dominated by Arabic writers who kept alive the writings of the Greeks and Romans, and their influence and books spread from Baghdad in Iraq to Cordova in Spain. One of the reasons for this was the supply of good quality paper. The first Arabic paper making factory was set up in Baghdad in CE 794, the manufacturing process having been learned in China. Thus, the writing and the copying of manuscripts and books increased and spread to Spain via Syria and North Africa. Libraries were set up and students moved to places of learning. Arabic became the lingua franca. During this time the system of medical education became developed and formalised. Medicine became more of a profession and seen as a scholarly pursuit.

By the end of the period, medical education had begun its European progress, first at Salerno them moving northwards. Medical schools in a recognisable modern form were set up and examinations, curricula and the development of the universities formed part of this progress. New knowledge was limited, and teaching and learning methods did not develop greatly, other than in an expansion of the role of the book and libraries.

MEDICINE AND THE ARAB WORLD

The later half of the first Millennium saw a flourishing of the arts and sciences in the Arabic world. While the language was Arabic, the work was based mainly on Greek sources and the authors, while generally of Arabic origin, were also Christian and Jewish. The main work was carried out in the 8th–11th centuries CE.

In the period between the fall of Rome until the 9th century, Byzantine and Christian scribes kept books alive. The early Christians were not positive about doctors and health. The human body was sacred and thus not to be dissected or studied. The best brains were in the Church, and their feelings against medicine came to a head in CE 391, when Christian fanatics set light to the library at Alexandria. Therefore, little was contributed to medicine or to the experience of medical learning during this period from Christian sources.

One of the earliest and best known of these early Arabic scholars was Hunayn (CE 809–873), a Christian and also known as Johannitius. He promoted professional ethics and standards, and produced a series of books, the best known of which was *Masa il Hunayn*, written for medical students. The approach was a familiar one of question and answer and was catechismal in nature, easy to learn and remember and providing students with a way of reading and preparing for examinations. Hunayn's books were based on the works of Hippocrates and Galen, and the paradigm was that of humours and elements. Hunayn also helped in reviewing and correcting the Arabic translation of Dioscorides' great work on sources of medicines from plants.

One of the most famous physicians of the time was Abu Bakr Muh al-Razi (Rhazes) (circa CE 845–930). He was not a devotee of Galen and wrote 15 books. The largest and most famous of these was *Liber Continens*, a comprehensive treatise which brought together his personal collection of cases for teaching and for reference. He reviewed the aphorisms of Hippocrates and organised them so as to be easier to remember. He made his reputation as a clinician, and there is a story recorded of a patient who was vomiting blood, whom no one could diagnose or help. Al-Razi noted that the patient had drunk water from a stagnant pool and prescribed a substance which made him sick. The patient vomited up a leech, the source of the bleeding, and a legend was born. It is interesting to note that he began the study of medicine at the age of 40, and would today be considered a mature student.

Al-Razi noted the special relationship between the doctor and the patient. He encouraged doctors to ask questions in a friendly way and provided a checklist for action:

+ To define the disease from the symptoms and clinical examination.

+ To find the reasons for this particular type of illness.

+ To deduce from causes as well as symptoms whether the particular case involves one or more diseases or types and to define them.

+ To distinguish adequately one type from another.

+ To recommend treatment by diet, drugs or both.

+ To gain the patient's confidence and his readiness to respond willingly to his physician's advice and also to build up the patient's general attitude and morale.

+ To forecast what was going to take place and thus warn the patient of what might happen before it does, as suggested in Hippocratic prognostics.[2]

Al-Majusi, from the same country (Iraq) as Al-Razi, also produced a checklist—this one for the successful author. He judged that an author has the responsibility:

+ To make clear the author's objectives and motives for writing it.

+ To explain the benefits that might be derived from reading it.

+ To have a title relevant to the subject matter.

+ To spell out the methods, concepts and doctrines adopted by the author.

+ To name the author.

+ To explain the concepts and validity of his writings.

+ To have proper organisation.[3]

In the same text he urges that the physician's only aim should be to relieve the patient's suffering and to care for and promote his health without divulging the patient's secrets.

These two lists (quoted from Sami Hamarneh's chapter in O'Malley) are remarkably modern, both from a medical and a teaching perspective. The first observation is that they set out a systematic approach to diagnosis and treatment. Multiple pathologies are seen to be possible, and differential diagnosis is important. Getting the patient's confidence is also a part of the process in order that the advice given can be taken more readily. Finally, the prognosis and the doctor's responsibility to discuss this with the patient is of interest. The patient is to be warned about what might happen, and this should mean being honest with the patient in order to set out the possible implications. All very modern. The second list is also of relevance, and readers may judge for themselves how successful this present volume has been in achieving its objectives.

Ethical issues were regularly considered. Ishaq al-Ruhawi wrote a complete text on the subject and included sections on the high calling of the physician and the trust which results from such qualifications. Another manuscript from the thirteenth century contains a chapter on the knowledge and training needed by anyone entering the health professions. The person should study the essentials of logic, anatomy, geometry, astronomy, mathematics, meteorology, optics and music. He should know what the philosophy of each medical school was and what it stood for. After academic requirements are met, the physician should have regular attendance at hospitals, examining and visiting patients. This must be one of the earliest examples of continuing professional development and emphasises the breadth of knowledge required.

One example of an ethical dilemma is recorded in Browne's *Arabian Medicine*. It is the story of a knight who fell ill and was at the point of death. A Christian priest of great authority was asked to help with the patient. He asked for wax to be brought and softened it to make plugs. He then pushed the wax into the patient's nostrils. The knight died. When asked to explain, he said that the knight was suffering and he had plugged his nostrils so that he might die and be at peace.[4]

In this same manuscript there is a section on the testing of competence. Sinan ibn Thabit ibn Qurra (c. CE 880-943), an eminent physician in Baghdad, convinced the caliph al-Muqtadir (CE 908–932) to issue and enforce an edict that all physicians in Baghdad should take and pass an examination (set by Sinan himself) before receiving a licence to practice medicine. Some 860 people submitted to the examination.[5] In Spain, where Arabic culture was strong, teaching was by seminars and debates on medical issues. Later in Europe, such practice was used to defend theses and provide intellectual rigor to the work.

Browne's *Arabian Medicine* also offers a splendid example of examination leniency. One of the candidates presenting to Sinan was a dignified and well-dressed old man. He was treated with consideration and respect, and when the other candidates had been dismissed Sinan asked to speak to the old man further, and in particular to ask who was his teacher. At this the old man laid money on the table and said that he could not read or write, nor had he had any education, but that he had a family to support by his 'professional labours'. Sinan said that he could continue on the condition that he would not treat a patient with a disease that he knew nothing about, and that he would not prescribe phlebotomy or any purgative drug save for simple ailments. The old man agreed. The following day a well-dressed young man appeared. He was asked with whom did he study and replied that it was the old gentleman who had been yesterday. He was then asked if he followed his methods, and upon replying 'yes', he was asked not to go beyond them![6]

Ibn Jumay (1153–1198 CE) was physician to the ruler Saladin and became very famous for his medical skills. He wrote a fascinating treatise, *On the Revival of the Art of Medicine,* for Saladin, in which he complained about the deplorable state of medicine. In this treatise he offers a very clear exposition of the purpose of medicine.

> *As to the art of medicine, its material is the human body and its parts in so far as they can be affected by health and disease, its objective is to maintain health in them by preserving it when they are healthy and by restoring it to them when they are sick and unhealthy, through actions that it performs on them, such as nourishment, administration of medicines, bleeding, cutting, cautery and incision. Therefore the Ancients counted medicine amongst the practical arts.*[7]

> *Medicine is difficult not only after acquiring all the knowledge, for much skillfulness and long training in the treatment of the sick. That is the physician, after encompassing all the knowledge mentioned above and establishing it firmly in his memory so that he can recall it easily whenever he wants to, possess the capability to apply all the general laws he knows*

to individual cases and adjust them to the patient and the treatment.[8]

The art of medicine is difficult…it is possible only for someone endowed with good character, a well guided intellect, sufficient time and competence to study, and patience to bear with long hardship and work and who is fortunate enough to be apprenticed to a skilled master, well prepared for the method of discipline and for the long practice of medicine in the proper way.[9]

He notes that in the time of Hippocrates the move began to teach not only those in the family but others. He considers three areas of concern: teachers, students, and the examination of practitioners. He says,

Teachers—selecting them from persons of excellent knowledge and masters skilled in practice, teach them the works of the old masters. Educate the students and train them in the treatment of the sick under their supervision.

Selecting students—excellent mind, well guided intelligence, a character disposed to the good, desire for excellence, steadfastness in toil and study, abstinence from pleasures.

Examination of physicians—examine the condition of his mind. Ask him all the information the art of medicine comprises.

In this respect the physician is like a captain skilled in the management of a ship. Just as the captain skilled in the management of ships will not wait for the winds to spring up and for the sea to become agitated, but recognises that long before it happens.[10]

Fine words which bear repeating a thousand years later.

Aphorisms also remained important in this period and Isaac Judaeus, an Egyptian Jew, wrote: 'Ask thy reward when the sickness is at its height, for being cured the patient will certainly forget what you did for him'.[11]

Arabic physicians were highly regarded for their skill and expertise. El Hakim in Sir Walter Scott's *Talisman* is a wise physician with magical powers.[12] He is able to penetrate the court of King Richard the Lionheart and cure him and several other characters. It is possible that El Hakim was in fact Saladin, which makes the story even more interesting.*

Another possible model for El Hakim was Maimonides, a Jew born in Cordova (CE 1135–1204) and another key figure in the development of medical education at this time. A recent translation of his *Book of Knowledge* gives insight into the ways in which teaching took place, and how the physician should present himself. Maimonides was likely the son of a distinguished scholar who gave him early instruction, and he was well grounded in the arts and sciences, being familiar with the works of Hippocrates and Galen, and a follower of Aristotle's teaching. He must have read Avicenna's *Canon of Medicine*, and he was a pupil of Averroes in Cordova. After the invasion of southern Spain by the Moors, he became a refugee and wandered across North Africa and settled in Cairo where he became physician to Saladin. He visited Palestine, which was in Christian hands at the time, and when he died his body was brought to Tiberius where his grave is an important monument to this day.

The *Book of Knowledge* is an important theological work, and indeed it is best known for this. But within the pages are some

*As an interesting footnote, Sir Walter Scott's *Talisman* was also based on an interesting account of Sir Simon Locard, who at the battle of Teba took prisoner an emir of wealth and distinction. He took possession of a stone which was said to be more valuable than silver and gold. The story is taken up in the *History of the Lockharts of Lee and Carnwath*[13] (1976, Carnwath) by Simon MacDonald Lockhart. 'It was said to be a remedy for bleeding fever and the bite of a mad dog, and sickness in horses and cattle. The charm is red in colour and triangular in shape and mounted on a silver coin which hangs from a silver chain. The coin has been identified as a groat from the reign of Edward IV (1422–1483)…The penny is used by dipping it in water with "twa dips and a swirl". The water can then be drunk or used to wash the wound or to bathe the patient. No words must be spoken in the process or the cure will be ineffective.' The stone has numerous cures to its credit and is still in the possession of the family in Scotland.

fascinating examples on medicine and teaching. For example, on health, Maimonides describes the appropriate diet to keep well, not to eat too much and to be moderate with wine. On being a proper scholar he notes that 'he must not go about with his head in the air and outstretched neck or on tiptoe slowly like conceited women'. The dress ought to be pleasant and clean and not allowed to have a spot or grease mark. He should not dress in purple and gold, neither must he be seen in poor clothes which disgrace the wearer.

Methods of learning are also of interest in the book:

Although it is commanded to study both day and night, man learns most by night. As far as teaching is concerned, the rabbi (teacher) should sit at the head and his pupils around him like a crown in order that all may see him and hear his words. The teacher does not sit on a seat and the pupils on the ground, but either all sit on the ground or all on seats. He has an affinity for students. The sages said "let the honour of your students be cherished like your own".[14]

For one must take care of the students and love them like one's own children. Pupils add to the master's wisdom and broaden his heart. The sages said "Much wisdom I have learned from my masters, more from my friends, but most from my pupils. Even a small twig kindles a great fire so a little pupil stimulates the rabbi and there goes out from his questions marvellous wisdom".[15]

This phrase, quoted at the beginning of this chapter, is one of the most moving and profound in learning and teaching. It was repeated a thousand years later in a different form by another rabbi, Martin Buber in his book, *I and Thou*, which describes the fundamental relationship between teacher and pupil. Buber traces the relationship developing until the pupil surpasses the teacher in scholarship and creativity. For the teacher this is one of the most exciting moments in the whole relationship, to see the pupil do better than the master.[16]

Maimonides gives an interesting account of his daily life:

My duties to the Sultan are very heavy. I am obliged to visit him every day, early in the morning; and when he or any of his children or any of the inmates of his harem are indisposed, I dare not quit Kahira, but must stay during the greater part of the day in the palace. It also frequently happens that one or two of the royal officers fall sick, and I must attend their healing. Hence as rule I repair to Kahita very early in the day, and even if nothing unusual happens I do not return to Misr until the afternoon. Then I am almost dying with hunger. I find the antechambers filled with people, both Jews and Gentiles, nobles and common people, judges and bailiffs, friends and foes—a mixed multitude who await the time of my return.

I dismount from my animal, wash my hands, go forth to my patients, and entreat them to bear with me while I partake of some slight refreshment, the only meal I take in twenty four hours. Then I attend to my patients, write prescriptions and directions for their various ailments. Patients go in and out until nightfall and sometimes even, I solemnly assure you, until two hours or more into the night. I converse with and prescribe for them while lying down from sheer fatigue, and when night falls I am so exhausted that I can scarcely speak.[17]

Not much thought then of measures such as the European working time directive restricting doctor's hours.

Public knowledge of medicine was also widespread. Browne's *Arabian Medicine* quotes the story of the slave girl Tawaddud (from *Arabian Nights*) who was offered for sale by her bankrupt master. The Caliph offered her freedom if she could answer questions on theology, law, medicine and astronomy. Talwaddud answered them all and even asked questions back which her interrogators could not answer.[18]

By the beginning of the 11th century, development in medical education within the Arabic world was slowing down but still influential. By this time there were three types of medical schools available. The first were those associated with hospitals, such as at Baghdad, Damascus or Cairo. Such centres had lecture theatres, libraries, pharmacists and facilities for the preparation of drugs, and were ideal for running courses. Second were private medical schools, such as those run by al-Razi. As his fame was considerable he attracted students from far and wide, and his school was filled with students. Third was the apprenticeship system where students would be linked to a well-known doctor and would be instructed by the master in medicine and ethics.

Arabic culture and medicine also flourished in Spain, especially in surgery with a major centre in Cordova. In the 10th century the two sons of Yunis al Harrani travelled from Cordova to Iraq to obtain medical training, returning to Spain ten years later: a good example of the extent of education and the concept of the 'medical magnet' drawing students from a great distance for training.

The influence of Arabic medicine eventually waned. There are perhaps two reasons for this: first was the influence of religious factors, and second was a strict adherence to the writings of the ancients. These writings were accepted as the truth and little was done to challenge this paradigm. The culmination came with the writings of Ali al-Husayn Ibn Sina (Avicenna, CE 980-1037), one of the greatest Arabic scholars.

Avicenna was an infant prodigy and wrote poetry and books on a wide range of subjects. He became the great authority, and his very substantial output of books, especially the *Qanun* (*Canon of Medicine*), were read, copied and recited. His writings were based on Hippocrates and Galen, and the *Canon* was one of the most influential books ever written. Eventually in the 12th century his teaching was criticised by others but little changed. His writings were used for centuries. Indeed, the *Canon* was still being used in Montpellier in 1650, and until the Renaissance was the text to read. The Unani medicine in India and Pakistan has survived to the present day and is based on Avicenna's teaching.

When Baghdad was sacked in CE 1258 by the Mongols, the influence of the Arabic world was considerably lessened, though it survived in Granada for another 200 years.

Because of the importance of Avicenna it is useful to note some of the ways in which he taught medicine, as set out in the *Canon*. He divides medical knowledge into the theoretical and the practical. He then sets out the principles to follow and how to treat individual diseases. The whole book is systematic and well laid out. He defines medicine as:

> *...the science by which we learn (a) the various states of the human body, in health and when not in health, (b) the means by which health is likely to be lost and when lost how it can be restored. In other words it is the art whereby health is conserved and the art whereby it is restored after being lost.*[19]

Note the emphasis on 'learning' as the key process in becoming a doctor.

He further notes that 'theory' of medicine is that which when mastered gives us a certain kind of knowledge, apart from any question of treatment. 'Practice' of medicine is not the work that the physician carries out but is that branch of medical knowledge which, when acquired, enables one to form an opinion upon which to base the proper plan of treatment.

These two comments show the method by which Avicenna set out the curriculum and the way in which, in a very systematic form, the student should learn. There are numerous sections on definitions of terms such as 'cause', 'symptoms', 'illness' and 'malady', and how they relate. Whether or not the knowledge base was accurate, the pedagogy was clear and remains so today: a theoretical base and practical aspects linked to the treatment required. There was also a strong sense that preserving health is as important as treating disease, and an emphasis on knowing the cause of disease before giving treatment. Again, while the 'causes' set out now seem strange, it was the process of trying to understand illness and disease which is perhaps most important and which was then communicated to the student. Avicenna makes the point that in the 'practical' side of medicine there are two parts:

1. Hygiene—the science of regulating a healthy body so as to maintain it in health.

2. Healing—the science of ruling the sick body so as to enable it to return to a state of health.

There are some detailed passages on the management of specific symptoms, for example pain. This section includes a discussion on the 'theory of the nature of pain', and lists the types of pain which may occur. These include: boring, compressing, corrosive, dull, heavy, incisive, irritant, itching, pricking, relaxing, stabbing, tearing, tension and throbbing. Such a list must have ensured that when a student saw a patient with pain an attempt would be made to analyse and manage it accordingly. He concludes that pain 'dissipates bodily strength and interferes with the normal functions of the body'. There is a full section on sleep and the waking state which is fascinating. As far as treatment is concerned, he advocates three methods: regimen and diet, the use of medicines, and manual or operative interference.

The *Canon* is remarkably easy to read in translation and must have been easy to follow and to remember. As the knowledge base did not significantly change over a very long period it is easy to see why this book would become the bestseller it turned out to be.

Arabic medicine was at its height between the 9th and 11th centuries though it survived until the 14th century. The contribution was enormous, but like other systems of medicine before and since, it did not change and evolve and was taken over by other paradigms which developed new knowledge and ways of improving health. Educational systems also progressed from blind faith in the ancients to the discovery of different methods of learning and assessing the outcome of the educational process.

We now move to the next section of this history, and developments in Europe beginning in Salerno and spreading across the continent until the Renaissance and the invention of printing completely changed the knowledge base and the methods of its dissemination. But first a detour to England.

MEDICINE IN ANGLO-SAXON ENGLAND

While there was little new knowledge in this period, the flame was kept alive in centres of learning in England as elsewhere. For example, Bede in 7th century Northumberland was a scholar of European significance, and created a centre of learning with a library and pupils. The writings of Bede contain numerous references to illness and disease, and to remedies and miracle cures, such as those found in his *De Naturum Rerum*. In addition, there was an Anglo-Saxon literature on health and medicine which was brought together in the wonderfully titled *Leechdoms, wortcunning and starcraft of early England*. The original manuscripts were translated by the Rev. Oswald Cockayne in three volumes between 1864 and 1866. There are extensive references to herbs and their use in a wide range of conditions. For example:

> *If a mans head be broken, take the same wort, betony, scrape it then rub it very small to dust, then take two drachms weight, and swallow it in hot beer, then the heads will heal very quickly after the drink.*[20]

Names of some of the 'leeches' or practitioners are referred to in the text, for example 'Dun taught us'. The works were designed for someone with knowledge, and there may have been a school operating. Frequent reference to the phrase 'as leeches know' suggests a group of professionals. The manuscripts in the volumes were written between 900 and 1100 and may have been used in the form of a commonplace book. The herb section relates to the writings of Dioscorides, indicating the spread of knowledge during this so called 'dark age'. A key figure in the manuscripts is Bald, whose leech book is translated. Interestingly the books, in addition to herbs, cover charms, dream interpretation and superstitions.

Roger Bacon, born in 1214 was an important figure in this period, having studied at Oxford and Paris. He had a particular insight into science, especially experimental science, which went against church teachings. For example, he noted:

> *Experimental science has three great prerogatives over the other great sciences; it verifies conclusions by direct experiment; it discovers truth which they otherwise would not reach; it investigates the course of nature and opens to us a knowledge of the past and of the future. We have three means of knowledge—first authority, which by enforcing opinions on the mind without enlightening it, induces belief but not comprehension; second, reasoning, by which we cannot distinguish a sophism from a demonstration except by verifying the conclusion by experience and practice; and third, experience, which is the end of all speculation and the queen of the sciences, since it alone can verify and crown their results.*[21]

A remarkably powerful statement of the philosophy of science and the experimental method for a 13th century scholar, and it is perhaps understandable why he did not receive the credit he deserves.

THE RISE OF THE UNIVERSITIES

One of the most significant developments in the whole history of medical education was the creation and rise of the universities. Beginning in Salerno in southern Italy, the concept spread across Italy to Bologna and Padua, to France (Montpellier and Paris) and to England (Oxford and Cambridge), and across Europe. By the 15th century, even a small country such as Scotland, on the fringes of Europe, had three universities, at St Andrews, Glasgow and Aberdeen.

The *Universitas* denoted a collection of scholars, and for a time the term was not restricted to groups of scholars but was also applied to corporations or guilds. Often there were no buildings to begin with, and homes were used for teaching. In some universities, masters and pupils both sat on straw on the floor, the master having a sack to sit on to appear more dominant.

Universities, as communities of scholars, brought together a range of academic interests, mainly theology and philosophy but also professions such as medicine and law. They provided a place of study and libraries for the students. Some students came from significant distances and were attracted because of the fame of the university or of the teacher. For example, Harvey studied at Padua. Universities formalised the teaching and the outcomes, and degrees were awarded, often with particular rituals and ceremonies, many of which endure today. Much was about honour and dignity, and maintaining the greatness of the guild. For example, little in the oath taken in Paris in 1441 referred to duties to patients. Universities were communities with privileges, guarded jealously. Funding was by patronage and endowments, and by student fees. They were places of debate on current issues, and these discussions were often passionate. The inclusion of medicine as one of the professions associated with a university was an important factor in its development as a profession and as a scholarly pursuit. In almost all instances it would be expected that those training to be medical doctors had a first degree in the arts. As we will see later, it tended to focus on the book learning aspects of medical practice, as it was never quite comfortable with surgery, a much more practical art. It emphasised the difference between the

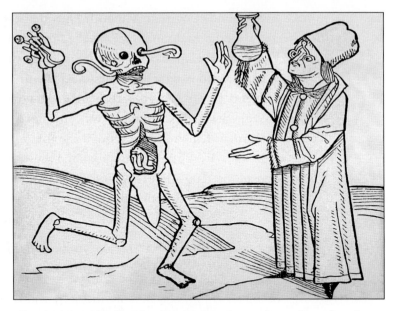

The physician, identified by the piss pot, tries to charm the patient from death, but to no avail. Todendanz, Mainz, 1491

medicus (the artisan or craftsman) and the *magister medicinae* (the scholarly physician).

One of the most important consequences of the universities was that following graduation as a master it was seen as a privilege to teach: a responsibility to the craft or guild and to the university. This responsibility was jealously guarded and this fundamental consequence set the pattern for hundreds of years. Perhaps medical education at present sees more tensions; more work to do, more things to learn, more paper work to cope with, more demanding patients. All of these factors are pushing the doctor (from the Latin *docere*, to teach) out of the role as teacher. Another lesson to consider at the conclusion of this book.

Salerno, the beginnings

Salerno was perhaps the first organised medical school in Europe and lasted from 1096 until 1270. Crucially, it was said to have been founded by four masters, Elinus the Jew, Pontus the Greek, Adale the Arab, and Salernus the Latin. It was open to all, irrespective of religion, and while it was closely associated with the nearby monastery at Monte Casino, it was a lay foundation. Of course, it had a library and the manuscripts were available to physicians. Its founding was attributed to Duke Robert, a Norman Knight who captured the town in 1075. It had a range of very distinguished alumni whose fame and writings spread the reputation of the school.

It developed a curriculum and students were publicly examined.

> *No one could proceed to the study of medicine until he had attained the age of 21, had proved his legitimacy and had studied logic for five years. The medical course lasted for five years, with an additional year under the supervision of an older practitioner. The candidate having passed the examination took the oath to uphold the school, to attend the poor gratis, to administer no noxious drug, to teach nothing false, and not to keep an apothecary's shop. He then received a ring, a laurel wreath, a book, and a kiss of peace, after which he was entitled to call himself Magister or Doctor, and to practice medicine.*[22]

This quotation reveals much about early medical education: the process of selection, clinical supervision, the examination, the responsibilities of the doctor and the symbolism of entering the profession. All of this was carried out in a scholarly community and in an atmosphere of religious tolerance. There was no restriction on nationality. It was in Salerno that the medical graduate was first called doctor, and degrees awarded. Teaching may well have taken place in the house of the Magister and consisted of the pupil being given a copy of a text for his own use.

One of the most famous products of the school was a book: the *Regimen Sanitatis Salernitanum*. This handbook of medicine was said to have been written for Robert, Duke of Normandy, son of William the Conqueror who stayed at Salerno in 1100 suffering from a wound on his way home from the crusades. The book, written in rhyme is dedicated to Robert.

The Salerne school doth by these lines impart
All health to England's King and doth advise
From care his head to keep, from wrath his heart
Drink not much wine, sup light and soon arise[23]

It is a remarkable poem, light-hearted yet full of wisdom, 300 Latin Leonine verses long. The translation by Sir John Harrington, published in 1607, is the text used here. After these first few words of introduction, some of the most famous lines in medical education appear, memorable, relevant and practical:

When meate is gone, long fitting breedeth smart
And afternoone still waking keep your eyes
When moou'ed yourselfe to natures needs
Forbeare them not, for that much danger breeds
Use three physicians still; first doctor Quiet
Next Doctor Merry-man, and Doctor Dyet.[24]

As we have discussed before, the absence of readily available books and the itinerant nature of the medical practitioner meant that remembering was a key part of learning, and what better way than in verse. The book (poem) has lots of wisdom on the herbs to use, and when to use them. It is a very practical poem and it is perhaps not surprising that it lasted so long as a learning resource. It was copied all over Europe and used widely. As an example of this, consider the following verse from Harington's translation.

Rise early in the morne, and straight remember
With water cold to wash your hands and eyes,
In gentle fashion retching every member,

And to refresh your braine when as you rise

In heat, in cold, in July and December

Both comb your head, and rub your teeth likewise

If bled you have, keep coole, if bath' keepe warme;

If din'd, to stand and walk will do no harme

Three things preserve the sight, grasse, glasse and fountains

At eve'n springs, at morning visit mountains.[25]

Compare this now with a manuscript in the keeping of the Macbeaths, physicians to the Lords of the Isles and the King of Scotland. It is written in Gaelic and is from the 16th century, or earlier. The Macbeaths (or Beatons) practised on the Island of Skye, on the furthermost reaches of Europe. It is entitled *Regimen Sanitatis* (*The Rule of Health*) and will be considered in more detail in a subsequent section, but note the similarity of the English translation below compared with that above in the Harrington translation.

Of the Order of diet or the eating of food. This is it, that is when a person rises in the morning let him stretch first his hands (arms) and his chest and let him put clean clothes on and let him then expel the superfluities of the first digestion, and of the second digestion and of the third digestion by the mucus and superfluities of the nose and chest for these and the superfluities of the third digestion and then let him rub the body if he has proper time because of the remnants of sweat and of dust which are on the skin, for the skin is porous and it will draw towards it everything that is near according to Galen in the first book of Simplici Medicina. And then let him comb his head and wash his hands and face out of cold water in the summer and out of hot water in the winter and let him wash his eyes with water which has been held in the mouth and warmed there....And then let him rub his teeth with the leaf of the melon in the summer and with the skin of the yellow apple in the winter.[26]

Although expanded in the Gaelic version, the resemblance is clear. The ideas and applications of Salerno transported across Europe and finding practical application in northwest Scotland. What more could a school of medicine wish for in the establishment of a reputation?

We know a little about the approach to the patient as practised in Salerno. In a quotation from an anonymous writer cited by Corner:

> *When you are called to see a patient...at your entrance inquire of him who greets you what the sick man suffers from and how his illness progresses; this is advisable in order that when you come to him you may not seem entirely uninformed as to the illness...entering the sick room you should have neither a proud or a greedy countenance...you may resume the conversation with a few remarks in which you praise the neighbourhood, commend the arrangements of the house or compliment the liberality of the family...then turning to the patient you may ask him how it goes for him and have him put out his arm. At first there may be differences between your state and that of the patient, either because he is excited at you arrival, or because he is worried about the size of your fee, so that you find the pulse rather confusing.[27]*

The writer goes on to consider examination of the urine, and to count the pulse for at least 100 beats. Finally, he urges not to turn a lingering eye upon the patient's wife, daughter or maid servant.

Of particular interest in the history of the Salerno school was Constantine the African. He was of Arabic descent and came to Salerno about 1077, where he stayed for some time, translating medical works from Arabic and Greek into Latin. He thus performed a most important function in bringing to light a wide range of literature from the ancients. Commentaries on such works were an important part of the work of the school and became part of the medical curriculum. By the 12th century, the full development of the school, based on a curriculum with a range of standard texts together with anatomical demonstrations, had been established. Instruction was by a teacher to groups of students, and there was a loose organisation into some form of guild. It was Frederick II in 1231 who established the first official regulation for the granting of a medical licence by the passing of a public examination before the masters. It is important to note that surgeons were required to have studied the anatomy of the human body, but is likely that this was done by the use of animals.

Of particular interest is the role of women in the Salerno school. Various names are recorded, the most famous of which is Trotula. Her writings were extensive, and she had a major work on diseases of women, *De Passionibus*. Thus, Salerno pioneered the role of women teachers in medicine.

Another interesting work from the Salerno school is a range of *Prose Salernitan Questions* which have been translated from a manuscript in the Bodleian Library in Oxford (edited by Brian Law, 1979). Presented are several hundred questions on a range of scientific and medical matters, with the answers given. Again, an excellent way of recording and remembering relevant areas of knowledge which could be taken along into the wider world. It was written by an Englishman in around 1200, and examples of questions include:

Q. How does menstruation occur?

A. Any woman, since by nature she is cold in make-up, and cold is opposed to heat, cannot fully burn up the food that is in her stomach, and there remains certain superfluities which nature expels month by month, so that this is called menstruation. But when she has conceived, her warmth is increased by her foetus, and so the food is better digested and such great superfluities do not arise; and from those which remain the offspring of her womb is nourished, for it is increased by her menstrual blood. Therefore the blood which ought to be emitted outside is retained inside as food for the foetus. And so women who are carrying in the womb do not have menstruation.[28]

Q. Why do the nerves have feeling when the brain does not have feeling?

A. The brain because of its softness, as has been said, does not receive the motion of this kind. But the nerves, even though they proceed from the brain at no great distance from it, are somewhere in the middle between softness and hardness, and so receive change of this kind.[29]

An unusual 15th century commonplace book

One of the most fascinating sources for the study of the learning habits of doctors is the commonplace book, and one of the most interesting is that described by Jones in *Manuscript Sources of Medieval Medicine*.[30] It is the commonplace book of Thomas Fayreford, a 15th century medical practitioner, and is written as a collection of sections recorded on different occasions over time. Fayreford allotted each section heading its own share of blank paper, then added to these sections at different times. He was probably educated at Merton College Oxford and lived in Devon. He lists over 100 cases, the ailments and in some cases the cures. He examines these systematically, and in the medical 'Practica' begins with the ailments of the head and works down through the body. The surgical section does the same though not as systematically.

An interesting question to ask is where the knowledge and information came from? In some instances this was from Fayreford's own observations and practical experience. In others the experience of other practitioners is cited. Lastly, he copied from other texts such as *Gilbertus Anglicus*. Interestingly, in many of the recipes there were *experimenta*, a term he uses when he describes a remedy which produces a cure but unsupported by the authority of ancient medicine. These were not covered in books and must have come from personal experience or that of colleagues. Some of the prescriptions are in middle English (indicating a literature in this area), as well as in Latin. This fits well into the previous section on leech books written in this way.

Such a commonplace book is very modern. Built on the practitioner's own experience, those of others and from written sources, it comes together as a practical record of experience and could provide other practitioners with a reference source. Log books and case notes provide the same today, and require the same connection with the wider literature for comparative purposes and for learning. Such commonplace books provided a splendid source of learning, problem-based and student-centred.

Jones[30a] also describes the use of folding calendars, fastened by a tassel to the belt. They were used to contain astrological reference material and notes, and several have survived and are available at the British Library and Wellcome Library. They were made of folded parchment and sewn together. They listed information, prognostic details and treatment—a highly efficient, portable compendium and the equivalent of today's handheld computer.

Surgery and medical education

In contrast to the physician's art which was essentially a re-working of previous writing, surgery was much more active and this resulted in a series of books which were practical and based on very real experience. Surgery moved forwards while medicine remained very much the same. One of the negative aspects of this, and something which lasted for many centuries, was that surgery was seen to be inferior to medicine, and surgeons were kept at a distance from the seats of medical power. Yet their impact was considerable. The physician was learned, the surgeon less so, and associated with trade and barbers. This error was pointed out at the time by Guy de

Chauliac, a surgeon of distinction, and has been commented on since.

It is interesting to note that in Garrison's *History of Medicine* (1913) the author considers the principal outcome of the school at Salerno was the work of two surgeons, Roger and Roland.[31] Roger's *Practica* was written around 1170 and was an independent work. It was re-edited by Roland between 1230 and 1240. Roger's work became a standard text and he was familiar with cancer, prescribed ashes of seaweed and sponge containing iodine for goitre, introduced suture of the intestine over a hollow tube, taught the use of styptics and sutures and ligatures for haemorrhage, and the healing of wounds by second intention (laudable pus). There is also a description of the many instruments available to the surgeon.

Henri de Mondeville (1260–1320) was another original surgeon, who emphasised cleanliness when dealing with wounds. He had been trained by the Parisian scholastics and his writings were verbose but full of good practical sense. He was also capable of stinging aphorisms, as Garrison quotes:

> God did not exhaust all his creative power in making Galen.
>
> Many more surgeons know how to cause suppuration than heal a wound.
>
> Keep up your patients spirits by music of viols and ten stringed psaltery.[32]

Guy de Chauliac was perhaps the most distinguished of the surgeons (1300–1368) and the most eminent authority in the 14th and 15th centuries. He was educated at Toulouse, Montpellier and Paris and took a special course in anatomy in Bologna. He considered human anatomy to be essential for the surgeon and wrote on such subjects as cancer, ulcers, fractures and described a method of anaesthesia, introduced by Theodoric. The extension treatment of fractures by the use of traction with pulleys is said to have been introduced by de Chauliac, and there are some splendid illustrations on the use of such apparatus. In spite of his experience, he still felt that the healing of wounds should be assisted by surgical interference, using salves and plasters rather than leaving the wound to heal naturally.

De Chauliac set himself high ethical standards and was seen as a gentleman and a scholar (he was also a medical historian). Perhaps that is why he was concerned about the separation of medicine from surgery. His main work, *Inventarium et Collectorium* (*Chirurgia Magna*), was written in 1363. It passed through many editions and translations and was used as late as the 16th century in a shortened form. He was a reformer and earned the title 'Restorer of Surgery'. His advice to surgeons was, 'a good surgeon should be courteous, sober, pious, and merciful and not greedy of gain, and with a sense of his own dignity'.[33]

Two of the most interesting saints in surgery are associated with this period of history. Cosmos and Damian were brothers living in Asia Minor and were said to have had great healing powers. After terrible martyrdom, their chief miracle credits them with the first transplant when the gangrenous limb from a white patient was removed and the black limb from a dead Moor transplanted. Numerous paintings show the patient with limbs of different colours.

Mythic or not, such vignettes describe early surgeons and their work, and there were many more of them such as John of Arderne and Bernard de Gordon. However, the important issue for this book is how such ideas were put into practice and how surgeons in the 12th to the 14th century were trained. Surgery was a practical art, and much of it based on real experience rather than a discussion of Galen or Hippocrates. Roger's writing, for example, was divided into four books, each dealing with practical aspects of surgery. His own experience is evident, and in addition to treatment there are sections on diagnosis. Roland, who re-edited Roger's *Practica*, notes that this book is not just for those who are already surgeons, but for those learning. Roland was a teacher, and he points out his method in the second part of his book.

Let no one accuse me of prolixity or crude style, for often brevity leads to obscurity rather than to compendiousness. I write not only for those who are already proficient, but also for others. And therefore whatever I heard in private or public from the admirable doctor (Roger) and whatever I have been able to glean from his writings, I have put into order, so that his ideas may more clearly be grasped.[34]

Here is someone who has thought about learning, trying to explain the procedures in a straightforward way. Much of the practice of surgeons would be from injuries at work or in battle, and there are sections in most of these works, for example, on how to deal with arrow injuries. The methods of teaching are also interesting. William de Congenis, who taught at Montpellier around 1200, is quoted by one of his pupils in the following way:

Master William gave lectures to the University students at least twice a year, at Christmas and Easter, when all other lectures finished. Now this was his method of teaching. He had the book on surgery by Roger before him, but instead of merely repeating the text, he followed the order of the chapters and showed how he himself operated, sometimes approving of what Roger said, at other times changing it for something better, and sometimes even discarding it, as contrary to ordinary surgical practice.[35]

The instruction was not just by lectures but by watching operations 'because only in this way can the student obtain full comprehension of operating, and besides this he gates courage, because in surgery boldness is essential.' William and his pupil did not condemn itinerant surgeons, as they realised that practical experience was key. The pupil also notes that having once seen a failed operation on the eye he found a simpler and more successful way of performing it. All of this reflects the need to be able to learn from experience and to observe and understand the operations and their advantages and disadvantages.

Learning by doing, recording the results and auditing them was part of this. The need to have the experience is well illustrated by a few lines from Theodoric at the end of his book:

> *I have not put anything into this book which I have not tested, for I did not wish my work to contain more of other men's ideas than my own. For it would be useless to bring out a new book if equally good or better ideas could be found in other books. I have also striven to be brief, for I do not wish to make my book tedious to read.*[36]

Knowledge of the works of Roger and Guy de Chauliac spread around Europe, carried by pupils to wherever they practised. Surgeons, especially surgical teachers, have always had to be good practitioners and skilful operators first, to remain credible in the eyes of their peers. It is from this that their effectiveness as teachers depends.

Other developments and personalities in the Middle Ages

This chapter has so far concentrated on Arabic medicine, Salerno, and some developments in English medical education. However, much more was happening in medical education in the Middle Ages, and developments in the universities of Padua, Bologna, Montpellier and Paris were of great importance. Padua, for example, was founded in 1222 and had a college of doctors by 1250. It had a formal degree structure and an elaborate process of examination and graduation. In a similar fashion to Salerno, graduates were given a book, ring and cap, and the ceremony was followed by a feast paid for by the graduate, together with gifts to the Bishop and promoters of the student. These were often in the form of gloves. The great period of Padua began in the 15th century and this will be detailed in the next chapter.

Montpellier had a medical school around 1137. While some of the schools were restrictive in that teachers could only be drawn from graduates of the particular school, Montpellier was different. In 1180, Guillem VIII decreed that no one should have a monopoly of teaching in the natural sciences: 'I will not grant concession or prerogative to any one person who shall have the sole right to teach and hold schools in the Faculty at Montpellier...and therefore I decree that anyone, from wheresoever he comes, may teach the natural sciences at Montpellier'.[37]

Bologna was equally important as a centre of medical education, with many famous teachers such as Theodoric (who favoured a sponge impregnated with mandragora and opium as an anaesthetic), Henri de Mondeville and William of Salicet. Teaching methods were similar to those in Salerno and Padua, though the organisation of the university was different in each case.

Paris was the other major centre, and perhaps the most interesting of them all. Students came from all over Europe to study. While the teaching was highly organised, there were no university buildings as such, and until 1742 it was situated in houses on the rue de la Bûcherie and the rue des Rats.

Writers of this time demonstrate and expand two other features of medical education. The first is that of medical questions, which were set out to assist learning. For example, in the late 12th or early 13th centuries, Henry of Winchester wrote a text entitled *Medicinales Questiones*. He was probably associated with Montpellier, and his book was compiled from many texts. The purpose is clearly set out in the opening sentence: 'The purpose of the present book is to go briefly over medical questions, so that disputants may have an easier entrance and the complex difficulty of the texts may be clearer'.[38] A very relevant purpose for a textbook. The second feature is that of the compilation. Gilbertus Anglicus, for example, confesses in the opening words of his *Compendium Medicinae*: 'Here begins the book of diseases, particular and

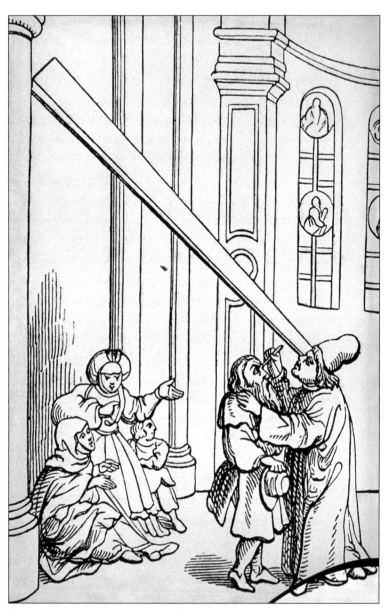

The doctor, pictured removing a foreign body from the patient's eye, is unable to do so because of the large mote in his own eye. Augsburg, circa 1540.

universal, written by master Gilbert, extracted and excerpted from all the authors and from the practical manuals of the masters'. He quotes from a very wide range and the book made his name (he is quoted in Chaucer's 'Doctors of Physic' tale).

These two examples illustrate one of the main features of this period. There was complete domination by the ancients. Contemporary writers complied, commented on and set questions from 'ancient' texts. There was little new knowledge and thus the learning outcomes of the practitioner varied very little. What determined where one went to learn medicine was partly related to the quality and reputation of the teacher and partly on the learning resources, the library.

The guilds were also important in some places. For example, in Florence the medical guild was sixth in precedence. Admission to the guild was a formal procedure, and in 1349 a law was passed by which all practitioners were obliged to attend public lectures and discussions at the medical school. There were penalties for non-attendance. By 1372, a provost was chosen every 3 months, and twice a month a topic was chosen and notified to doctors 3 days in advance for debate.

Guilds also regulated members' private lives. For example, they were forbidden to carry out a conversation or to drink in a public tavern. But there were benefits. They were allowed to wear pantaloons of Alexandrian velvet, white silk stockings and shoes of morocco leather with gold buckles.

Medieval textbooks of medicine

In Riesman's book[39] there is a fascinating section on the textbooks found in the libraries of early medical schools. For example, between 1395 and 1516 in the library of the Faculty of Medicine in the University of Paris, there were 26 books including the works of Alexander of Tralles, Aristotle, Averroes, Avicenna, Constantin Africanus, Galen, Gilbertus Anglicus, Hippocrates, Rhazes and Simon of Genoa. Such books were a real treasure, and it was only with the invention of printing (to be discussed in the next chapter) that more widespread availability occurred. Books were at the heart of the university and community. They provided the source of information and of debate. They allowed teaching to take place and commentaries to be written. As will be seen in all subsequent chapters, until the late 20th century, books were the mechanism by which knowledge was disseminated and by which reputations were gained. The teacher was important and his tool for distant learning was the book. In subsequent chapters, we will see how this has changed over the centuries.

A student perspective

Books for students were also in great demand. Rashdall[40] notes that:

> ...the first business of a student, in coming up, was to provide himself with books. Odofredus quotes, apparently as a sort of typical piece of undergraduate extravagance, the case of a man who on coming up with an allowance of 100 librae from his father, 'Fecit libros sous babuinare de literis aureis'

The father is clearly concerned that he does not buy too many expensive books (monkeyed up with golden letters) and perhaps try second-hand ones.

The *Pecia* system

It is often assumed that manuscript copies of books were difficult to produce. However, a system of production did exist and the author is grateful to Richard Marshall for the following note:

The rapid expansion of the European Universities in the 13th century created a large body of lay readers and a need for an efficient, secular, book trade. While previously books had, on occasion, been unbound for rapidity of copying, by the middle of the century a process was in place for the mass production of student texts.[i] Sections (or *peciae*) of a book were hired out by members of the book trade (the *librarii*) to many different scribes at once, who copied the portions in turn.[ii] The Universities naturally began to take an interest in and responsibility for this scholarly book trade, and rules drawn up for the regulation of *librarii* specified such things as the quality of texts provided and rates for the hire of *peciae*.[iii] An 'accredited' *librarius* was known as a *stationarius*, not only implying that he enjoyed a 'fixed place of business' (from *statio*), but also with connotations of holding an official appointment.[iv] The system apparently worked remarkably well, being adopted throughout Europe, able to satisfy demand and flexible enough to adapt to changes in curriculum. The quality controls placed upon exampla not only ensured, for the first time, that scholars has access to standardised versions of texts (preventing the misunderstandings caused by textual deviation), but also allowed for some re-editing.[v] But most important of all from a student's perspective, their books were now cheap and easy to come by, no longer hidden away in ecclesiastical libraries or produced bespoke by church scribes. The intellectual renaissance of Europe could continue apace, uninhibited by a scarcity of sources.[vi]

Bibliography

Bataillon L, Guyot B, Rouse R (eds). La production du livre universitaire au moyen age: exemplar at pecia. Paris: Éditions du Centre National de la Recherche Scientifique; 1988.

Denifle H Chatelain E (eds). Chartularium Universitatis Pariseinsis (4 vols). Paris; 1889–1897.

Reynolds L D, Wilson N G. Scribes and scholars: a guide to the transmission of Greek and Latin literature. Oxford; 1991.

Notes

[i]The earliest books produced using the pecia system apparently date from the previous century (c. 1150–1180). However, it took time for the method to spread and become established. (In Schooner H. 'La Production du Livre par la Pecia', in La Production du Livre Universitaire au Moyen Age: Exemplar et Pecia, pp. 24–27.)

[ii] Rouse R, Rouse M. 'The book trade at the University of Paris, c. 1250–1350'. In La Production du Livre Universitaire au Moyen Age: Exemplar et Pecia, p. 44.

[iii] The earliest of these book provisions is that of the University of Paris, drawn up in 1275 (CUP No. 462 = Charlularium Universitatis Parisiensis vol 1, pp. 532–534). One of similar date survives in Bologna. See Rouse n. 20, p. 104.

[iv] Rouse, p. 43.

[v] cf. ms. Paris, Bibliotheque Nationale, lat. 15350, ff. 169r, 181v 184r, etc.

[vi] Reynolds L D, Wilson N G. Scribes and scholars: a guide to the transmission of Greek and Latin literature. Oxford; 1991; pp. 114–118.

Literacy

One obvious inference from this is the ability to read. We saw this in relation to Egyptian medicine, the physician often depicted with a pen, and so it was in the Middle Ages. While books were scarce, they were available and the writing of notes and commonplace books provided a way in which knowledge could be transmitted. Schools were therefore essential if this transmission was to be continued. Europe at the time had certain advantages to allow the dissemination of knowledge, in that it had one religion, one learned language and one social system. It was only by the late 14th and early 15th centuries that vernacular languages were generally used for the training of practitioners, though they had been used in local settings. There was distinction granted by scholarship and it could be obtained by those who were of humble birth. It gave an important social lift up the ladder. Widening participation and its advantages are not new.

SOME CONCLUSIONS

In this chapter we have covered a very considerable period of time, from the fall of Rome until the early 15th century. We began with a review of the monastic and early Christian healing work and then moved into Arabic medicine. This period saw the consolidation of writings from ancient medicine and commentaries on the work of such medical men as Hippocrates and Galen. The development of medical school organisation began, with examinations and rituals of graduation.

However, it was the rise of the universities in the 11th and 12th centuries that proved crucial in the development of medicine as a scholarly venture, with examinations and ceremonies. The responsibility of the new doctor to teach and be part of the school was central to this process. However, not much changed in terms of the knowledge base. The teaching and learning was still based on the ancients, although pupils were not passive and took part in discussion and debate. However, there were some interesting signs of change. For example, the use of the commonplace book in recording actual practice and the outcomes of treatment. The surgeons led the way in challenging authority and in presenting a practical and robust learning based on experience and outcomes. In that sense they pre-empted the Renaissance in their challenge to authority.

By the end of the period there were numerous medical schools all over Europe, each different and each having teachers who attracted pupils. It is interesting to note that in the 15th century, Padua drew 30–40% of its pupils from northern Europe, reinforcing the concept of the 'medical magnet'. Part of the attraction was the books and libraries of the universities, and the notion of such schools as places of learning—as communities of scholars. Books and a common language provided the medium for the transmission of this knowledge. The curriculum was established as was the length of time taken to become a doctor. There was debate on significant issues of medical behaviour, and the beginnings of an ethical framework.

REFERENCES

1. Maimonides. The Book of Knowledge. Translated Russell H M, Weinberg J, Edinburgh: Royal College of Physicians of Edinburgh; 1981; 63.
2. Sami Hamarneh S. In: O'Malley C D, ed. The history of medical education. Los Angeles: University of California Press1970; 51.
3. Ibid.
4. Browne E G, Arabian medicine. The Fitzpatrick Lectures 1919-20. Royal College of Physicians. Cambridge: Cambridge University Press; 1962; 70.
5. Ibid, 41.
6. Ibid.
7. Jumay I. Treatise to Salah ad-din on the revival of the art of medicine. Translated by Hartmut Fahndrich. Weisbaden: Kommissionsverlag Franz Steiner GMBH; 1983; 8.
8. Ibid, 13.
9. Ibid, 16.
10. Ibid, 27–32.
11. Guthrie D. A history of medicine. London: Thomas Nelson & Sons; 1958; 90.
12. Scott W. Talisman. Everyman Edition; 1906.
13. History of the Lockharts of Lee and Carnwath. Private printing; 1976; 5–8.
14. Maimonides, 58.
15. Ibid, 63.
16. Buber M. I and Thou. 2nd edn. Translated by Smith R G. Edinburgh: T and T Clark Ltd; 1958.
17. Riesman D. The story of medicine in the middle ages. New York: Paul B. Hoeber; 1936; 63.
18. Browne, 31–33.
19. Gruner O C. A treatise on the Canon of Medicine of Avicenna. London: Luzak & Co; 1930; 25.
20. Cockayne O. Leechdoms, wortcunning and starcraft of early England. London: Longman & Co.; 1864–66; 71
21. Riesman, 78–79.
22. Guthrie, 107.
23. Regimen Sanitatis Salerni. Translated by J Harrington. Salerno: Ente Provinciale per il Turismo; 1966; 22.
24. Ibid.
25. Ibid.

26. Gillies H C. Regimen Sanitatis. A Gaelic manuscript from the 16th century. Glasgow: Alex MacLaren; 1911; 38–39.

27. Corner G W. Treatise of medicine at Salerno in the 12th century. Ann Med Hist 1931; 3:14–15.

28. Lawn B, ed. Prose Salernitan questions. London: Oxford University Press for the British Academy; 1979; 12–13.

29. Lawn, 106.

30. Jones P M. In: Schleissner M R. Manuscript sources of medieval medicine. New York: Garland Publishing; 1995; 35.

30a. Jones P M. Medieval medical miniatures. London: British Library in association with the Wellcome Institute for the History of Medicine; 1984.

31. Garrison F H. An introduction to the history of medicine. 4th edn. Philadelphia and London: WB Saunders Company; 1929; 152.

32. Ibid, 156.

33. Thorndyke L. History of magic and experimental science. New York; 1934–41, Vol iii; 518.

34. Talbot C H. Medicine in medieval England. London: Oldbourne Books; 1967; 91.

35. Talbot, 93.

36. Ibid, 99.

37. Ibid, 56.

38. Ibid, 62.

39. Reisman, 345–354.

40. Rashdall H. The universities of Europe in the middle ages (vol 1). Oxford: Oxford University Press; 1895; 417.

4

Renaissance and reformation: books, bodies, blood and branding irons

Studies serve for delight, for ornament, and for ability. Their chief use for delight, is in privateness and retiring; for ornament, is in discourse; and for ability, is in the judgement and disposition of business.

Francis Bacon, in an essay 'On Studies'[1]

INTRODUCTION

*T*his chapter deals with a major point of transition in medicine and medical education. The Renaissance and the Reformation were movements which challenged authority and re-set culture, authority and governance for generations. These movements re-discovered roots and gave confidence to challenge and see afresh some of the problems of society. In one sense, as has been remarked by others, it was strange that it took so long to recognise that things could change and that the writings of the ancients were not the end to wisdom. Yet as has been described in the previous chapter in relation to medicine, for almost 1000 years the work of Galen and Hippocrates was interpreted, commented on and re-interpreted, but never really challenged. The physician–translators or medical humanists, such as Niccolo Leoniceno, Thomas

Linacre and, latterly, John Caius, were key to this challenge as they made available to the medical world the writings of the Greeks. The speed by which such 'new' writings appeared in medical school curricula varied, as might be expected.

The period to be discussed in this chapter covers the middle of the 15th century until the middle of the 17th century, a period of around two hundred years which changed the pattern of medical knowledge and its practical implementation for the benefit of patients and the public. All of this happened in the context of a flowering of art and science which was astonishing in its breadth and scope. These broader developments will be described only briefly as a backdrop for the changes in medicine. Neither, as has been mentioned before, is this a history of medicine, rather that of medical education, and examples of change will be given, rather than a complete review. Other excellent books on this topic are available. The key issue is how medical education evolved in the midst of this revolution in thinking. How was the education of doctors modified as a result of the broader developments in knowledge and understanding of the world?

The Renaissance was a time of great names in medicine, philosophy and science: Vesalius, Paracelsus, Culpeper, Harvey, Willis, Boyle, Descartes, Van Leeuenhok, Browne, Glisson, Sydenham, Locke, Bacon, Copernicus, Galileo and many others. The period also saw the founding of the Royal Society in London, with a flourishing of interest in nature and its understanding. The Royal Society originated as an 'invisible college', whose members began meeting in the 1640s to discuss the ideas of Francis Bacon; its official founding date was the 28th of November, 1660. Its founding members, several of whom were medically qualified, came from all backgrounds to form a 'Colledge for the Promoting of Physico-Mathematicall Experimentall Learning'. Two words stand out in this title in the context of this book. The first is 'Colledge', a forum where people could meet and share new and developing knowledge, and which would encourage experiment. The second is

'Learning' as one of the objects of the exercise—something which is at the very heart of this book.

In addition to the great movements of the Renaissance and Reformation, there are four specific issues which are discussed here, and which will be developed further in this chapter. First is the invention of movable printing type by Johannes Gutenberg in Mainz in 1452. This provided a means by which knowledge could be disseminated and debated in a way not previously possible. It meant that books, until then limited in availability, became easier and cheaper to acquire, and that knowledge grew more transportable. It is interesting to note that one initial concern with this new technology was that there might only be a single book, by a single author on chemistry or anatomy etc., and that room for different views would be limited. This was quickly disregarded and shown to be false. In educational terms it was a huge advance.

The second major issue relates to bodies, and the development of anatomy. The publication in 1543 of the *De humani corporis fabrica* (usually shortened to *Fabrica*) by Vesalius completely changed the view of the body and made its study appropriate and important. It is relevant to remember that Galen performed dissections on animals, and that the church forbade a study of the body by dissection. The work of Vesalius and those who followed showed just how much there was to learn and understand. The examination of human anatomy began the relentless process of new knowledge acquisition which continues today at an even faster pace. It meant that the medical curriculum had to take this new information into account and ensure that doctors were aware of the implications.

The third general issue relates to blood and the way in which Harvey in his great book *Exercitatio anatomica de motu cordis et sanguinis in animalibus* (shortened to *De motu cordis*) demonstrated the circulation of the blood. While this was short of a full experimental process, it showed that with careful observation and measurement it was possible to begin to understand the functions of the body; thus began the study of physiology. It did not matter that the final piece of the puzzle, the discovery of capillaries, was not revealed until microscopes were developed (an outstanding development in its own right). Once again there were profound implications for medical education.

The fourth issue relates to branding irons, and the ways in which surgeons were learning to manage and treat injuries and wounds. The writings of Ambrose Pare, Peter Lowe and others show how much development there had been and how direct observation, often in battle conditions, meant that it was possible to change and improve practice. Anaesthesia and antisepsis were still a long way off but much could still be done. The education of surgeons was progressing through books and the long established processes of lectures, demonstrations and apprenticeships.

There is one additional issue worth picking up in this introduction—the rise in medical guilds, colleges and faculties. All across Europe such organisations were developing as a means of bringing doctors together for mutual support and learning. They also functioned as closed shops with strict membership requirements, often to limit the practice of others. Such developments were important for educational purposes but also had negative and inward-looking consequences, often degenerating into professional disputes and feuds. These were not edifying and did not necessarily assist in improving patient care. In almost all instances, the surgeons were separated from the physicians, and the 'rounded doctor', someone who could practise in a variety of situations, became more difficult to find. The establishment of the Faculty of Physicians and Surgeons in Glasgow in 1599 was perhaps the exception to this.

These are the major themes which will be developed in this chapter. Toward the end of the chapter is a consideration of many of the other names in medicine and in philosophy who contributed to changes in this period. Finally, there will be an analysis of the impact and implications of such changes for medical education.

THE RENAISSANCE

Beginning in 14th century Italy, the Renaissance was a remarkable movement, an escape from Scholasticism into a new world of creativity and invention. Florence was the birthplace, and the forerunners were Dante and Petrarch. For the first time, the middle class (as a merchant class) had sufficient wealth to challenge the aristocracy and to commission and champion art, literature and music. As discerning patrons they supported a huge outpouring of creative works, by some of the world's greatest-ever artists.

There was a re-discovery of the works of the Greeks and a return to humanism through writers such as Aristotle and Plato. The medical humanists translated Greek medical works into Latin and allowed them once again to be read and debated. For example, the Aldine Press in Venice printed a translation from Greek of Galen by Thomas Linacre in 1525. There was a feel for the finer things, and the wish to create something as good as the past. In medicine, the writings of Hippocrates in the original were re-discovered and translated into Latin. New thinking was everywhere, and artists and scientists were interchangeable. The building of the new Florence showed a civic confidence, and artists such as Leonardo da Vinci dissected the body and discovered the ventricles of the brain by injections of wax. Art and anatomy were as one in artists such as Michelangelo, Raphael, Dürer, and da Vinci. All of this activity paved the way for medical discoveries and, in particular, those in anatomy.

The Renaissance spread beyond Italy in the 16th and 17th centuries, taking with it the spirit of change and challenge. This was as true of science as it was of art, philosophy and other disciplines. For example, the writings of Copernicus on the motions of the earth and sun laid the foundations for those to come, such as Newton. However, such discoveries were not always welcome to those in authority, and there was often a price to be paid. Excommunication, banishment and death were some of the penalties paid for being at the leading edge.

THE REFORMATION

This was the second great movement which occurred around this time. The players in these revolutions were interchangeable, and, as an example, Copernicus was medically qualified and a contemporary of Martin Luther. When Luther nailed his 95 theses to the church in Wittenberg in 1517, his intention was not a break-up of the church but an internal reformation; it was an attack against the state of the church at the time. But what resulted was a complete schism in the organisation of the church and the creation of several different sects and denominations which broke from the Catholic church of Rome. This brought far-reaching consequences, including the loss of a unified Europe, held together by language and religion. From then on Latin would gradually cease to be the lingua franca, and there would be a steady rise in vernacular tongues, within which books and papers would be translated. Authority in the shape of the church was also challenged and this allowed, over a period of years, freer thinking and opened the door to dissection and experimentation. There was still a God, and he could be worshiped in a more personal way, but the authority had been challenged.

It was also a time of great scholarship. The Dutch theologian and scholar Erasmus (1466–1536) was a European leader although he did not want to be caught up with the politics of the Reformation. Francis Bacon and later Descartes were active and these individuals and others explored new ways of learning and identifying how society and science worked.

GUTENBERG AND THE PRINTED BOOK

At the heart of these huge social upheavals came an invention which transformed much and gave impetus to the process of change—the printed book. Johannes Gutenberg was born circa 1400 in the German city of Mainz. He was the son of a merchant. It is probable that he went to Latin school and then university at Erfurt. After a series of disasters and journeys, he arrived again in Mainz, where he borrowed enough money to print the 42-line Bible in 1452. Using movable lead type it became possible to print a whole book, and to do it repeatedly.

It was a huge success and over the next few decades printing presses were set up all over Europe. It provided, for the first time, a means for mass communication and dissemination of knowledge. Books became less costly and available to a much wider group, and the middle, merchant classes were eager to have their own collections.

Gutenberg's contribution to learning cannot be over-emphasised. It was immense and is only now, 600 years later, being challenged by the computer, the web and the grid.* From humble beginnings and a difficult start, he was given a place at court and his death is recorded as the 3rd of February, 1468.

As has been said several times, much of the history of medical education has been the history of the book. Its production and use, its writing and destruction, its power and its ability to change. Osler, writing in the early 20th century, makes the valuable point that the book brings the 'mind of the reader and the mind of the author together'.[2] In the words of Walter Scott in *Harold the Dauntless*, 'the romancer's tale becomes the reader's dream'.[3] Books are so important that their future will be discussed in the conclusions of this text.

BODIES AND ANATOMY

A pre-requisite to improving medical skill in order to change the patterns and natural history of disease was an understanding

---

*Just as this chapter was being finalised, plans were announced to digitise all of the books of the great libraries of the world and make them available on the internet to anyone. How interesting to note that there was once a time when books were in short supply and only affordable to those who were rich, and now almost anyone can view any book.

of the structure and function of the human body. The breakthrough came in 1543 with the publication of *Fabrica* by Andre Vesalius. It was a remarkable book. Vesalius was born in Brussels in 1514 and studied medicine in Louvain and Paris in 1533, which at the time was a strong centre of Galenism. Anatomy then was based mainly on animal dissection and Galen was the established authority. Vesalius was an enthusiastic dissector, and in 1537 he moved to Padua, where the authorities allowed for a supply of human bodies. Dissections were public and Vesalius lectured to a classroom of 500 people. He entered into a very active phase of his life and in 1538 produced the first six tables, *Tabulae Anatomica Sex*, illustrating the human body. By 1543 he had completed the atlas *Fabrica*, which was a magnificent volume. Those who have only seen copies will not fully appreciate the size, quality and range of the plates and illustrations from this book as seen and touched at first hand. They are magnificent. It was probably illustrated by John Stephen of Calcar, a pupil of Titian. It was drawn on the basis of direct observation, and exploded some of the inaccuracies of Galen's work. Vesalius himself makes the obvious point:

> *How much has been attributed to Galen, easily leader of the professors of dissection, by those physicians and anatomists who have followed him, and often against reason!…Indeed, I myself cannot wonder often enough at my own stupidity and too great trust in the writings of Galen and other anatomists.*[4]

In a similar vein, Realdo Colombo wrote in 1559 that 'a man learns more in a day by the dissection of a dog than by continually feeling the pulse and studying Galen's writing for many months together'.[5]

Interestingly, the *Fabrica* was followed by the *Epitome*, which was a shortened version for students. The atlas had a profound impact, and in particular on Vesalius' successors in Padua, Fabricius and Fallopius, through which a direct route can be traced to Harvey, later a student in Padua. Vesalius did little more and was hounded because of his book. He went to Jerusalem on pilgrimage and was shipwrecked on the Greek island of Zante, where he died in 1564. All his key work had been carried out in a 3–4 year period.

Following Vesalius, as mentioned above, two important anatomists give a direct link to Harvey and the circulation of the blood. First is Gabriele Fallopio (Fallopius) who was professor of anatomy at Pisa (1548) and then Padua (1551). He carried out significant research and his name is commemorated in the term, Fallopian tubes. More particularly, he was the teacher of Hieronymous Fabricius of Aquadapente. Fabricius worked as a surgeon and became professor in 1565. He was interested in embryology and described the valves in veins, and was an important precursor of Harvey who studied in Padua in the late 1590s until 1602. Fabricius retired in 1613. He has one other important claim to fame, in that he used some of his considerable wealth to build a magnificent lecture theatre in Padua, circular and tiered to allow viewing of dissections.

BLOOD AND ITS CIRCULATION

The discovery of the circulation of the blood by Harvey was one of major significance. Harvey was born in Folkestone in Kent in 1578 and was educated at Kings School, Canterbury, and Caius College, Cambridge, where he obtained a BA. He then moved to Padua and studied under Fabricius and graduated as a doctor of medicine in 1602. He had a glowing testimony at Padua and on his Diploma is written: 'He conducted himself so wonderfully well in the examination and had shown such skill, memory and learning that he had far surpassed even the great hopes which his examiners had formed of him'.[6]

While others had considered the Galenic view that blood did not circulate, he was the first to show that this was not true and provide an alternative view. On returning to England he had a distinguished career, becoming a Fellow of the Royal College of Physicians in 1607, physician to St Bartholomew's Hospital in 1609 and, in 1618, physician to James I. He was later appointed physician to Charles I and was elected Warden of Merton College Oxford in 1645 when he was 67. He was the Lumelian Lecturer in the College for 40 years, and his notes can still be seen at the British Museum. Although elected to the Presidency of the Royal College of Physicians in 1654, he declined on the grounds of age and ill health.

Even in his old age, Harvey continued to learn and said: 'I myself, though verging on my 80th year and sorely failed in bodily health, nevertheless feel my mind still vigorous, so that I continue to give myself studies of this kind, especially connected with the sacred things of Apollo'.[7]

Like much good research, it was carried on a part-time basis, and he eventually published it in book form in 1628 as *De Motu Cordis et Sanguinis in Animalibus* (*On the motion of the heart and blood in animals*). Like many discoveries before and afterwards, there was strong opposition to the proposals for many years, perhaps best illustrated by this quotation from Molière in *Le Malade Imaginaire*, as Monsieur Diafoirus discusses the prowess of his son:

> *What pleases me most about him—and in this he is follow-*
> *ing my example—is that he holds blindly to the opinion of*
> *our ancients, and has never wished to understand or listen*
> *to the so-called discoveries of our century on the circulation*
> *of the blood and other opinions of the same kind.*[8]

One of Harvey's first actions was to point out Galen's errors: 'It is absolutely necessary to conclude that the blood in the animal body is impelled in a circle, and is in a state of ceaseless motion'.[9]

Harvey's discovery was of significance in a number of ways. He did not approach the problem as a modern scientist, and he still believed in vital forces and spirits. But he had to be sure that his case for circulation was a good one and, while not using a completely hypothesis–driven model, tried to provide evidence for circulation. For example, one of the propositions from Galen was that blood was made continuously in the liver. Harvey measured the volume pumped out each beat, 60 cc which amounted to 250 litres per hour, impossible to produce at such a rate. His experiment with ligatures on the arm to demonstrate the venous valves and their one way movement of blood was another key piece of evidence. He noted that poisons circulated rapidly, again in favour of circulation, and that the various blood vessels were of different thickness, those nearest the heart having the greatest thickness to withstand high fluid pressures. All of this added up to blood circulating and confirmed the heart as a pump. However, Harvey's view was different from that of Descartes who clearly viewed the body as a machine and the heart as not just a pump:

> *So the heart is the beginning of life, the Sun of the microcosm ....by whose virtue, and pulsation the blood is mov'd perfected, made vegetable, and is defended from corruption, and mattering: and this familiar household-god doth his duty to the whole body, by nourishing, cherishing, and vegetating, being the foundation of life, and the author of all.* [10]

Not just a pump then. With the development of the microscope the final piece of the jigsaw was filled in with the discovery of the capillaries.

What then was the educational significance of Harvey's discovery? First it added to the knowledge of the body, which, with the great developments in anatomy, began to change the curriculum for the student. It established that problems could be solved by careful experiments and measurement. It changed the way in which doctors thought about the body. It did not have any immediate therapeutic implications (that was some time away), but it did alter perceptions of the working of the body and paved the way for many more anatomical and physiological discoveries.

Harvey was a great benefactor and gave the College a large library and museum of anatomical works. His estate was used to endow an annual feast where benefactors were to be praised and the fellows exhorted to mutual love and affection and to 'Search and study out the secret of nature by way of experiment'.[11] He changed the profession and gave medicine a new model.

OTHER PHYSICIANS

While Harvey has been given pride of place for his discovery of the circulation of blood, there were many others who changed the way medicine was practised. The following summary is no more than that, but it records some individuals and events of particular importance in education.

Paracelsus (1493–1541)

Theophrastus Phillipus Aureolus Bombastus von Hohenheim has sometimes been called the 'Luther of medicine' because of his protest against authority. He used the name Paracelsus to mean 'surpassing Celsus'. He was one of the most controversial figures of his age and began his medical career in Basel. He saw himself as a prophet or apostle, defining the moral character of medicine. He was a wandering student and had no real curriculum in his studies, but as he said himself: 'When I saw nothing resulted from (medical) practice but killing and laming, I decided to abandon such a miserable art and seek the truth elsewhere'.[12]

His writings were a mixture of religious and medical, and he saw his cause associated with reformation. He wrote numerous pamphlets that had considerable influence over the public, many of which set out predictions of civil and political unrest. He produced two pamphlets on syphilis and used the opportunity to attack the incompetence and greed of medical practitioners. He was particularly concerned about the medical care of the poor, and the woodcut from the front page of one pamphlet illustrates the contrast between the rich doctor and the poor patient. He condemned the ancients and publicly burned the works of Galen and Avicenna on the eve of St John's night, 24th June, 1527. He aimed to replace the medical theories of the past with a new theory based on a search for specific treatments, though it was mostly based on a biblical and theological infrastructure. He believed in the doctrine of signatures, in which cures similar to the appearance of the disease were used. He taught in German and wore a pharmacist's apron rather than an academic gown. He was outspoken and had a particular interest in chemistry, which he considered the way forward in medicine.

Hieronymous Fracastorius (1483–1553)

Fracastorius was a well-known physician who composed a long poem, *Syphillis, sive morbus Gallicus*, on syphilis and wrote one of the first works on epidemiology. In 1546, he wrote *Di Contagion*, a text on infection, and included a classification of the spread of infection by direct contact, fomites and from a distance.

Thomas Linacre (1461–1524)

Linacre trained as a physician at Bologna and returned to England and petitioned Henry VIII in 1518 to give patent letters to establish a body of physicians, which in 1551 become the Royal College of Physicians of London. He became its first president and the original college met in his house. The prestigious Linacre Lecture and Fellow are named after him.

John Caius (1510–1573)

Caius learned medicine in Padua and lived in the same lodgings as Vesalius. He returned to England to co-found Gonville and Caius College in Cambridge in 1557.

Nicholas Culpeper (1615–1654)

Culpeper is included, not because of his *Herbal* (*The Complete Herbal. To which are now annexed The English Physician, enlarged, and Key to Physic with rules for compounding medicine according to the true system of nature forming a complete family dispensatory and natural system of physic to which is also added upwards of fifty choice receipts selected from the author's last legacy to his wife*), nor because of the system of medicine used (mainly astrological), but for the way in which it criticises the establishment. It is also one of the earlier books directed at the public to assist them in treating disease.

Culpeper began practising medicine in Cambridge but had no university degree. He first produced his book as a *Physical Directory, or a translation of the London Dispensatory* in 1649, an unauthorised translation of the College of Physicians Latin *Pharmacopoeia*. He had several run-ins with the College of Physicians, who were equally venomous about him. He accused them of writing in Latin and being too expensive, so he produced his book of cheap and affordable remedies. Indeed from then on most books were produced in the vernacular.

In the preface he notes that he cannot trust any other authors, so consults 'my two brothers Dr Reason and Dr Experience and took a voyage to visit my mother nature, by whose advice, together with the help of Dr Diligence, I at last obtained my desire; and, being warned by Mr Honesty, a stranger in our days, to publish it to the world, and I have done it'.[13] But why does he have to write this book? 'To this I answere, neither Gerrard not Parkinson, or any that ever wrote in the like nature, ever gave one wise reason for what they wrote, and so did nothing else but train up young novices in Physic in the School of tradition, and to teach them just as a parrot is taught to speak.'[14]

Thomas Sydenham (1624–1686)

Sometimes known as the English Hippocrates, and the father of English medicine, Sydenham's particular interest was in the practice of medicine at the bedside, and with clear observations and good record keeping, he attempted to classify and analyse disease. He still held to the theory of the four humours and his works went through numerous translations. He writes:

> ...the art of medicine was to be properly learned only from its practice and exercise; and that in probability, he would be the best skilled in the detection of the true and genuine indications of treatment, who had the most diligently and the most accurately attended to the natural phenomenon of disease...with nature as my guide, I should swerve not a nail's breadth from the true way.[15]

He was educated at Oxford, but his studies were interrupted by the English Civil War. He eventually settled in Westminster where he remained for the rest of his life. Some of his most important works were on epidemiology, particularly on fevers (1666), which was dedicated to his friend Robert Boyle. He suffered badly from gout in his latter years, and his treatise on gout is a major piece of work. He read widely but was sceptical of bookish knowledge. When asked to recommend a book in preparation for medical studies the famously replied: 'Read Don Quixote; it is a very good book; I still read it frequently'[16]. It was Boyle who inspired Sydenham to pursue his epidemiological studies, while another friend, John Locke (1632–1704), wrote a poem in his honour, and they were both close while Locke was writing his *Essay concerning Human Understanding*.

Locke was also medically qualified and may have been Sydenham's student. Locke also wrote *Some thoughts concerning Education* in 1693. It is an interesting work, particularly on the education of children. He has a fascinating section on 'curiosity' arguing that it should be encouraged. Questions should be answered and the issues explained in understandable language.[17] Locke also comments on medicine as follows:

> *And thus I have done with what concerns the body and health, which reduces itself to these few and easily observable rules. Plenty of open air, exercise, and sleep; plain diet, no wine or strong drink, and very little or no physic; not too warm or strait clothing; especially the head and feet kept cold, and the feet often used to cold water and exposed to wet.*[18]

Sydenham's book *Medical Observations* (1676) is a classic and was used extensively. It contains notable observations and continually refers to the power of nature and the need to restore balance. For example:

> *A disease, however much its cause may be adverse to the body, is nothing more than an effort of nature, who strives with might and main to restore the health of the patient by the elimination of the morbid humour.*[19]
>
> *Why! The fever itself is nature's instrument.*[20]
>
> *Here I cannot but break out in praise of the great God, the giver of all good things, who hath granted to the human race, as a comfort in their afflictions, no medicine of the value of opium, either in regard to the number of disease it can control, or its efficiency in extirpating them.*[21]

And on Gout, Sydenham comments:

> *Gout attacks such old men as, after passing the best part of their life in ease and comfort, indulging freely in high living, wine and other generous drinks, at length, from inactivity, the usual attendant of advanced life have left off altogether*

the bodily exercises of their youth. Such men have generally large heads, and are of a full, humid and lax habit, and possess a luxurious and vigorous constitution, with excellent vital stamina.[22]

The victim goes to bed and sleeps in good health. About two o'clock in the morning he is awakened by a severe pain in the great toe; more rarely in the heel, ankle or instep. The pain is like that of a dislocation, and yet the parts feel as if cold water were poured over them...now it is a violent stretching or tearing of the ligaments, now it is a gnawing pain, and now a pressure of tightening. So exquisite and lively meanwhile is the feeling of the part affected that it cannot bear the weight of bedclothes nor of the jar of a person walking into the room. The night is spent in torture.[23]

What wonderful clinical descriptions, easy to recognise and remember, easy to learn. Sydneham also had a splendid sense of humour, as the following quotation reveals: 'The arrival of a good clown exercises a more beneficial influence upon the health of a town than twenty asses laden with drugs'.

Sydenham emphasised the clinical aspects of illness and the importance of nature. He influenced generations of doctors by his teaching and accurate clinical observations.

Marcello Malpighi (1628–1694)

Malpighi was professor at Bologna and provided microscopic evidence of capillaries, corroborating the work of Harvey.

The Chamberlens

William Chamberlen was a Huguenot refugee who settled in England in 1569 and died in 1596, leaving two sons who practised surgery. Peter is credited with the invention of the obstetric forceps, which the family kept as a secret and did not reveal until Hugh Chamberlen died in 1728, when patents were taken out. This is an extraordinary example of a secret remedy, in this case a surgical instrument, which was kept within a single family for 150 years.

The Beatons

Another famous medical family were the Beatons, the hereditary physicians to the Lords of the Isles in western Scotland (referred to in the last chapter).[24] Every monarch in Scotland from Robert I to James VI had a Beaton for a doctor. This spanned the period 1300–1700, and 76 Beatons have been identified. When Martin Martin (a graduate of Padua) visited the island of South Uist in 1695 he noted that 'the following Irish Manuscripts in the Irish character to wit; Avicenna, Averroes, Johannes de Vigo, Bernardus Gordonus and several volumes of Hippocrates. The Regimen Sanitatis and Lilium Medicinae were translated into Gaelic'.[25] It is interesting to note how they dealt with disagreement: 'It does not become us to contradict the pronouncements of the doctors but to bury them with honour'.[26] They seemed to have remained staunch Arabians and there are almost no references to Paracelsus, Paré and Vesalius in their writings. It is worth noting that Gaelic thus joined Greek, Latin and Arabic as one of only four languages in which this body of knowledge was formally and systematically studied from Hippocrates to Riverius. The break-up of the clan system in Scotland in the 17th century put an end to this classical tradition.

Robert Boyle (1627–1691)

Boyle was a remarkable person; born in Dublin of very rich parents he was able to indulge his interests with ease. He visited

Florence in 1642 at the time of Galileo's death just outside the city. He was much influenced by this and read Galileo's works, and it has been suggested that this influenced his interest in science. He was instrumental in the formation of the Royal Society. He was a friend of Sydenham and, indeed, suggested remedies to him. While he had no medical or scientific degrees, he was a pioneer of chemistry and laboratory medicine. He had sufficient private means to have his own laboratory in Oxford and joined a group of scientists there, though he was never a member of the University. His main book was *Usefulness of Experimental Natural Philosophy*, which had as its major theme the contention that experimental science was a proper way to proceed and that Galenism was not tenable. As did Paracelsus, he believed chemistry was the way forward. He shared with Sydenham a vision of the moral duty of the physician to improve medical practice. He wrote on many other topics, including the *Skeptical Chemist* (1661), in which he argued that matter was made up of corpuscles. Many of his ideas were taken up by others, including Descartes.

He notes that: 'The physician is to look upon the human body as an engine that is out of order'[27] interacting with the environment. He reflects some of the views of Francis Bacon (see later) when he writes:

I look upon a good physician not so properly as a servant of nature, as one that is a counsellor and friendly assistant, who, in his patients body, further those motions and other things, that he judges conducive to the welfare and recovery of it; but as to those he perceives likely to be hurtful, either by increasing the disease, or otherwise endangering the patient, he thinks it is part to oppose or hinder.[28]

He was particularly concerned with hypothesis and experimentation, and for broadening the base of medical knowledge. To Sydenham, observation was what mattered, while Boyle looked for hidden causes in nature. He hoped that systematic investigation and data collection would yield insights into the basic workings of nature. The two friends thus disagreed, in that Sydenham felt that all that was knowable was already waiting to be collected, while Boyle was interested in how nature worked. Boyle believed that physicians would benefit from organising their subject in a rational way. Such changes, with the gradual incorporation of new knowledge, would reform medicine without it losing its status.

In essence, Sydenham was the clinician and Boyle was the medical scientist, a distinction which has lasted through the centuries and is fundamental to medical education. What kind of doctor do we want and need? The scientist or the clinician? This will be discussed further in the final section of this book, but it would be fair to say at this point that the distinction is an artificial one—we need both, and all doctors need both attributes.

BRANDING IRONS AND WOUNDS

In the midst of these momentous developments in anatomy and physiology, the surgeons were progressing with equal intensity. Paris was the centre of activity and Ambrose Paré (1510–1590) was the doyen and father of modern surgery. Much of his work and those of other surgeons was based on practice in war, and there was plenty to do. Wounds were a particular issue, and the standard treatment was with a branding iron and the use of a 'digestive' and 'hot oil'. Paré discovered that a simple dressing was just as effective, and used that phrase 'I dressed him, and God healed him' to describe the process.[29] He worked at the hôtel-Dieu in Paris, and in spite of having no Latin was admitted to the Surgical College of St Come.

His writings describe his methods in detail, practical and tested. He considered that the duties of the surgeon should be '…to remove what is superfluous, to restore what has been dislocated, to separate what has grown together, to re-unite what has been divided, and to redress the effects of nature'.[30]

Parè wrote a series of reminiscences, *Journeys in diverse places* (*Voyages faits en divers lieux*), in which he tells his own story, full of incident and excitement. He wrote them in a reply to an attack on him by Etienne Gourmelen, Dean of the Faculty of Physicians of Paris: a reflection on the rivalry between the two branches of medicine. The physicians were annoyed that a surgeon should write on a wide range of subjects, and also to do so in French, not Latin. One of his replies to Gourmelen, whom he used to call ironically 'mon petit maître', says it all: 'Dare you teach me surgery, you who have never come out of your surgery? Surgery is learned by the eye and the hands. You, mon petite maître, know nothing else but how to chatter in a chair'.[31]

His aphorisms are always worth repeating, and show how practical he was and how others learned from his experience.

He who becomes a surgeon for the sake of money will accomplish nothing.

Mere Knowledge without experience does not give the surgeon self confidence.

A remedy thoroughly tested is better than one recently invented.

It is always wise to hold out hope to the patient, even if the symptoms point to a fatal issue.[32]

Parè was one of the surgical greats. His influence was enormous and his impact on changing surgery considerable. His writings and his ability to communicate his own experience point to a teacher of exceptional ability, and this in spite of the limitations under which he operated: no anaesthesia and antisepsis, and limited anatomy, physiology and pathology.

At about the same time as Parè, John Halle (1529–1568) gave his definition of the characteristics of a good surgeon: 'The heart as the heart of a lion, eyes like the eyes of a hawk, and his hands as the hands of a woman'.[33]

Other surgeons of note in that period were Thomas Vicary, who wrote the first anatomy text in English, and Peter Lowe, who wrote *A Discourse of the Whole art of Chirurgerie*, the first surgical text in English in 1597. This volume is of particular interest as it illustrates several educational issues. First is the link between Lowe and the Paris school of surgery (medical magnets, see p. 471). He was trained in Paris and worked there during the wars with Spain. Second is the very practical nature of the text. For example, it describes operations and wound dressings, and provides illustrations of surgical instruments, including a set for carrying 'in a little case'. Third is the dialectic approach of the text: the dialogue being between John Cointret, Dean of the Faculty of Surgery in Paris, and his scholar, Peter Lowe.

Lowe confirms the importance of Paris as a centre of excellence in surgery: '…where the professors are learned, wise and grave men who are so careful of the weal-publique that they admit no man into their Colledge except that he hath past his whole course in the science of Chirurgerie'.[34]

He sets out his intention to pass on his knowledge, mentioning again his 'secrets':

> *I impart to you my labours, hidden secrets and experiments by me practised and dayly put to use to the great comfort, ease and delight of you and such as have occasion to use my helpe in France, Flaunders and elsewhere, the space of 22 yeares: thereafter being Chirurgian major to the Spanish Regiments at Paris, 2 yeares: next following the French King my Master in the warres 6 yeares.*[35]

He notes that: 'I applied myself to the studie of chirurgerie, which is by the consent of all learned men not only a science very profitable and necessary to all sorts of people but also most ancient and honourable'.[36]

The dialogue itself is fascinating. Here are a few extracts (CO is John Cointret and LO is Peter Lowe):

> *CO. Seeing all doctrine whatsoever is founded on reason should begin at the definition into the end we may better understand…first may I ask you what is Chirurgerie?*

LO. It is a science or art that sheweth how to worke on mans body exercising all manual operations necessary to heal men in as much as is possible by the using of most expedient medicines.

CO. How many operations useth the chirurgian most commonly?

LO. Five.

CO. Which may they be?

LO. The first is to take away that which is hurtful and superfluous, as to take away tumours, warts and cancers and such like. Secondly to help and add to nature that which is wanteth, as to put in an artificial ear, nose, eye, hand, a leg, a plate in the roof of the mouth. The third is to put in the natural place that which is out of place, as to put the guts in the caule or net that covereth the guts called the epiplon or omentum, after they have fallen into the scrotum, to put bones in their own place being out of joint. The fourth is to separate that which is contained as in opening aposthumes, opening a vein, applying of horse leaches, cutting a ligament under the tongue, cutting two fingers growing together. The fifth is to join that which is separated as in healing broke bones, healing of wounds, ulcers, fistules and such like.[37]

The reader will note the similarity with the writings of Ambrose Parè. Indeed, Lowe acknowledges over 80 ancient authorities he has drawn upon for the book. He has some interesting words on how to learn surgery when asked by Cointret: 'Aristotle, the Prince of Philosophers counselleth us to begin at general things, thereafter to proceed to things more particular, from easy and facile things, to obscure and difficult, as is observed in all other sciences'.[38] No specifics are given but the principle is clear: start at the beginning and proceed forward.

Finally, one small practical note: when asked how many instruments the surgeon should carry, Lowe responds: 'Six.

A pair of sheers, a razor, a lancet, a sound, a triball and a needle'.[39] This could be the same response today.

These extracts show how practical surgery was and how, with an apprenticeship and exposure to numerous cases, a young surgeon might learn quickly.

GUILDS, COLLEGES, MEDICAL SCHOOLS AND REGULATION

In this period of medical history there were many professional rivalries and very large numbers of unqualified practitioners. The rise of the guild or college was an attempt to set standards of practice and maintain a body of doctors who were learned scholars and university educated. They only partly succeeded in this, and it was to take several more centuries and numerous fights and legal battles to achieve this.

In Europe, guilds, faculties or colleges were formed to bring together medical practitioners in particular areas. They acted as regulatory bodies, admitting only those who had satisfied certain standards. To that extent they were conservative and defensive, upholding the status quo. For example, the London College of Physicians was founded in 1518 by Henry VIII on the agreement that only those with degrees from Oxford or Cambridge were accepted into the College and allowed to practice in London. Hence, this was part of the reason why many students went to continental schools to become doctors.

Colleges and guilds did set up examinations and provide libraries and lectures, and a place for doctors to meet and discuss medical issues. They set standards and tested those who wished to practice, but they were small. The London College of Physicians had only around 20–30 fellows during the 17th century, while there were many more 'unlicensed practitioners' serving the population.

The Royal College of Surgeons of Edinburgh was established in 1505 as an 'Incorporation of Barber Surgeons with examinations in anatomy and the nature and complexion of man's body'. Prospective surgeons had to read and write, and the college provided an executed criminal for dissection each year. In England, the Royal Company of Barber Surgeons was established in 1540 by Henry VIII, and in Glasgow the Faculty of Physicians and Surgeons was established in 1599. This latter Faculty, now a College, ends each meeting to this day with the words '…and the poor were treated gratis, and the Faculty adjourned'.[40] A sentiment reflected in many of the guilds and colleges.

More details on the charters of the Royal Medical Colleges are discussed in Chapter 11.

MEDICAL SCHOOLS IN EUROPE

Medical schools sprang up all across Europe in the Renaissance period, the most famous ones being Padua, Bologna, Paris and Montpellier. They attracted students from near and far, and graduates returned home to spread medical knowledge. In this section, three medical schools—Paris, Padua and Vienna—have been chosen as case studies to illustrate the curriculum and the learning methods. In addition there is a note on non-university practitioners based on the work of Pelling and Webster,[41] together with a brief reference to the founding of the University of Leiden.

The medical school at Padua

In the 16th century and into the 17th, Padua was the location of perhaps the most famous medical school of all— Shakespeare's 'nursery of the arts'.[42] Harvey trained there, Vesalius published there, and an astonishing number of distinguished alumni spread the school's renown all over Europe. Padua was the place to be. It emphasised clinical instruction, and the first botanical gardens for medical purposes were founded there in 1545. It was still using the *Canon* of Avicenna well into the 17th century. But things were changing and gradually the Greek masters were introduced, and Hippocrates and Galen displaced the Arab teachers.

Padua was organised as colleges of doctors. The usual form of public examinations were employed including the writing of a dissertation. A hat, ring and books were given and the expenses paid by the graduate. The great advances in the medical school were mostly related to clinical teaching. In 1543, Giovanni Battista da Monte was the first to give lessons at the bedside of patients in the wards of St Francis' Hospital. First, the student was to observe the patient's appearance and then talk with him about his symptoms, then note his pulse and observe everything necessary to gain knowledge of the illness. This was a revolution, changing the scholastic nature of medical education to a practical one. It was eventually taken up across Europe, especially by Dutch graduates and in particular Jan van Heurne of Utrecht, who returned to Leiden. This was carried forward by van Heurne's son Otto, then Silvius de Boe and Herman Boerhaave and disseminated across the world.

Classes at Padua were organised on a strict hourly routine, announced by a bell in the tower of the Bishop's Palace. Teachers who failed to heed the bell were subject to a penalty. Of particular interest was the anatomical lecture theatre built in 1594 by Girolamo Fabrici d'Acquapendente. It is a magnificent theatre which still stands in 'il Bo', the old medical school. Anatomy began here with the work of Vesalius and was carried on by a very distinguished group of scholars. The Hall in 'il Bo' contains portraits and insignia of the greats in medicine at the time.

It is interesting to note that John Aubrey wished to go and study in Italy, and asked the advice of William Harvey who had graduated in Padua 40 years before. His response is illuminating. 'He bid me go to the fountain head and read Aristotle, Cicero and Avicenna, and did call the neoteriques (modern authors) shitt-breeches.'[43]

Paris and early modern France

France was one of the great centres of medical education in the 17th century. Paris was pre-eminent (followed by Montpellier); graduates had to take a second degree if they wished to practise in the city. The profession at the time was described as a 'penumbra', with the university graduates at the centre and the others, such as surgeons and unlicensed practitioners, filling the shadow. It is possible that the general public found this latter category more useful than the former.

Students were expected to follow the lectures in the faculty for a specified number of years and then to supplicate to be bachelors of medicine. Bachelors had to demonstrate their learning by giving a series of lectures, undergoing a number of oral examinations and serving a practical apprenticeship. They were then licensed by the bishop and received the right to practise in the local community and world wide (*hic et ubique*). Finally, the licentiates were incorporated into the select body of doctors and given the mark of respect, the doctoral cap.

Students were expected to read the ancients, and as late as 1516 the 'Commentaries' of the medical faculty of Paris record an admonition to three bachelors of medicine who had read books other that those assigned and, in consequence, were reprimanded for opposing the views of their teachers. The influence of Galen was especially strong in Paris and remained so well into the 17th century.

Particular medical men to note were Jean Fernal, who invented the Latin words physiologica, pathologica and therapeutics, and Laurent Colot (1520–1590). Colot developed adult lithotomy and (as with the Chamberlens, p. 103) passed the knowledge to his heirs where it remained in the family for eight generations until 1727—another example of 'secret' medicine. There was a rise in the importance of chemistry, and the book *Course de Chimie*, by Nicolas Lemery, became a classic.

The curriculum consisted of a teaching programme in five parts: physiology, semiology (the study of signs and symbols), pathology, hygiene and therapeutics. There were additional courses in anatomy, botany, surgery and pharmacy. Clinical supervision was poor and there was no practical course. Students were expected to graduate first and then pick up practical knowledge. In the words of Diderot: 'As a result the young doctor makes his first essays on us, and only becomes skilful by dint of murder'.[44] In the small towns around Montpellier, the large number of unsupervised bachelors were said to learn medicine by 'filling their first graveyard'. By the 17th century, professors were expected to give practical courses on the causes, progression and treatment of disease. The most famous course was by Lazarus Riverius, at Montpellier in 1640, and used his text *Praxis Medica*.

The medical school at Vienna

Another example of a medical school (outside Italy) which was also changing is Vienna. By the 19th century it would be one of the most famous in the world, but in the 16th century it was still small. Durling has reviewed its early days, along with the publication of an early manual for medical students and practitioners, the first printed introduction to the study of medicine (*Liber do modo studendi seu legendi in medicina*).[45] The medical faculty at Vienna was established in 1389, with a small number of staff and students. The statutes which set out the functions of the faculty might be traced to Padua, where one of the founding professors had studied. The *Liber* was written in 1520 at the request of students, and was not officially commissioned by the faculty. The faculty itself was well organised and listed the requirements for a bachelor's degree in medicine: a candidate had to have studied for a fixed number of years and at his examination would reply to two doctors in the presence of all of the doctors. His knowledge, character and station had to be assessed before he could be given the unanimous support of the faculty. There were various fees to

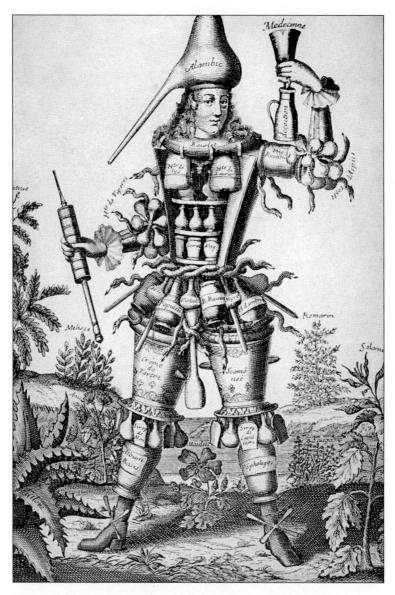

The apothecary: a man surrounded by pills and potions and the
instruments to deliver them to patients. These include a special
instrument for administering enemas. French, 17th century.

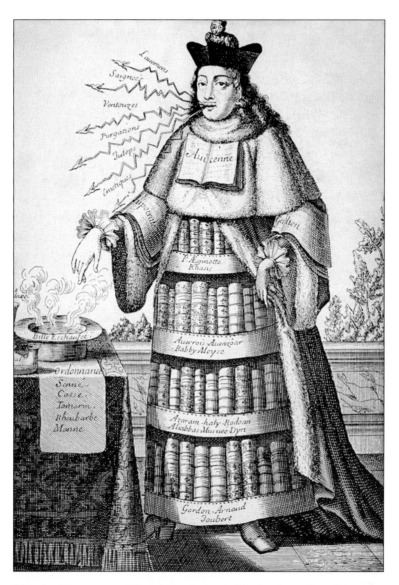

The physician: a man of learning, surrounded by books and speaking words of wisdom. Note the references to Hippocrates and Galen on the sleeves, and the names of Avicenna, Gordon, Arnoud, Joubert and others on the gown. French, 17th century.

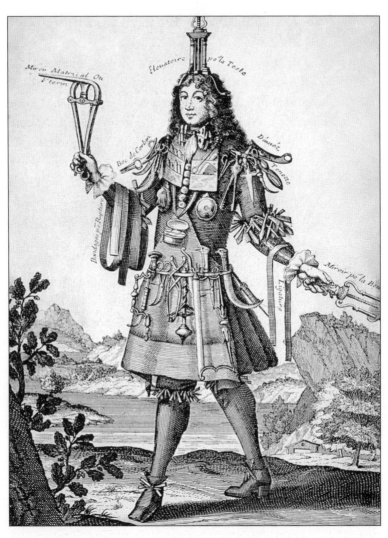

The surgeon: a man of action with a series of instruments for performing operations, including knives, scissors, bandages and ligatures. French, 17th century.

pay, and for doctoral status, the candidate had further conditions to satisfy.

To be granted an MD, the licentiate would be solemnly conducted to St Stephen's Cathedral by his promoter, accompanied by all the available doctors and others in the faculty. In the church the licentiate would 'determine' one further question, after which the beadle read the oath. Having sworn to lecture in the faculty for at least one year, he would then be recommended by his promoter. He would then praise the science of medicine and cite a chapter of Avicenna, Galen or Hippocrates. These texts would prompt further questions to which he would respond. As usual the graduate ended up entertaining all of the faculty.

The faculty also had the responsibility for the regulation of doctors in Vienna, and in this they had the support of the bishop, though it was difficult to enforce. There are a number of examples of this enforcement, including banning clerics from dispensing medicines or examining urines.

The key person in the production of the *Liber* was Martin Stainpeis, who matriculated in Vienna in 1476 and died in 1527. He lived through some momentous events in central Europe, and was elected Dean on eight occasions. The *Liber* is a quarto of 136 numbered pages and was printed in Vienna and dedicated to the Bishop of Vienna. In the dedication, Stainpeis expresses the hope that the bishop will demand that all former alumni practise according to the manual. The *Liber* is divided into seven books. The first sets out how the medical student should plan his reading. The second enumerates the books the graduate should peruse, and the third the reading for apothecaries. The fourth lists the errors in the latter, and the fifth lists simple and compound medicines in common use. The sixth outlines the correct style of practice, and the seventh book contains data the physician should always keep before him while visiting patients. The detail in each of these books is considerable and follows the student through the five years of the course. A remarkable list of books is given and a wonderful range of non-medical books (*Aesop's Fables*, for example) is included to keep up the habit of reading.

There are some splendid commonsense notes for the student: for example, make marginal notes of the most memorable passages, write down any tried remedies in a personal 'vade mecum', and collect all chapters on different diseases into one book and list at the end references to each book. The student should obey the fourteen rules in his daily practice (shortened here for brevity):

1. Pray regularly to God and be reminded of the words of Galen: 'Nature is the worker of all things, the physician is only her servant'.

2. The physician should be honest and not promise what he cannot deliver.

3. The physician should be dignified in his consultations.

4. He must not be a party goer.

5. He must have a pure conscience.

6. He must at all times be clean.

7. He must be a perpetual student.

8. He must keep aloof of civil cares.

9. He must dress according to his station.

10. He must live chastely and honestly.

11. If the physician wishes to take a wife he must be circumspect, let him marry his equal and not someone older than himself.

12. Because of the tremendous variety and complexity of work, he who professes medicine can become perplexed. Let him therefore study book 7 (*Speculum visitationis practicae*) in order that he might become calm and consoled.

13. Never send out a prescription without first checking it.

14. Let the doctor always have in his study a picture of Our Lord or the Virgin Mary to pray to in moments of stress.[46]

Finally, there is a section encouraging the doctor to be

...of good character and good memory, well formed, well behaved, daring in diseases where nothing is to be feared, circumspect in dangerous cases, let him flee severe diseases, be gracious to the sick, peaceable with his colleagues, cautious in prognosis, chaste, sober, pious, compassionate, not grasping or extortionate, but in accordance with his own labours and resources of his patient, the quality of the end sought and his own dignity, let him receive moderate recompense. [47]

Such early books give a clear message of the material to be learned and the methods used. The immensely practical nature of the work, the interaction of the student with the learning materials, working out his own 'vade mecum', is true problem-based learning.

Non–university educated practitioners

One of the features of this period was the number of non-university educated practitioners. Pelling and Webster have written on this subject with some excellent examples outside of London. The Royal College of Physicians at this period was very small and had little influence at the time, especially in the provinces. The number of fellows was around 30 and the number of candidates between six and eight.

The surgeons had a different system through the Royal Company of Barber Surgeons. Pelling and Webster record that in 1514, 72 surgical licences were issued in London, and at other times there seem to have been around 70–100 surgeons. By this period, surgeons were men of learning and widely read. They seem to have made more of a positive contribution than the physicians.

However, for many of the citizens of London, medical care would have come from the lower echelons of the barber surgeons, apothecaries or midwives. Most medicine came from family, neighbours, priests and a wide range of unlicensed male practitioners or wise women, having no formal authority from ecclesiastical or civil body to practise. The scale is difficult to assess but between 1550 and 1600 there were proceedings recorded against 236 individuals, and this must have been the tip of the iceberg. In the eyes of the College, all those outside its remit were considered ignorant, and we have seen how Culpeper replied to this.

Pelling and Webster note that:

> ...*the great majority of practitioners possessed no licence and only a limited education. They relied on their natural gifts. Many were simple tradesmen. Critics were fond of reciting the catalogues of "honest trades" deserted by intended medical practitioners. Some had been painters, some glaziers, some tailors, some weavers, some joiners, some cutlers, some cooks, some bakers, some chandlers...with other like rotten and stinking weeds...in town and country...abuse both physic and chirurgery.*[48]

It is interesting to note that in today's climate of widening participation, such trades would be welcomed into medical school.

Women were recognised as playing an important part in medical practice. They were apothecaries and surgeons, and a Mrs. Cook was appointed as resident surgeon apothecary to Christ's Hospital. Twenty-nine female practitioners were reprimanded by the College of Physicians between 1550 and 1600.

In a disunited profession in London, Pelling and Webster have estimated that there were around 50 physicians, 100 surgeons, 100 apothecaries and 250 other practitioners. If the population was around 200,000 in 1600, there would be one practitioner for every 400 people, not counting midwives, nurses and public health officers. Perhaps because of this confusion it is not surprising that people did not opt for a prolonged period of education. Yet there were those who wanted to have the qualifications and collected them in the way that we do today.

To investigate the situation in the provinces, Pelling and Webster used the example of Norwich, which was likely to be typical of others in the country. It was an important centre of trade and had a population second only to London. It had a cathedral, and a stable population ideal for study. It also had good records. Many of the physicians had doctorates, or more frequently licences from Oxford, Cambridge and the continental universities. From the 1550s there was a guild of barber surgeons and physicians, perhaps typical of other centres. It is important to note that the Norwich practitioners provided for a compulsory lecture every 3 weeks. York also included procedures for dissections. The guild had a warden who changed every 2 years. Like other organisations, there were special duties to treat the poor. As the Norwich Company also included the apothecaries by 1571, it predated the Glasgow structure by almost three decades. Women practitioners were important enough to be treated separately, and the constitution of the Company makes reference to 'brothers and sisters', indicating equality.

Pelling and Webster give considerable detail of the practitioners in Norwich and their daily work and case load. They show clearly that much was happening outside London and the two universities. Links with the Continent were strong, and all branches of the profession could be included in the process. Postgraduate and continuing education was thriving, medical care was being delivered cheaply and the care of the poor was given a special place. The number of practitioners indicates a ratio of 1 per 400 head of population (or perhaps less), a significant number if to this is added nurse midwives and others. The system was able to operate effectively without the control of the university trained physicians because of the strong community bonds which grew up. Unity in the profession nationally was to take much longer to achieve.

The University of Leiden 1575

This university is included here because of the manner of its founding. In one of the most remarkable choices ever given to a city, William of Orange rewarded the city of Leiden for its help in withstanding a long siege against the Spanish by offering either a remission of taxes to all citizens for 10 years, or the founding of a university. To their credit, the citizens chose a university. This story could not be confirmed on a personal visit to Leiden but one senior academic confessed that he still liked to tell it to students. In the late 17th and early 18th centuries, it was to become the centre of European medicine. It was open to all regardless of religion and established one of the earliest botanic gardens in 1590. Leiden's professor of anatomy, Nicholas Tulp (1593–1674), is forever remembered in Rembrandt's depiction of the anatomy lesson.

OTHER SIGNIFICANT INFLUENCES

Throughout this period there were a number of other significant influences on medicine. Some of the scientists have already been mentioned and, as the community was small, there was considerable overlap. In addition, there were scholars, playwrights and philosophers who all reflected or shaped medical practice. Some were medically qualified, others were acute observers of human behaviour.

Two playwrights

Two playwrights of the period had particular interests in medicine, though many others could have been chosen: Ben Jonson, Webster or Marlowe. However, Shakespeare and Molière are particularly interesting. Shakespeare's work keenly reflects the times and the role of doctors; Molière showed with great insight the nature of medical practice.

Shakespeare

Shakespeare demonstrated considerable knowledge of medical practice and health. His son-in-law, Dr. John Hall, may have been an influence, and Hall's case notes are of particular interest.

References to medicine abound in Shakespeare's works. For example, in *Twelfth Night*, Sir Toby says: 'Does not all our lives consist of the four elements?'[49] Fabian in the same play also recognises the use of urine in diagnosis: 'Carry his water to the wise women'.[50]

In a broader reference to diagnosis, Macbeth says

If thou couldst, doctor, cast

The water of my land, find her disease

And purge it to a sound and pristine health

I would applaud thee to the very echo

That should applaud again...

What rhubarb, senna, or what purgative drug,

Would scour these English hence.[51]

He was familiar with poisons, apothecaries and the use of drugs. He describes the poor state of the apothecary and the fascinating range of products available. In *Romeo and Juliet*, in particular, drugs are of special importance, and one is described which causes the person who takes it to appear dead. At the heart of the play is the message sent to Friar Lawrence who is unable to deliver it because:

While suspecting that we both were in a house

Where the infectious pestilence did reign

Seal'd up the doors, and would not let us forth

So that my speed to Mantua there was stayed.[52]

The plague and quarantine prevent the delivery of the message and lead to the consequent death of the two lovers.

Shakespeare records seven doctors in his plays, and one is referred to but does not appear. For a full account, the reader is referred to Simpson.[53] He never portrays a bad doctor, though there are some references to the doctor's love of money and, occasionally, his ineffectiveness. For example, in *Timon of Athens*, Timon says:

> *Go suck the subtle blood o'th' grape*
> *Till the high fever seethe your blood to froth*
> *And so scape hanging. Trust not the physician*
> *His antidotes are poison,*
> *And he slays more than you rob.*[54]

Surgeons are described on several occasions, and not always with approbation.

Molière

Molière is much more scathing about doctors. A quotation from one of his plays has already been given, but others provide a real flavour of medical practice and the education of doctors.[55] For example, in *Le Malade Imaginaire*, Monsieur Diafoirus, who is also a doctor is proud of his son's education:

> *He never showed signs of a lively imagination, nor of a quick intelligence you find in some; but these were qualities which led me to foresee that his judgement would be strong, a quality essential to the exercise of our art...Eventually after much hard slog, he succeeded in graduating with glory; and I can say without vanity that, in his two years on the benches, no candidate has made more noise than he in the disputes of our school. He has made himself formidable, and no thesis can be advanced without his arguing the opposite case to its ultimate extreme.*[56]

In *L'Amour mèdicin* there is a splendid comment on how doctors quarrel and the need to keep this from the public:

They should have contented themselves with the perpetual discrepancies in the opinions of the principal master and ancient authors of this science which are known only to those who are well read without showing the common people as well the controversies and inconsistent judgements.[57]

In a mock graduation at the end of *Le Malade Imaginaire*, the candidate answers all questions on the treatments for different ailments with the same responses, Clysterium donare, postea seignare, ensuitta purgare. The school in Paris at the time believed only in enemas, bleeding and purging; there was no other remedy!

As Calder notes:

…the strategy of Molière Paris doctors is to keep their body of theories and codes of practice intact. Too this they reduce the whole field of medicine to a verbally self-contained system; they banish the world of phenomena and experience from their discipline with a self referential linguistic code. When asked to explain why opium induces sleep, the graduand answers:

'Quia est in eo
Virtus dormitiva
Cunjus est natura
Sensus assoupire.'

The answer tells us nothing of the chemical composition of the opium or of the body's responses to it. Instead it is a perfect circle of words. Opium brings sleep "because it contains sleep-making properties whose nature is to induce drowsiness in the senses."

The response from the masters is 'Bene, bene, bene, bene respondere, dignus, ignus est entrare, In notsro docto corpore'. Roughly translated as 'he replies well and is worthy to be admitted to our learned body'. Everyone agrees![58]

Finally, Molière's last words on stage and his last words on medicine are revealing:

Vivat, vivat, vivat, vivat, cent fois vivat

Novus doctor qui tam bene parlat!

Mille, mille annis at manget et bibat

Et seignet et tuat![59]

Again in translation: 'Long live, long live, long live, long live, a hundred times long live the new doctor, who speaks so well! For a thousand and a thousand years may he eat, drink, bleed and kill!' This is a remarkable commentary on the experience in medical school in France (and no doubt elsewhere), supporting comments earlier in this chapter from Paris and Montpellier.

The philosophers

A number of Renaissance scholars and philosophers contributed to thinking in medicine and to our understanding of learning. Erasmus was perhaps the most distinguished, and John Locke's work on education has already been discussed. However, there are three others who merit special mention: Sir Thomas More, Francis Bacon and Renè Descartes.

Sir Thomas More (1478–1535)

More's classic, *Utopia*, was written in 1515 and details a perfect community and how it is governed. In describing the work to his friend Peter Giles, More apologises for being late in delivering the manuscript. He gives his excuse in words which will be very familiar to busy people:

> *For when I am home I must commune with my wife, chat with my children, and talk with all my servants. All the which things I reckon and account within business, for as they must of necessity be done; and done must they needs be, unless a man will be a stranger in his own house.*[60]

He makes a particular plea to deal with poverty and the issue of equity in Utopia, and that education is a priority. When there is spare time, a series of lectures is available, and most of the population are free attend. There is a spirit of cooperation and all work together for the common good, with public service in the community.

Within the city there are four hospitals which are large, wide and ample so that there is no crowding even if many have to be admitted. They are well appointed and have 'cunning physicians' present continually and remark is made that there is no one who would rather lie at home ill, than be in the hospital. They all agree that health is a 'most sovereign pleasure' and that sickness is grief, which is the enemy of pleasure. While no nation needs doctors less:

> ...physic is nowhere in greater honour because they count the knowledge of it among the goodliest and most profitable parts of philosophy. For whilst they search out the secret mysteries of nature, they think themselves to receive thereby not only wonderful great pleasure, but also obtain great thanks and favour of the author and maker thereof.[61]

Perhaps most controversially, More recommends euthanasia for those in continual pain and anguish and incurable disease:

> ...the priests and the magistrates exhort the man, seeing he is not able to do any duty of life, and by overliving his own death is noisome and irksome to others, and grievous to himself, that he will determine with himself no longer to cherish that pestilent and painful disease. And seeing his life is to him but a torment, and that he will not be unwilling to die, but rather take a good hope to him, either to despatch himself out of that painful life, as out of a prison, or a rack of torment, or else suffer himself willingly to be rid of it by others.[62]

There are some in Utopia who can devote themselves to learning and are exempt from all labours. But most of the people throughout their whole life give their spare time to learning, and they are taught in their own native tongue. They have access to all of the learning of the past.

More's stress on education, community and the importance of health and wellbeing are of significance, as is his acknowledgement of the role of euthanasia. *Utopia* has been widely read over the past centuries and its influence is considerable.

Francis Bacon (1561–1626)

Bacon was a complex individual. He was Cambridge educated and over his career acted as Solicitor General, Lord Keeper and Lord Chancellor, and was created Baron Verulam in 1618 and Viscount St Albans in 1621. He sought to create a new system of philosophy and was an inspiration for both scientists and philosophers. The 'Invisible College', the forerunner of the Royal Society, originally met to discuss his writings. His best known works are *The Advancement of Learning* and *Organum Novum*, together with a series of essays.

In *The Advancement of Learning*, Bacon considers the pace of learning (and the rather poor salaries of teachers). He also emphasises the importance of philosophy, 'so if any man consider philosophy and universality to be idle studies, he doth not consider that all professions are from thence served and supplied'.[63] This was an important statement, and for generations it was considered relevant to have an arts degree before studying medicine. There are those who would advocate the same today.

Bacon then considers human learning and concludes that man's understanding, as the seat of learning, consists of three parts:

history to his memory
poesy to his imagination
philosophy to his reason.[64]

History in this sense is about the world, natural history and the study of mechanical things. As far as knowledge of the body is concerned, it is divided into four aspects: health, beauty, strength and pleasure. 'So the knowledges are medicine, or art of cure; art of decoration, which is called cosmetic; art of activity which is called athletic; art of voluptuary—educated luxury.'[65]

The art and success of medicine are difficult to measure:

> ...for almost all other arts and sciences are judged by acts or masterpieces, as I may term them, and not by the successes and events. The lawyer is judged by the virtue of his pleading, and not by the issue of the cause. The master of the ship is judged by the directing of his course aright, and not by the fortune of the voyage. But the physician, and perhaps the politique, hath no particular acts demonstrative of his ability, but is judged most by the event; which is ever as it is but taken: for who can tell, if a patient die or recover, or if a state be preserved or ruined, whether it be art or accident?[66]

This issue of the measurement of the quality of the doctor's work and his or her competence is another issue which reverberates through this book. The role of the physician is not only to restore health but to relieve pain and suffering, and not only when this may improve the patient, but 'when it may serve to make a fair and easy passage'.[67] This latter sentiment is similar to that expressed by More in *Utopia*.

In *Organum Novum*, Bacon considers the interpretation of nature and man. It begins with a classic statement of the role of man in science:

> Man, as the servant and interpreter of nature, does and understands as much as his observations on the order of nature, either with regard to things or the mind, permit him, and neither knows or is capable of more.[68]

He also makes the clear statement that 'Knowledge and human power are synonymous. Since ignorance of the cause frustrates the effect'.[69] Knowledge is power! He goes on to say that discoveries are due to chance and experiment, and that present sciences are just arrangements of matters already discovered. The present sciences are useless for discovery of effects. He considers that there are two ways in which the truth can be investigated. The first is from our senses, using the information to develop general theories and principles. The second is to use these axioms to construct even more general ones. He argues for the use of reasoning and for imagination to see new things and relationships, for induction as well as deduction in our understanding of nature. However, he recognises that new ideas will not be easy to introduce.

> *Again, in the habits and regulations of schools, universities, and the like assemblies, destined for the abode of learned men and the improvement of learning, everything is opposed to the progress of the sciences; for the lectures and exercises are so ordered, that anything out of the common track can scarcely enter the thoughts and contemplations of the mind.*[70]

> *But by far the greatest obstacle to the advancement of the sciences, and the undertaking of any new attempt or department, is to be found in men's despair and the idea of impossibility.*[71]

This reflects another theme of this book, the introduction of new knowledge and ideas.

Bacon's *Essays* provide a fascinating glimpse into his wider interests. In particular, the essay 'On Studies' reflects his interest in learning. The quote at the beginning of this chapter comes from this essay. Study helps those who have natural abilities to improve and cultivate themselves. 'Read not to contradict or confute; nor to believe or take for granted; nor to find talk or discourse; but to weigh and consider.'[72] There then follows his memorable statement on the value of books.

> *Some books are to be tasted, others to be swallowed, some few to be chewed and digested: that is some books are to be read in only in parts; others to be read but not curiously; some are to be read wholly and with diligence and attention. Some books also may be read by deputy, and extract made*

of them by others…Reading maketh a full man; conference a ready man; writing an exact man.[73]

It is perhaps not difficult to see how the writings of Bacon stimulated so much debate and discussion, providing as they do a focus for new thinking and new ideas.

René Descartes (1596–1650)

René Descartes was educated at the Jesuit College at La Flèche, and like many others he wanted to find a new way of thinking by inventing a new way of reasoning. He travelled widely, testing himself and reflecting on his experiences. His main work, *Discourse on Method*, contains much that is relevant to education, and to medical education in particular. He considers first the mind and makes the statement 'it is not enough to have a good mind, rather the main thing is to apply it well'.[74] His comments on books reflect those of others, 'that to read good books is like holding a conversation with the most eminent minds of past centuries, and, moreover, a studied conversation in which these authors reveal to us only the best of their thoughts'.[75]

He set out four rules to observe:

the first was never to accept anything as true that I did not know to be evidently so

the second to divide each of the difficulties I was examining into as many parts as possible and necessary in order best to solve it

the third, to conduct my thoughts in an orderly way, beginning with the simplest objects and easiest to know, in order to climb gradually, as by degrees, as far as the knowledge of the most complex

and the last, everywhere to make the most complete enumerations and such general reviews that I would be sure to have omitted nothing.[76]

His dictum 'Cogito ergo sum' ('I think therefore I am'), was the beginning of his method. I know I exist, how can I explain everything else?

Descartes discusses the work of Harvey on the motion of the heart and goes wider and raises issues about other parts of the body. He eventually concludes that the body is a machine, albeit made by God and much better than any made by man. This section is of critical importance in the description of the body and was the foundation for a new way of understanding its function. It changed ideas and, not surprisingly, was contested. It set out a new philosophy, *Cartesian logic*, which has had a long and distinguished pedigree.

Descartes recognised how much was still to be known in medicine:

> *It is true that the medicine now practised contains little of notable use; but without intending to do it any dishonour, I am sure there is no one, even amongst those who practice it, does not admit that what is known of it is almost nothing compared with what remains to be known.*[77]

The final paragraph in the *Discourse* notes that he 'has resolved to devote the time left to me to live to no other occupation than that of trying to acquire some knowledge of nature, which may be such as to enable us to deduce from it rules in medicine which are more assured than those we have had up to now'.[78]

The discussion of Bacon, More and Descartes was to allow a broader consideration of the state of learning in the 16th and 17th centuries. Other examples could have been chosen, but these three illustrate the depth of the changes which were occurring, and which had a considerable influence on medical thinking and education.

SOME CONCLUSIONS

The 16th and 17th centuries were times of great change. The Reformation and the Renaissance set the wider context and the social and cultural patterns which challenged authority and the ancient writers. Scholars and philosophers began to think differently and this was reflected in medicine and medical education. The environment within which medicine was learned changed, not only because of the increasing knowledge but in new ways of thinking.

The increase in knowledge was considerable, particularly in anatomy and physiology, and the role of chemistry was beginning to be appreciated. In medical schools, the curriculum was changing, in some faster than others. Methods of learning were also changing. The printed book had a huge impact, perhaps the greatest of all. Lectures were being delivered in different ways, as the grand lecture theatres in Padua and elsewhere show. Anatomy was taught by those who knew the body, and not from a distance based on the writings of Galen. This alone was a considerable shift. Clinical experience was seen to be essential and the teachings, particularly of surgeons such as Ambrose Parè, demonstrated this. The techniques of learning remained similar, whether it was the question-and-answer method used by Peter Lowe, or the poetic rhymes of Fracastorius in his description of syphilis. But learning was there, and not only confined to the universities and medical schools, but to local guilds, companies and colleges, which provided a focus for learning and the development of professional practice.

Secret learning, already mentioned in this book, was also apparent, and the examples given of the Chamberlens and Colot show how deeply ingrained it was. The profession was not united and there were considerable rivalries between the various branches. The examination structure and qualification in medicine was essentially similar to that in the Middle Ages. Selection for university, and for some of the guilds and colleges, was partly related to the ability to read and write. The significant rivalry between the physicians and surgeons was unhelpful and perpetuated a distinction which was to last for several more centuries. The surgeons, on the whole, seemed to be more progressive and had learned much from experience.

But perhaps the most important issue was the change in attitudes to medical practice, expressed in the writings and teachings of many of those described in this chapter. Paracelsus is a prime example, burning the books of the ancients. Harvey begins to investigate the working of the heart and shows that Galen was wrong, and overturns a whole conception of the body. This is taken up later by Descartes who describes the body as a machine. New technologies such as the microscope are introduced, extending the human senses.

The role of the doctor is also explored, and the differences between Sydenham, the physician, and Boyle, the experimental medical scientist, are exposed. The question for medical education would be which model would be developed? This is a foretaste of the debate at the beginning of the 20th century, sometimes called the Osler–Flexner debate, on the kind of education to be delivered to aspiring medical practitioners. Again this debate continues.

This period in the development of medical education changed everything. Yet the fruits of the changes in terms of patient care were less than might have been expected, as the knowledge base had a long way to go, though much had been achieved.

REFERENCES

1. Bacon F. On studies. In Pitcher J, ed. The essays. London: Penguin Books; 1985; 209.
2. Osler W. Principles and practice of medicine. 9th edn. New York: Appleton; 1920. In preface by T McCrae.
3. Scott W. Harold the Dauntless. Oxford: OUP; 1913; 518.
4. Porter R. The greatest benefit to mankind: a medical history of humanity from antiquity to the present. London: Harper Collins; 1997; 181.
5. Colombo R. De re anatomica, Venet. 1559 Lib xiv; 258.
6. Sloan A W. English medicine in the seventeenth century. Durham: Durham Academic Press; 1996.
7. Ibid.

8. Molière J P. Le Malade Imaginaire.

9. Porter, 214.

10. Porter, 210.

11. Royal College of Physicians Annals, IV, f; 63a

12. Porter, 202.

13. Culpeper. The complete herbal. 1653, page vi.

14. Ibid.

15. Lathan R G. The works of Thomas Sydenham. London. See Vol I, page 4.

16. Blackmore R. A treatise on syphilis. 1723, page xi.

17. Locke, J. Some thoughts concerning education. 1693; para 118.

18. Locke, para 30.

19. Sydenham. Vol 1; 29.

20. Ibid, Vol 1; 54.

21. Ibid, Vol 1; 173.

22. Ibid, Vol 2; 123.

23. Ibid, Vol 2; 129.

24. Bannerman J. The Beatons: a medical kindred in the classical Gaelic tradition. 1998. Edinburgh: John Donald Publishers Ltd; 1998.

25. Ibid, 89.

26. Ibid, 91.

27. Kaplan B B. Divulging of useful truths in Physick. The medical agenda of Robert Boyle. Baltimore: Johns Hopkins University Press; 1993; 73.

28. Ibid, 125.

29. Guthrie D. A history of medicine. London: Thomas Nelson & Sons; 1958; 90, 146.

30. Porter, 158.

31. Guthrie, 144.

32. Guthrie, 148.

33. Porter, 186.

34. Lowe P. The Whole Course of Chirurgerie, 1597. Facsimile edn. Classics of Medicine Library; 1981; 82.

35. Lowe P. A discourse on the whole art of Chirurgerie. 1612.

36. Ibid, B.

37. Ibid, chapter 1.

38. Ibid, B3.

39. Ibid, chapter 1.

40. Gibson T. The Royal College of Physicians and Surgeons of Glasgow. Edinbugh: MacDonald Publishers; 1983; 19.

41. Pelling M, Webster C. In: Webster C, ed. Health, medicine and mortality in the sixteenth century. Cambridge: Cambridge University Press; 1979; 165–235.

42. Shakespeare W. The taming of the shrew. Act 1, scene 1.

43. Aubrey J. In: Clark E, ed. Brief lives. Oxford: Clarendon Press; 1898; Vol 1: 300.

44. Brockliss L B, Jones C. The medical world of early modern France. Oxford: Clarendon Press; 1997; 500.

45. Durling R J. An early manual for the medical student and newly-fledged practitioner. Martin Stainpeis' Liber de modo studendi seu legendi in medicina, Vienna 1520. Amsterdam: Clio Medica; 1970; 7–33.

46. Ibid, 22–23.

47. Ibid, 23.

48. Pelling and Webster, 185–6.

49. Shakespeare W. Twelfth night. Act 2, scene 3.

50. Shakespeare W. Twelfth night. Act 3, scene 4.

51. Shakespeare W. Macbeth. Act 5, scene 2.

52. Shakespeare W. Romeo and Juliet. Act 5, scene 2.

53. Simpson R R. Shakespeare and medicine. Edinburgh; E and S Livingstone; 1959.

54. Shakespeare W. Timon of Athens. Act 4, scene 3.

55. Calder A. Molière. The theory and practice of comedy. London: The Athlone Press; 1993.

56. Molière. Le Malade Imaginaire.

57. Molière. L'Amour mèdicin.

58. Calder, 133.

59. Calder, 137.

60. More T M. Utopia. Knoxville: Wordsworth Classics; 10.

61. Ibid, 95.

62. Ibid, 97-8.

63. Bacon F. The advancement of learning. 1605. In: Encyclopaedia Britannica. Chicago; 1952; 30.

64. Ibid, 32.

65. Ibid, 50.

66. Ibid, 51.

67. Ibid, 52.

68. Bacon F. Organum novum. In: Encyclopaedia Britannica. Chicago; 1952; 107.

69. Ibid, 107.

70. Ibid, 124.

71. Ibid, 125.
72. Bacon F. In: Pitcher J, ed. The essays. London: Penguin Books; 1985; 209.
73. Ibid, 207.
74. Descartes R. Discourse on method (1637). Harmondsworth, England: Penguin Books; 1968; 27.
75. Ibid, 30.
76. Ibid, 41.
77. Ibid, 79.
78. Ibid, 91.

5

Knowledge begins to grow: the 18th century

But why think. Why not trie the expt.[1]

John Hunter to Edward Jenner

How selfish soever man may be supposed, there are evidently some principles in his nature which interest him in the fortunes of others. And render their happiness necessary to him, though he derives nothing from it except the pleasure of seeing it.[2]

Adam Smith, *The Theory of Moral Sentiments*

INTRODUCTION

Several factors influenced 18th century thought in relation to medical education. It was an age of revolution—in America (1776) and in France (1789). A spirit of change charged the air, and books such as Thomas Paine's, *The Rights of Man* (1792), set the scene. It was also the age of Enlightenment, especially in Scotland with people like David Hume, Adam Smith, Dugald Stewart and Francis Hutcheson exploring new ways of thinking. In England, Jeremy Bentham (1748–1832) was writing about utilitarianism and the promotion of happiness.

It was the age of the polymath, when it was possible to be involved in a range of disciplines: science, medicine and the arts. Typical of this was Erasmus Darwin (1731–1802), an Edinburgh medical graduate from Lichfield who not only practised medicine, but wrote poetry (including the lengthy *The Temple of Nature*) and invented mechanical devices, including a speaking machine and a copying machine. His interests ranged across all of the sciences, and he established the Lunar Society of Birmingham, which often met at his house in Lichfield, and whose members included Franklin, Wedgwood, Boulton and Watt. By the end of his life he was recognised as one of the great English poets and is known to have influenced Blake, Wordsworth, Coleridge and Shelley. Another polymath was Sir John Pringle. He had an outstanding undergraduate career, graduating MD from Leiden in 1730. He settled in Edinburgh and was appointed professor of moral philosophy but continued to practise medicine. He became part of the army and advised the government and wrote *Observations on the Diseases of the Army* in 1752. It is of interest that a year later James Lind (1716–1794), another Edinburgh graduate, published his book *A Treatise on Scurvy* in 1753.

It was an age of great collectors, including the two Hunter brothers whose collections in London and Glasgow still remain significant. Sir Hans Sloane (1660–1753) amassed the great collection which would form the basis for the British Museum. James Cook (1728–1779) made a voyage of discovery around the world, bringing back exotic species. He was accompanied by Joseph Banks, another great collector who was a long-term friend of John Hunter.

It was a vibrant time in the fine arts. Theatre, writing, poetry and the visual arts all flourished in the 18th century.

Changes in health were also evident. England may have escaped the plague rife in southern Europe but numerous infections, such as smallpox, ague and fevers reduced the population to 5,200,000 by 1731, the lowest for almost 100 years. Deaths exceeded births. Johann Peter Frank was beginning to develop a major interest in public health, and the publication of his great work *System einer vollstandigen medizinischen Polizey* in nine volumes (1779–1827) was a major initiative. Medical practice continued much as before but there were some important discoveries which had an impact on medical education and these will be discussed later. Latin was the universal language of learning until the middle of the century when lectures began to be given in the vernacular. In many places, examinations were conducted in Latin until the 1830s and in Edinburgh until 1833. Private or extramural medical schools flourished in most medical centres. Teaching was given in the wards of hospitals, and, for example, Percivall Pott at St Bartholomew's Hospital gave lectures privately and used the wards for teaching. The same was the case in many provincial cities across Britain. One of the greatest of these private schools was that of William Hunter, which will be described later in this chapter. Teachers were not well paid and depended on the fees of students, which in some cases could be considerable. In 1771, Alexander Monro II wrote of his father that he had around 300 students, each of whom paid him 3 guineas.[3]

Many distinguished people, such as Diderot, Voltaire and Rousseau, studied medicine but did not practise; it was the mark of being part of a cultured and elite group. While medicine was practised in towns, there was a considerable rural population served by a variety of medical and non-medical practitioners. William Buchan wrote his book, *Domestic Medicine* (1769), in an attempt at educating the public about medicine. There was little regulation of medical practice (this really began in the 19th century and will be discussed in Chapter 6). In educational terms, the major shift was in the more systematic presentation of the subject, and while it was still possible to choose both the subjects studied and the teacher, there was more structure to the process. Students often complained that there was no guide to their subjects. In some places, cadavers for dissection were scarce. Students began to want more than just a dry lecture.

In the course of the century, there were three main centres of education which attracted students from all over the world: Leiden in Holland, Edinburgh in Scotland, and London in England. It is interesting to note that the last two were dominated by four Scots who all knew each other and were born in Lanarkshire within 30 miles of each other, within a period of 30 years: Cullen, Smellie, and the Hunter brothers. By the end of the century, the great development in clinical teaching was beginning in France and this will be discussed more fully in the next chapter.

The history of medicine in this period has been extensively documented and, indeed, just listing the names is like a roll-call of the greats in medicine: Hermann Boerhaave, Bernhard Albinus, William Cullen, John Gregory, Stephen Hales, William Hunter, John Hunter, Albrecht von Haller, Erasmus Darwin, Joseph Black, Henry Cavendish, Joseph Priestley, Antoine-Laurent Lavoisier, William Heberden, Giovanni Morgagni, Mathew Baillie, Edward Jenner, Thomas Percival, Johann Peter Frank, Sir John Pringle, James Lind, William Withering and many others. Their contributions are well described in text-books of the history of medicine.

Several important discoveries were made in the period, including that of aspirin from willow bark (Edmund Stone) in 1763, digitalis from the foxglove in 1785 (William Withering) and the discovery of and use of vaccination in 1798 by Edward Jenner (1740–1823). There were improvements in surgery, with the better handling of wounds, and cutting for the stone (to remove from the bladder) and cataracts.

However, the feature which characterises this period most is the clear ability of some institutions and individual teachers to attract students from all over the world. These we have already referred to as 'medical magnets'. To illustrate the concept, three places and four people will be examined in some detail, and from this a series of characteristics will be drawn out and discussed later in Chapter 10. They are Boerhaave (1669–1738) in Leiden, Cullen (1710–1790) in Glasgow and

Edinburgh, and William Hunter (1718–1783) and John Hunter (1728–1793) in London. The process could be applied to many other professions and at almost any period of time. It would have also been possible to choose others here, but these names and places exemplify the issues particularly well.

STUDENT LIFE

Much of the teaching of medicine in the 18th century was by way of apprenticeship.[4] The master accepted the pupil, who paid for the privilege and was taught and instructed in the methods and secrets. Apprentices needed to be literate and numerate, and the agreement was a formal one. Generally, the apprentice lived in the master's house and had to keep the rules, including not gambling or going into taverns or theatres. In *The adventures of Roderick Random* by Tobias Smollett (1721–1771), who had been a surgeon's apprentice, the hero confirms that he was able to 'bleed and give a clyster, spread a plaister, and pre-pare a potion'.[5] Smollett was a friend of both of the Hunter brothers, and in Roderick Random some of his experiences are related.

Roderick begins his career in a northern university and studies Greek, mathematics, moral and natural philosophy, but does not like logic. He has an interest in belles-lettres and has a talent for poetry. Following his studies, he joins Mr Lancelot Crab a surgeon in town as an apprentice. He claims knowledge of pharmacy and a little surgery and, while this is inadequate, the surgeon needs him to do all the dirty jobs. He leaves this post and goes to London taking with him some clothes, 'a case of pocket instruments, a small edition of Horace, Wiseman's surgery and ten guineas in cash'. He decides to enter the Navy as a surgeon and has first to pass the examination at Surgeons Hall. When he arrives for the examination a young man has just come out and the crowd succeed in finding out all of the examination questions. At length the Beadle calls his name

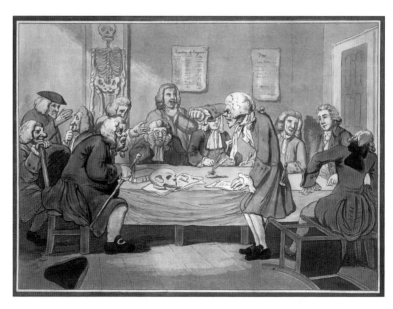

Roderick Random (a licentiate from Scotland) facing a board of examiners at Surgeons Hall. 1800. Reproduced courtesy of the Wellcome Library, London.

and he enters the Hall to be faced with a dozen grim faces sitting at a long table. He was first asked where he was from and when he answered Scotland the reply was 'we scarcely have any other countrymen to examine you here—you Scotchmen have overspread us of late as the locusts did Egypt'. The questioning proceeded and included one on how to deal with wounds of the intestine. This ended up with the examiners arguing with each other, and he was sent from the room. Happily he passed.

Lane has calculated the number of surgeon apothecaries in England in 1783 as 2607, or 82.3% of the medical workforce.[6] Medical families were common, often lasting for several generations. While there were and are advantages to apprenticeship, the disadvantages relate to the lack of a proper curriculum, and the inflexibility of the training. It would not be difficult to be out of date, and the apprentice was likely to see only a limited range of conditions.

Being a student was not easy. For many it meant travel and financial hardships. Bonner has nicely captured the spirit of the age.[7] Students were often young, in their teens as apprentices or even as students at university. Even then, they were a rowdy and coarse lot, callous and cynical. They behaved badly in classrooms, hissing and booing, and throwing things, even firing pistols. In general, however, medical study was hard work with long hours, especially as an apprentice. Student societies were set up: the Royal Medical Society in Edinburgh in 1734, the Guy's and St. Thomas's Hospital Physical Society in 1771 and the Medico–Chirurgical Society in Glasgow in 1801. Students were often unwell, and recorded their ills in letters home. But good teaching kept them awake and interested. For example, Benjamin Brodie said of John Abernethy at St. Bartholomew's Hospital: 'He kept our attention so that it never flagged and what he told us could not be forgotten'.[8]

BOERHAAVE

Herman Boerhaave was born in 1668, the son of a minister, and entered University of Leiden with the intention of becoming a theologian. He graduated Doctor of Philosophy, and while temporarily employed as a librarian, read all of the books in the library, including those on medicine. He submitted an MD to the University of Harderwyck in 1693. He published his *Institutiones Medicae* in 1707, and his *Aphorismi, Aphorisms Concerning the Cure of Diseases* in 1708. He became professor of botany and medicine and, in 1718, chemistry. His textbook on chemistry, *Elementa Chemicae*, was the best book on the subject throughout the 18th century. His acolytes and pupils went everywhere: Albrecht von Haller founded the school in Göttingen, Gerhard van Swieten went to Vienna, Linnaeus (Carle Linne) went to Uppsala, and the Edinburgh connection will be discussed in more detail later. He was called Cummunis Europae Praeceptor; the common teacher of Europe. He was seen as a master and friend, and corresponded widely. His pupils turned up in many guises: Thomas Secker (MD Leiden 1721) was a curate in Houghton-le-Spring in County Durham and became Archbishop of Canterbury in 1758. Martin Martin from Skye in Scotland graduated in 1710 from Leiden and wrote a book on the Western Isles of Scotland which was used by Johnson and Boswell doing the same journey years later.

The examination system in Leiden was similar to that in many other places. The student was examined on Hippocrates and Galen, and if he passed this he could ask the rector to be 'promoted', which included the printing of the thesis in Latin. Most graduations were in public and included the defence of the thesis. The 'promoter' then conferred the degree of Doctor of Medicine. To be promoted by Boerhaave was a special honour and one not to be forgotten; it was often recorded in obituary notices. Boerhaave was so famous that it is said that a letter from China addressed to Mr Boerhaave, Europe was delivered to Leiden. He held strong Christian beliefs, and when he gave up the Church he did not give up studying theology. He was still a Calvinist, searching for the truth in nature. He loved music and hosted performers at his country home near Leiden.

Boerhaave never stopped studying and continued to shape and change his mind with what he read. For example, his *Institutiones* of 1707 was Cartesian in philosophy, while his great volume on chemistry in 1732 had a non-mechanical ethos. His motto was '*Simplex veri sigillum*': 'Simplicity is the sign of truth'.

Boerhaave did not make any new discoveries, or conduct ground-breaking experiments; his teaching was the source of his renown. In Leiden during the time of Boerhaave, the lecture theatre (*theatrum anatomicum*) was well equipped and used for public dissections as well as for student lectures. Boerhaave's lectures were turned into books and transported across the world. James Houston was a young Scot who was in Leiden in 1710 and wrote about his stay there. He notes:

I can no more judge of the genius of the Dutch, than if I had never lived amongst them, for I know no Dutchman than my professors; but, if I am allowed to take Dr Boerhaave for a sample of the whole, I do say, that he is the most extra-ordinary Man of his Age, perhaps in the whole world; a clear Understanding, sound Judgement, with Strength of memory that nothing could exceed, and indefatigably labor-ious: it is true, he had not that brightness of Invention, that some authors may have: but with these talents he has done more Service to the World in the Knowledge of Physick, than all his predecessors in the Whole World put together; by digesting a huge Heap of Jargon and indigested stuff into an intelligible, regular, and rational system.[9]

Boerhaave was able to synthesise, clarify and put knowledge into a systematic form. Leiden at the time was a small town, tolerant and with a city council bent on improvement. Like Edinburgh, they made the key decisions and Boerhaave was the person to take things on. He held four different university chairs at the same time. His *Institutiones* covered the workings of animals, diseases, signs, preserving health and the cure of disease. There was a large botanic garden and a hospital in which to teach. His breadth of reading was considerable, and he had the ability to change his mind when faced with new ideas. He hated Descartes, but thought that Hippocrates and Sydenham were excellent.

Above all he was a teacher and inspired a generation of students from around the world. Some of these have been mentioned already but others have documented the extensive spread of Boerhaave's influence across Europe and America; they idolised him. William Hillary (Leiden MD, 1723) in his book, *An Inquiry into Improving Medical Knowledge* (published in London in 1761), says of Boerhaave:

Blessed with great penetration, a sane judgement, and the strongest of memory, all of which he applied with indefatigable industry, to obtain a perfect knowledge of all the learned,

and many of the modern languages, and all the sciences; an
able philosopher, the greatest anatomist, chemist, botanist
and the most eminent physician of this or any other Age.[10]

Another notebook from a student gives an insight into the
life of a student in Leiden.[11] Sinclair (1711?–1767) was from
Caithness, in the far north of Scotland. He had his early training
in Edinburgh with an Edinburgh surgeon and apothecary,
George Young, whose shop was in the Lawn Market. Sinclair
probably studied in Edinburgh before his trip to Leiden in
1736. In 1737 he went to Paris and graduated MD at Rheims
in 1738. His notebook describes the trip to Holland and the
expenses he incurred. At the time there were many Scottish
students at Leiden, which was noted to be a clean and quiet
town where there were many students from other lands,
including from far away 'Muscovy'. They could ride and fence
as well as study, and there was even a Scottish Minister to look
after them. They travelled around Holland, saw the sites and met
other fellow students.

Sinclair was busy. There were public and private lectures by
Boerhaave and Albinus, and he attended up to four public
lessons each day and four private colleges, in addition to the
time needed to write out the lectures. Perhaps the most
interesting pages record the books he bought and the money he
spent on them. He purchased 48 titles and spent one hundred
guilders on them. The range was considerable, and Leiden was a
great source of booksellers. They included in addition to medical
and science books, the works of Shakespeare, Dryden and Farquhar,
a remarkable and interesting small library to have collected.
Perhaps most interesting is the fact that Sinclair returned with
all his learning from Europe and his library and set up practice
in Thurso, a small town in the very north of Scotland.

Records show that between 1701 and Boerhaave's death
37 years later, there were 746 English-speaking students who
matriculated at the medical faculty (English 342, Scots 242,
Irish 120).[12,13] To show how powerful this influence was,

55 became fellows or licentiates of the Royal College of Physicians of London, including four presidents, and 45 were fellows of the Royal Society including Sir John Pringle who was president. They became royal physicians and men of distinction, and were important in developing the voluntary hospital movement. As will be discussed later, it was pupils of Boerhaave who established the medical school in Edinburgh, which would take on the mantle of Leiden as the great medical school of the later 18th century.

William Cullen, a pupil of Boerhaave and central to the development of the Edinburgh medical school, noted how he had been: 'taught to think the system of Boerhaave to be very perfect, complete and sufficient' and when he then dared criticise his hero, as we shall see later, he was advised to stop as his behaviour might damage himself and his university.[14]

Boerhaave corresponded widely with students and others. He wrote in Latin, French and Dutch. A regular correspondent for over 25 years was Sir Hans Sloane, who was President of both the Royal Society and the Royal College of Physicians in London. The last of his letters to Sloane (preserved in the British Museum) was delivered in July 1736 by the young Linnaeus. Boerhaave was asking Sloane, then in his 70s, a very special favour on behalf of Linnaeus:

> *Learn to know the man as I know him. You shall deign him worthy of your friendship, also worthy to reveal your treasures to; it is to inspect them that he greets you. That he should be granted this by you, I long for most ardently with all eagerness; and if you should have any trust in me, I shall be granted that wish.*[15]

What a remarkable letter from the doyen of medicine in Europe to the most senior member of the medical and scientific fraternity in England, delivered by the man who would define the classification of the animal and plant kingdoms.

Since the 18th century, the University of Leiden and the legacy of Boerhaave have grown. From an educational perspective, it is perhaps the 19th century which is of interest. Covering a small circular stair leading to the first floor is a series of cartoon drawings (Gradus ad Parnassum) depicting the life of the medical student. The first has the student leaving home and his tearful mother. In the second, the student is in debt and being tempted by wine, food and Venus. Next we see the student at study, and then finally as he is welcomed home by his father. At the top of the stairs is a room, the 'Zweetkamertje' or the 'Sweat Room'. Above the door is the legend, 'Abandon Hope all ye that enter' and the slogan 'hic sudavit sed non frustra'—'here he sweated but not in vain'. It was used as a waiting room for examinees in the 18th century and is covered in the signatures of past students. To this day, those who pass their doctoral examinations sign the wall to signify that their study was not in vain.

In the Boerhaave Museum in Leiden are four paintings which depict the four guises of doctors: the God, the angel, the man and the devil. They are beautifully painted and feature numerous clinical scenes, with both physicians and surgeons. In the first, the physician tends to a sick person, together with three other cases of doctors treating illness. The second sees doctors as ministering angels, and in the third the patients are on the road to recovery. The final scene, where the doctor is shown as the devil, gives the moral of the story. The patients are fully recovered and no longer remember how ill they were, and the doctors want paid. The bills are too high and the doctors are now seen as devils. A verse below the last print advises doctors 'laat de luyden u tellen, de wijl sy quellen', or 'get payment in advance while the patient is still in pain'.

CULLEN (1710–1790) AND THE MEDICAL SCHOOLS OF GLASGOW AND EDINBURGH

Scotland was the centre of medical education in 18th century Britain. The largest number of doctors were educated in Glasgow or Edinburgh: between 1750 and 1800, 2600 students received their degrees from Scottish universities, ten times the number from Oxford or Cambridge. While Oxford and Cambridge were educating the elite, the Scots were educating the middle and lower classes, and poor students were encouraged. The degree required 3 years of study, at least one of them in Glasgow or Edinburgh. They had a full range of courses: medicine, surgery and midwifery, and included practical work. The integration of medicine and surgery was of particular importance, given the separation between them in London (later broken there by the Hunter brothers). The colleges of physicians in London and Edinburgh refused to link with surgeons and midwives. Chemistry and botany were pioneered, and William Cullen persuaded the University of Glasgow to set up a chemical laboratory and began the first class in botany. He recruited Joseph Black who wrote to his father: 'I find every day that Chemistry is a branch of natural philosophy of the most extensive and solid use in all the arts but particularly in medicine'.[16] Black followed Cullen to Edinburgh. Black also notes one of Cullen's important features:

> *Dr Cullen about this time began also to give lectures on chemistry which had never before been taught in Glasgow and finding that I might be useful to him in that undertaking employed me as his assistant in the laboratory and treated me with the same confidence and friendship and direction in my studies as if I had been one of his children.*[17]

An interesting question is why it was Edinburgh and not Glasgow which became the centre of medical education in the 18th century. Both needed strong medical schools, but Edinburgh, with the support of George Drummond (1687–1766) the Lord Provost, was able to persuade the Council, and with the approval of the College of Physicians of Edinburgh, to approve posts, while Glasgow was more conservative and the higher echelons of the university were not interested. A hospital was built and clinical teaching flourished.

There is a message here to all university presidents about taking risks and being proactive.

The establishment of the Edinburgh medical school in 1726 is thus an interesting case study of why certain centres become important. Many Scots had been to Leiden to study, attracted by the teaching of Boerhaave and his colleagues. Alexander Monro primus (1697–1767) was already professor of anatomy and had studied with Boerhaave. Sir Robert Sibbald (1641–1772) had spent a year or so in Leiden, returning to become the founder of the Royal College of Physicians of Edinburgh (1681); he was first professor of medicine at the Town's College, later the university. The medical school was set up with Dr. Andrew Sinclair and Dr. John Rutherford as professors of the theory and practice of medicine, and Dr. Andrew Plummer and Dr. John Innes jointly as professors of medicine and chemistry. All four had been to Leiden. With the political instability in France, Edinburgh became an obvious place to have a medical school as part of the 'Town's University'. In 1750, a special ward was opened up for clinical teaching, the first in Britain. Supporting the University medical school there were numerous extramural classes, in Edinburgh and elsewhere. In Glasgow (which kept good records from 1803), 300–500 students enrolled each year and may have reached 1000 by the 1820s. In contrast, the number of graduations was between 5 and 15. Competition was fierce and lecturers were paid by the students following registration with a fairly small matriculation fee. This was the same in Hunter's London where the lecture fees were a crucial part of the income of the doctor. Students often arrived with letters of introduction and were generally poor. There was no real syllabus and students could choose as they wished.

Numerous guides appeared including one entitled: *A Guide for Gentlemen Studying Medicine at the University of Edinburgh* (1792, authorship disputed between James Hamilton and Alexander Hamilton, denied by both), which set out what was available. This book provides a way into the complex world of medical education, when the market was dominant and professors' fees came directly from students. It begins:

When young men, unacquainted with the extent of knowledge necessary for medical practitioners, are left to pursue their studies without a guide they must often be led astray with the enticing fields of fancy and speculation, when they ought to be attending other objects.

...Teachers and fellow students are often consulted about the plan of studying medicine; but as their opinions are generally biased by prejudice or motives of interest, it is obvious that their advice can never be depended on.

...The following sheets contain a concise description of all of the medical institutions at Edinburgh, with hints respecting the proper method for reaping benefits from them.[18]

The Author then gives some examples:

Anatomy. The plan of Dr Monro's course of lectures is much more extensive than any other teacher on anatomy, perhaps in Europe.

Chemistry. Dr Black, whose celebrity is so great that it is unnecessary to mention the important advantages which may be derived from attending his lectures.

Materia Medica. The medicines employed in the cure of diseases, have within these few years, been reduced to a small number, and, correspondingly, their history, qualities, appearances, and doses necessary to produce proper effects may be easily acquired. From this circumstance it has become fashionable for the young gentleman, studying at Edinburgh, to despise or neglect Dr Home's class.

Practice of Medicine. Dr Gregory, whose abilities are so well known, succeeded the celebrated Dr Cullen in this charge. As he has not yet made out a perfect plan of lectures, very little can be said respecting this course.[19]

This last statement was taken up by Dr. Gregory, who was clearly upset by this, and he produced a response in 1793 which was 152 pages long. Not surprisingly, Dr. Hamilton then gave an 86 page rebuttal to Dr. Gregory.

The author then gives his views on the numerous private schools and teachers:

> *In consequence of private teachers, the professors are stimulated to perform their duty with vigour, and are prevented from becoming inattentive. This advantage, however, is more than counter-balanced by the bad effects which have originated from the lectures of several private teachers.*[20]

Most interestingly, the author then sets out a plan of study for several different categories of student—a basic curriculum for them to follow. This included information for those who:

+ intend to complete their education at London or Paris
+ mean to take the degree of Doctor of Medicine at Edinburgh
+ wish to practise as surgeons or apothecaries immediately after leaving the College
+ wish to perfect themselves in the knowledge of the practice of medicine and surgery having served as an apprentice to a surgeon or apothecary
+ have already studied at another university and propose to graduate at Edinburgh
+ having obtained degrees of Doctor of Medicine at another university, attend the College of Edinburgh for the purpose of acquiring the opinions of the several professors on the different medical subjects.[21]

For each a plan is devised and, as an example, below is the advice offered to those students who wished to practice as surgeons or apothecaries immediately after leaving college:

> *First Year. Anatomy, Chemistry, Infirmary, Institutes of Medicine, Midwifery*
>
> *Second Year. Anatomy, Clinical Lectures, Infirmary, Materia Medica, Practice of Medicine*

Third Year. Anatomy, Infirmary, Lectures on surgical cases, Midwifery, Practice of Medicine.[22]

Other interesting information provided includes the library opening hours—10.00 am and 1.00 pm—and that in the first week of term most of the professors gave free 'taster' lectures to aid students to choose an appropriate course.

At this time Adam Smith was writing *The Wealth of Nations*, and in a letter to Cullen in 1774 Smith attributes the present acknowledged superiority of the Edinburgh course to the fact that professors received no salaries and had to rely on the diligence and success in their profession to attract students.[23] Smith based his ideas on an image of students which might be called idealistic and wrote in *The Wealth of Nations*:

Where masters really perform their duty, there are no examples I believe that the greater part of the students neglect theirs. No discipline is ever requisite to force attendance upon lectures which are really worth the attendance.[24]

Today, in an age of rising student fees, teachers may need to keep this in mind.

Alexander Monro secundus succeeded his father as professor of anatomy, and the triumvirate was completed by the appointment of Alexander Monro tertius to succeed him. Secundus was a major figure but tertius (1773–1859) did not live up to his predecessor's quality, who began his lectures with 'When I was a student in Leiden in 1719'.[25]

Cullen himself was born at Hamilton in Lanarkshire, where his father was a lawyer. He went to Glasgow University where there was no medical school and was apprenticed to a surgeon. He spent some time in London and travelled to the West Indies before settling back in his native Hamilton. He formed a friendship with the young William Hunter, who then went to London to study medicine. They corresponded on various ideas over the years, including the medical school at Glasgow. Cullen moved back to Glasgow, and at the age of 41 he was appointed professor, lecturing on medicine, chemistry and botany. He could well be seen as the father of the Glasgow Medical School before moving to Edinburgh in 1755. His lectures were in English rather than Latin. By the 1820s, Latin was no longer the language of the Scottish Universities and some thought it was unreasonable to continue to examine in Latin. George Jardine, professor of philosophy in Glasgow, noted:

> ...to discourse to the young men three or four years in English, without asking a single question in any other language; then all at once to mount upon their Latin stilts and come forward with the learning of a Celsus...[26]

Joseph Black was Cullen's assistant, who took over from him both in Glasgow and Edinburgh. Cullen wrote a popular textbook, *First lines of the Practice of Physic*, in 1777 but was not an innovator. He was well known as a teacher for the care he took of students and his interest in them. He was more than a good lecturer, he was a dedicated mentor to many, such as Black, Robert Willan, William Withering, John Rogerson, Gilbert Blane, John Letsom and others. He invited them to his home for supper and discussed medical and non-medical topics with them. He had a library of 3765 books, amongst which were a number of non-medical ones. Lisa Rosner, in *Medical Education in the Age of Improvement*, comments on the lives of the students.[27]

As a teacher, Benjamin Rush notes of Cullen:

> His constant aim was to produce in their minds (of the students) a change to an active from a passive state; and to force upon them such habits of thinking and observation as should enable them to instruct themselves.[28]

John Gregory, another teacher at Edinburgh, notes:

> ...[Cullen's] meaning plainly was that while he endeavoured to instruct his pupils in the well established and useful facts and principles of physic, which are often dry and tedious,

sometimes even disgusting, it was necessary to beguile and animate them on their weary way, by amusing them with more pleasing prospects, and engaging them in pursuits, which, by rousing them to active exertions, might quicken progress in their toilsome journey; even when they seemed to withdraw them farthest from the common beaten track.[29]

Rosner quotes from Samuel Bard who commented:

What I greatly admire is the manner in which Cullen gives these lectures. We convene at his house once or twice a week, where after lecturing for one hour, we spend another in easy conversation upon the subject of last evenings lecture, and every one of us is encouraged to make his remarks or objections with the greatest freedom and ease. I cannot help comparing him on these occasions to Socrates or some other of the ancient philosophers surrounded by his admiring pupils.[30]

Cullen had the ability to give his teaching a coherence which was helpful amidst the rather confusing situation in Edinburgh at the time, with lecturers competing and holding different views. He could engage people and, using stories, hold their attention. He took a broad view of the world and of his topics, and was concerned with relationships between them rather than the details. He wanted to incorporate new facts into his system yet maintain an established cohesion.

He was actively involved in the students' Royal Medical Society, founded in 1734 when six students got together to dissect the body of a woman who had died of a fever. The Society was given its Royal Charter in 1778. At the opening of the new Hall in 1775, Cullen gave the toast: 'May the professors and students always live in amity together, and sometimes drink wine together'.[31]

Cullen worked incredibly hard (one of the marks of a 'medical magnet') and with great efficiency. By 9 am each morning he had read all his letters, registered by an aide who noted the date, source, etc., and he dictated his replies before going on his visits. He would sign letters and write the appropriate prescriptions. All his correspondence, along with copied replies, were placed in folios for future reference. Most correspondence was answered within a day, and from 1781 he used a copying machine invented by James Watt. What could he have done with a computer and email?

Cullen's *Institutes of Medicine* rested on the three pillars: life and health (physiology), the causes of disease (pathology), and the prevention and curing of disease (therapeutics). He was concerned with the classification of disease and on some occasions was criticised for modifying Boerhaave's system. As Cullen notes, there was:

> *...an outcry against me...I promised to be cautious...as I truly esteem Dr Boerhaave as a philosopher, a physician and the author of a system more perfect that anything that has gone before, and as perfect as the state of science this time would permit of...I was however no violent reformer, and by degrees only, I ventured to point out the imperfections, and even the errors of Dr Boerhaave's system...*[32]

Students worked hard too. In a letter to his father, Thomas Ismay records that he rose:

> *...about 7, read until 9, then go to Dr Cullen's class, come back at 10 then breakfast and transcribe some notes which I have taken of his lecture. From 12 to 1 I walk in the infirmary, from 1 to 3 attend Dr Monro. Then come back and dine, as you may suppose I am very hungry. From 4 to 5 attend Dr Young from 5 to 6 transcribe notes I have taken from Dr Young and Dr Monro's lectures; from 7 to 9 transcribe the lectures I have borrowed and at 9 get supper; from 10 to 12 write lectures besides every Tuesday and Thursday from 5 to 6 o'clock I attend clinical lectures.*[33]

Cullen was a great teacher and had a passionate concern for his students. He worked incredibly hard and handed his learning on to thousands. With other colleagues in Edinburgh, he sent many graduates and students across the world. The first medical schools in America were founded by Edinburgh graduates: the University of Pennsylvania (1756) and Kings College New York, later Columbia University, in 1767.

WILLIAM HUNTER (1718–1783)

William Hunter was born at Long Calderwood in Lanarkshire in 1718, the seventh of ten children. He matriculated at Glasgow to study for the ministry but left without a degree. He became an assistant to William Cullen in Hamilton before moving to London. He went for a year to Edinburgh and attended the classes of Alexander Monro primus. He joined the renowned obstetrician William Smellie in London and lived with him for a while before moving to James Douglas, another anatomist and midwife, and then moved on to his own place. In 1743, he accompanied Douglas to Paris and attended Ferrein's classes in anatomy, the best in Europe at the time. This certainly widened his outlook, and he returned with the methods he was to use in London. It is of interest to note that when the anatomical drawings of Leonardo da Vinci were found in the library at Windsor Castle and were shown to William Hunter for his comments:

> I believe he was, the best anatomist and physiologist of his time; and that his master and he, were the first who raised a spirit for anatomical study, and gave it credit: and Leonardo was certainly the first man we know of who introduced the practice of making anatomical drawings.[34]

William Smellie (1697–1763) was born in Lanark, studied medicine at Glasgow and practised in his home town before going to Paris and settling in London. He became the leading obstetrician and teacher of his era; his book *Treatise on Midwifery* appeared in 1752. There was a large 'Scottish mafia' in London at the time and he knew them all; William Pitcairn, Tobias Smollett, John Armstrong, William Wilkie, John Pringle, Thomas Dickson and many others. He was a frequent visitor to Europe. In London as a surgeon and a man–midwife, he was not eligible to become a fellow of the College of Physicians and was rebuffed when he tried.

When William Hunter set up his own school, it was clear that he offered a more comprehensive course than any of the rival schools in London, and large numbers attended his lectures and had access to a body for dissection. This included London society of the day. In 1777, Adam Smith and Edward Gibbon attended a course of lectures and Hunter was acknowledged as an outstanding speaker. This was partly because of the major advances he spoke about in anatomy and obstetrics. He used lectures, rather than books, to communicate these advances; it was his knowledge and you had to come and hear it as delivered by him. In this sense he was like many others previously described in this book; the 'secret' knowledge had to be heard directly from the master rather than transmitted by others who had read books. Of course, there were good business reasons for doing this, but there was also a downside. William's publication rate was low, and he noted that some anatomists seemed to be writing up his discoveries and claiming the credit. This was particularly the case with Dr. Monro, the anatomist from Edinburgh. Hunter wrote his *Medical Commentaries* as a plain and direct answer to Professor Monro Junior—over 100 pages of arguments against Dr. Monro who may or may not have stolen the ideas behind his anatomical discoveries. In addition to some very detailed anatomy, it contains a list of testimonials from those who attended Hunter's lectures and who confirm the substance of his arguments.

William Hunter had an extensive obstetric practice, with very fashionable patients. He was Physician–extraordinary to Queen Charlotte, supervising her many pregnancies. In his favourite coffee house in London, he often gave the toast 'May no English noblemen venture out of this world without a

Scottish Physician, as I am sure that there are none who would venture in'.[35] By the end of the century, thanks to the work of Hunter and his contemporaries, the modern practice of non-intervention on uncomplicated births was established. Much of this was based on Hunter's mentor when he arrived in London, William Smellie, and to Charles White who practised in Manchester. Hunter's obstetric practice and lecturing gave him a considerable income, which allowed him to continue work on experimental physiology and anatomy, and build up his collections.

William also gave an interesting piece of advice to those aspiring to become doctors:

> Were I to place a man of proper talents, in the most direct road for becoming truly great in his profession, I would chuse a good practical anatomist, and put him into a large hospital to attend the sick, and dissect the dead.[36]

It is interesting to speculate on the kind of career advice Hunter would now offer. Would it include genetics, pharmacology, molecular biology or perhaps the arts and humanities or social sciences? The range is enormous, and it is difficult for the young doctor to choose the most appropriate. I suspect they use role models to help them on their way.

Other aspects of these *Two Introductory Lectures* are equally interesting. The whole of the first lecture (62 pages) is a history of anatomy from China, Greece, Rome and Arabia until the 18th century, a fascinating introduction for students. He includes latterly Vesalius, Harvey, Cheselden, Albinus and James Douglas, 'my old master and friend'. His second lecture is more concerned about the role of anatomy and its value. On page 67, he states:

> That anatomy is the very basis of surgery every body allows. It is dissection alone that can teach us, where we may cut the living body with freedom and dispatch…this informs the head, gives dexterity to the hand, and familiarise the heart

with a sort of necessary inhumanity, the use of cutting instruments upon our fellow creatures.[37]

What a wonderful human note in the last phrase!

He is scathing on those who do not think anatomy is valuable: 'Who then are the men in the profession, that would persuade students that a little anatomy is enough for a physician, and a little more too much for a surgeon? God help them'.[38]

An interesting facet of William Hunter's career was his role as professor of anatomy at the Royal Academy of the Arts; he was familiar with the artists Ramsay and Reynolds. The Royal Academy was established in 1768 and its foundation document decreed that 'there shall be a Professor of Anatomy, who shall read annually six public lectures in the Schools, adapted to the Arts of Design'. The Academy brought together the great British artists of the day for discussions and exhibitions. William's appointment was appropriate as both a distinguished anatomist and as an art collector. Zoffany's painting of him lecturing at the Academy is a classic. He began his lectures with a piece on the artist's role in depicting nature and the need to get close to nature and be 'life-like'. His statement at the opening of one of his lectures that 'The human body is so wonderfully complex that a man's whole life might be usefully employed in the study of it' is a comment on his own career.[39]

He also notes for the artist that 'All parts of the body, except the blood, are naturally a pale or white colour; and that the red, or purple, or blue which appears in the surface of living bodies is produced entirely by the red blood shining through the vessels and skin'.[40] He enjoyed giving the lectures and comments that 'I will endeavour to improve, to share in the pleasures of learning; and I shall think myself much obliged to any Members of the Academy if they will favour me with any useful hints, that may occur to them on the subject of my lectures'.[41] He covered poetry in these talks, as well as sculpture and painting.

After being in London and teaching for some time, Hunter commenced his own series of lectures on anatomy and advertised them as being carried out 'in the same manner as in Paris'.[42] In 1768, he eventually moved to premises in Great Windmill Street which contained 'a handsome amphitheatre and other convenient apartments for his lectures and dissections, there was one magnificent room fitted with great elegance and propriety as a museum'.[43]

As a testimony to William Hunter's teaching the following appeared in the *Gentleman's Magazine* obituary:

> *To consider him as a teacher, is to view him in his most amiable character: perspicuity, unaffected modesty, and a desire of being useful, were his peculiar characteristics; and, of most others, he was most happy in blending the utile with the dulce, by introducing apposite and pleasing stories, to illustrate and enliven the more abstruse and jejune parts of anatomy; thus fixing the attention of the volatile and the giddy, and enriching the minds of all with useful knowledge.*[44]

Brock quotes Simmons who said that Hunter was 'never happier than employed in delivering a lecture'.[45] And Hunter himself said: 'To acquire knowledge and to communicate it to others has been the pleasure, the business and the ambition of my life'.[46]

William Hunter led by example. In an oft quoted passage he says to his students:

> *I firmly believe that it is in your power not only to chuse, but to have, which rank you please in the world. An opinion the child of spleen and idleness, has been propagated, which has done infinite prejudice to science as well as virtue. They would have us believe that merit is neglected, and that ignorance and knavery triumph in this world. Now, in our profession it seems incontestable, that the man of abilities and diligence always succeeds. Ability, indeed, is not the only*

requisite; and a man may fail who has nothing besides to recommend him; or has some great disqualifications either of head or heart. But sick people are so desirous of life and health, that they always look out for ability; and surely the man who is really able in his profession, will have the best chance of being thought so. In my opinion, a young man cannot cultivate a more important truth than this, that merit is sure of its reward in this world. [47]

William had a major plan for a medical school in Glasgow and tried to encourage Cullen and Black to help: 'You, Black and I, with those we could chuse I think could not fail of making our neighbours stare. We should at once draw all the English, and, I presume, most of the Scots students. Among other reasons I should not dislike teaching anatomy near my two friends the Munros to whom I owe so much.'[48] The plan came to nothing, but Hunter's influence in Scotland was considerable.

JOHN HUNTER (1728–1793)

John was the youngest of the 10 Hunter children and left Long Calderwood to join his brother in London in 1748, just three years after the Jacobite uprising and the defeat of Prince Charlie in 1745. He rode to London with Thomas Hamilton, who would become professor of anatomy in Glasgow. His interest was in nature and when he arrived in London, William set him the task of dissecting an upper limb. It was clear that he was going to excel in this field. He commenced his study of surgery under Cheselden and Pott, and he could not have chosen two more distinguished surgeons under whom to learn. He recorded patients in his *Case Notes*, which ran to five volumes. He spent a brief period of 2 months at St Mary's Hall in Oxford. Because of possible tuberculosis, he enlisted in the army and was a surgeon in Belle Isle and Portugal. It was at this period he prepared work for the publication of his *Treatise on the Blood, Inflammation and Gunshot Wounds*, published many years later in 1794. When he returned to London he began his research in comparative anatomy and embryology, and began building up his collection which was eventually to become part of the Royal College of Surgeons of England.

John Hunter was very well known as a surgeon and operated on Adam Smith's piles when the great moral philosopher and economist came to England, staying in Wimbledon with his friend Henry Dundas and visited by the Prime Minister, William Pitt the younger. The operation was a success and even his bladder problems were relieved. The difference between the two brothers is evident in this story. Adam Smith presented William with a copy of *The Wealth of Nations*; John sorted out his haemorrhoids.

As his practice prospered, he married Anne (nèe Home), a poet who corresponded with Robert Burns and wrote a libretto for Haydn's *Creation*. It is interesting to note that one of Anne's closest friends, Alice Lee, married the American surgeon William Shippen, who had lodged with John in the winter of 1759–60. Shippen's contribution to American surgery was outstanding and will be discussed in another chapter. Anne's influence on John was considerable, though they seemed to live separate lives, he dissecting and she entertaining the cream of London society at their home. She even ensured that his portrait was appropriate and persuaded him to shave off his straggly beard before sitting for Joshua Reynolds. He moved from Jermyn Street to Leicester Square where he had his home, his consulting rooms, his lecture theatre and his museum. He lectured in his own home as staff at St George's refused to teach in the hospital. He had many pupils, one of whom was Edward Jenner with whom he corresponded regularly, including his famous line when discussing hedgehogs: 'But why think? Why not trie the expt?' Jenner practised in Berkeley in Gloucestershire and it was here that he vaccinated the boy James Phipps with pus from the hand of a dairy maid on the 14th of May, 1796.

London had a number of excellent surgeons at the time: John Abernethy, Sir Astley Paston Cooper and Philip Syng Physick, who became the father of American surgery. John Hunter's comments to the father of young Physick are memorable. When asked what books would be required, Hunter led him to the dissecting room and said: 'These are the books your son will learn under my direction: the others are fit for very little'. In pathology, there was Matthew Baillie (1761–1823), a nephew of Hunter and the son of the professor of divinity at Glasgow. The second was Giovanni Battista Morgagni (1682–1771), another outstanding pathologist. His great work *De sedibus et causis morborum* (*On the sites and causes of disease*) appeared in 1761 in five volumes. Marie François Xavier Bichat (1771–1802) was the third major figure in pathology, which was beginning to be seen as the science of disease.

John Hunter was, like his brother, committed to teaching. However, he was not fluent like his brother and did not attract such large audiences. He was diffident and self conscious and unable to trust his memory. But it was not how he said it, but what he said that mattered. In 1793 he wrote to the Governors of St George's Hospital: 'My motive in the first place was to serve the hospital and in the second to diffuse the knowledge of the art, that all might partake of it; this indeed is the highest office in which a surgeon can be employed'.[49] He was curious about things and recalled:

> *When I was a boy I wanted to know about the clouds and the grasses, and why the leaves change colour in autumn. I watched the ants, the bees, the tadpoles, and the caddis worms; I pestered people with questions about which nobody knew or cared anything.*[50]

Around 1774 he commenced a series of public lectures, and they amounted to around 100 in all. His broad interest in natural history meant that he wished to set up a school of natural history in London, and wrote to Jenner about it: 'My scheme is to teach natural history in which will be included anatomy both human and comparative'.[51] The idea was not followed through. It is not clear whether or not he was a good teacher, though he did have the ability to change his mind and think again. For example, he did not like his lectures to be quoted to him and said: 'Never ask me what I have said or what I have written, but if you ask me what my present position is I will tell you'.[52] And again: 'You had better not write down that observation for very likely I shall think differently next year'.[53] Perhaps most impressively, when it was pointed out to him that a statement he made conflicted with one he made last year he replied: 'Very likely I did. I hope I grow wiser every year'.[54] What a riposte for a media interview! He began his lecture course with the statement: 'In the course of these lectures I shall differ very much from what is taught in books on the subject of surgery. The ideas I have to communicate to you are mostly my own. I have reason to suppose they are true because they are founded on fact'.[55]

This is, in fact, John Hunter's legacy: he challenged everything and created an environment of curiosity, experiment and excitement. He was a thinker as well as a teacher. Hunter was often seen motionless waiting for inspiration and the 'flash of light'. His views on medical education are well recorded by Abernethy in his Hunterian Oration.

> *Medicine is one and indivisible, and must be learnt as a whole for no part can be understood if learnt separately. The physician must understand surgery; the surgeon, the medical treatment of disease. Indeed it is from the evidence afforded by external diseases, that we are able to judge the nature and progress of those which are internal.*[56]

As a Fellow of the Royal Society, he met and talked with the most distinguished scientists of the day. He set up a small group of Fellows who met in a coffee house in Dean Street and later at Young Slaughters in St Martin's Lane. Accounts suggest that these were noisy occasions on which ideas were discussed and debated. Hunter seemed to be the acknowledged chairman and members included a wide range of people, such as the Astronomer Royal, engineers, architects and mathematicians, a very good example of the contacts and links made by Hunter across all disciplines. His interests were very wide and included the natural world as a whole. He was curious about everything.

This was reflected in his lectures. Although titled 'The principles and practice of surgery', they were much wider than this and began with physiology and the concept of health. It was a very biological approach to surgical practice.

He was a very hard worker. William Clift, who was apprenticed to Hunter for seven years, wrote: 'I never understood how Mr Hunter obtained rest, when I left him at midnight it was with a lamp just rained for further study, and with the usual appointment to meet him at six in the morning'.[57] Another source records:

> ...from six in the morning or even earlier, until nine he was in the dissecting room; after breakfast he had patients at his house before going his round of visits. He dined at four, after which he slept for an hour; and when not lecturing he dictated to Bell his amanuensis till one or two in the morning, leaving only four hours for sleep.[58]

THE INFLUENCE OF THE HUNTERS

There were many pupils in London and elsewhere for whom contact and learning from one or other of the Hunter brothers was a crucial part of their education. In America, for example, both William Shippen and John Morgan were resident pupils with John Hunter and thus linked, with Cullen, to the developments in medical education in that continent. Philip Syng Physick (1768–1837) was a favourite pupil of John Hunter and is seen as the father of American surgery. They talked and shared experimental work between London and Philadelphia. He had learned from Hunter the value of the experimental method for establishing surgical principles. For example, he describes an experiment on a kitten in which the pleura is incised and a tube passed into the chest. The Hunters' influence on obstetrics and anatomy was also remarkable.

CONCLUSIONS

The four individuals discussed in this chapter illustrate some of the changes that medical education was undergoing in the 18th century. They all loved teaching, worked extraordinarily hard, and saw possibilities and opportunities in what they did. They wanted to change the world and to develop a 'system' to bring things together. John Hunter, for example, had a special interest in experimental work and his curiosity drove him. Students flocked to study with these 'medical magnets' and this is a theme which will be developed further in Chapter 10.

The two quotations at the beginning of the chapter signal the direction of medical education in the 18th century. The first is about curiosity and research, which is seen best in the work of John Hunter. It is a plea to challenge and experiment, and provide new ways of thinking. The second from Adam Smith (generally considered an economist but actually a professor of moral philosophy) highlights the philanthropic nature of medicine and the role of education and learning. The aim of medicine is to the benefit others, patients and the public, and this is what lies behind the purpose of medicine and of medical education.

REFERENCES

1. John Hunter to Edward Jenner. Correspondence date 2 August, 1775 in the archives of the Royal College of Surgeons of England.
2. Smith A. The theory of moral sentiments. Edition edited by Raphael D D, Macfie A L. Indianapolis: Liberty Fund; 1984; 9.

3. Bonner T N. Becoming a physician. Medical education in Britain, France Germany and the United States, 1750–1945 Oxford: Oxford University Press; 1995; 72–89.

4. Lane J. The role of apprenticeship in eighteenth-century medical education in England. In: Bynum W F, Porter R, eds. William Hunter and the eighteenth century medical world. Cambridge: Cambridge University Press; 1985; 57–103.

5. Smollett T. The adventures of Roderick Random (1748). Oxford: Oxford World Classics, 1979.

6. Lane, 57–103

7. Bonner, 61–102.

8. The Works of Benjamin Brodie. Dublin Quarterly Journal of Medical Science 1865; 40:134.

9. Houston J. Dr Houston's Memoirs of his own life time. Bickerstaff J, ed. London; 1747; 56–57.

10. Booth C C. Herman Boerhaave and the British, Part 2. Boerhaave and the development of medical education in Britain. J Roy Coll Phys of London 1989; 23:194–197.

11. van Strien K. A medical student at Leiden and Paris. William Sinclair 1736–38, Part 1. Proc Roy Coll Physicians Edinb 1995; 25:294–304.

12. Innes-Smith R W. English-speaking students at the University of Leyden. London and Edinburgh, Oliver and Boyd. E.A; 1932.

13. Underwood E A. Boerhaave's men at Leyden and after. Edinburgh: The University Press; 1977.

14. Cunningham A. Medicine to calm the mind. Boerhaave's medical system and why it was adapted in Edinburgh. In: Cunningham A, French R, eds. The medical enlightenment of the eighteenth century. Cambridge: Cambridge University Press; 1990.

15. Quoted by Booth op cit; 197.

16. Joseph Black to George Black. Correspondence dated 10 March, 1753. University of Edinburgh Archive.

17. Edinburgh University Manuscript Dc.2.76.

18. A Guide for Gentlemen Studying Medicine at the University of Edinburgh (authorship disputed James Hamilton or Alexander Hamilton both of whom denied authorship. 1792) London: Robinson; 1792.

19. Ibid, 2

20. Ibid, 5.

21. Ibid, 10.

22. Ibid, 15.

23. Adam Smith letter to Cullen. Correspondence dated 30 September, 1774. Cited in Thomson J. An account of the life, lectures and writings of William Cullen, MD (2 vol). Edinburgh: Blackwood; 1859; vol 1; 475.

24. Smith A. The Wealth of Nations. Vol 2. Campbell R H, Skinner A S, eds. Oxford: Oxford University Press; 1976: 764.

25. Comrie J D. History of Scottish medicine. London: Balliere, Tindall & Cox; 1932; vol ii: 493.

26. Jardine G. Outlines of philosophical education, illustrated the method of teaching the logic class in the University of Glasgow. Glasgow: Glasgow University Press; 1825; 469.

27. Rosner L. Medical education in the age of improvement. Edinburgh: Edinburgh University Press; 1991.

28. O'Donnell J M. Cullen's influence on American medicine. In: Passmore R, Doig A, Ferguson J, Milne I, eds. William Cullen and the 18th century medical world. Edinburgh: Edinburgh University Press; 1990; 241.

29. Gregory J. Additional notes to the managers of the Royal Infirmary. Edinburgh: Murray and Cochrane; 1803; 189.

30. Rosner, 58.

31. Cullen quoted in: Macarthur D C. The first 40 years of the Royal Medical Society. In: Passsmore R, Doig A, Ferguson J, Milne I, eds. William Cullen and the 18th century medical world. Edinburgh: Edinburgh University Press; 1990; 250.

32. Cullen quoted in: The Cullen Bicentenary exhibition. In: Passmore R, Doig A, Ferguson J, Milne I, eds. William Cullen and the 18th century medical world. Edinburgh: Edinburgh University Press; 1990; 250.

33. Ismay T. Letter from Thomas Ismay, student of medicine at Edinburgh, 1771, to his father. University of Edinburgh Journal 1936-7; 8:58.

34. Hunter W. Two introductory lectures, delivered by Dr William Hunter, to his last course of anatomical lectures at his theatre in Windmill Street: as they were left corrected for the press by himself. To which are added, some papers relating to Dr Hunter's intended plan, for establishing a museum in London, for the improvement of anatomy, surgery and physic. London; 1784; 37.

35. Porter R. William Hunter: a surgeon and a gentleman. In: Bynum W F, Porter R, eds. William Hunter and the eighteenth century medical world. Cambridge: Cambridge University Press; 1985; 18.

36. Hunter. Two introductory lectures; 73.
37. Ibid, 67.
38. Ibid, 68.
39. Kemp M, ed. Dr William Hunter at the Royal Academy of Arts. Glasgow: University of Glasgow Press; 1975; 34.
40. Ibid, 35.
41. Ibid, 37.
42. Finch E. The influence of the Hunters on Medical Education. Ann Roy Coll Surg 1957; 20: 216.
43. Ibid, 217.
44. Gentleman's Magazine obituary (LIII,I, 1793 365–6) Hunter.
45. Brock C H. In: Simmons S F, Hunter J, eds. William Hunter: a memoir. Glasgow: Glasgow University Press;1983; 6.
46. Finch, 206.
47. Porter, 13.
48. Finch, 237.
49. Finch, 206.
50. Finch, 208.
51. Finch, 221.
52. Moore W. The knife man. London: Bantam Press; 2005; 245.
53. Ibid.
54. Ibid.
55. Finch, 221.
56. Finch, 223.
57. Finch, 224.
58. Finch, 225.

6

Resistance and reform: the 19th century

I consider hospitals as the only entrance to scientific medicine; they are the first field of observation which a physician enters; but the true sanctuary of medical science is a laboratory; only thus can he seek explanations of life in the normal and pathological states by means of experimental analysis.[1]

Claude Bernard (1813–1878)

INTRODUCTION

The 19th century was another era of enormous change. Medicine at the end of the century would not have been recognisable to those practising at its beginning. The profession changed, society changed and the knowledge base was transformed. The typical physician at the beginning of the century was a cultured and highly educated person; by the end he was a clinical scientist, or at least many were. Until 1830, College Licence examinations in London were conducted in Latin. The structure of education was haphazard and unorganised. Attendance at lectures and walking the wards constituted the learning process. There was no real curriculum, and students could choose to attend subjects or not. It was generally believed that all that was needed to educate doctors were some hospitals and some private schools rather than a more formal organisation. Private schools (from the time of the Hunters) had flourished and continued to do so in London and in places like Edinburgh, Glasgow and Dublin, where the extramural schools were part of the provision for medical students. In particular, there was no regulation of practice or of standards, and most practitioners were unqualified. Anatomy became a major part of the curriculum at the start of the century, and cadavers were required, leading to body snatching and the infamous Burke and Hare murders in Edinburgh in 1827. All this had changed by the end of the century.

The situation in Scotland was a little different, and as Newman puts it:

> *Medical education in Scotland is a subject on its own, but its state at the beginning of the nineteenth century is obviously of importance to the history of medical education in England in that century, because Scottish education was so much better as to have been an example for imitation. It is extraordinary not only that it was not more imitated, but also that the infiltration of Scottish teachers into England, which is no new thing, did not lead to much wider adoption of Scottish methods. The English system must have been extremely tough to have resisted it, but resist it did, until in the present century features more Scottish than English have been adopted, having come from a common continental tradition, in which Scotland shared, from Germany, via Baltimore, USA.* [2]

Newman's book remains a remarkable source of information on 19th century medical education.

Medical societies were formed across the country and these will be discussed later. Medical journals were born. The *British Medical Journal* (*BMJ*) first saw light of day on Saturday, the 3rd of October 1840, and *The Lancet* was first published in 1823.

In assessing the educational changes, five themes emerge:

+ The importance of clinical examination.

+ Knowledge, science and pathology. Paradigms of disease.

+ Changes in the profession—regulation.

+ Public health and sanitary reform.

+ Students, the student life and women in medicine.

CLINICAL METHOD

At the beginning of the century, the lecture was the standard mode of imparting information. Hours were set aside in medical schools for the teacher to deliver a series of talks on a range of subjects. Clinical work consisted of history taking and prescribing. There was little or no teaching on clinical examination. But the situation soon began to change. One of the most significant of these changes was the establishment of the hospital as the prime focus for medical education. Hospitals became centres of medicine and learning. The 'clinic' and the ward became the place where advances were made and to which doctors from all over the world flocked for teaching.

France, and particularly Paris, exemplified this new way of thinking, and it was here, in the first decades of the 19th century, that advances were made in medical education. Hospitals became places of healing and development rather than refuges for those needing shelter. The hôtel-Dieu in Paris was at the heart of this. It all began in 1794 when after the Revolution a government report was presented which resulted in the setting up of three new schools of health (Ecoles de santè) in Paris, Montpellier and Strasbourg. Others were added and, by the second decade of the 19th century, Paris was the place to be if you wanted to become a doctor. Newman records that Cullen, Christison and Turner from Edinburgh were all in Paris at the same time in 1820.[3]

French medical education became integrated into a single system with licensing, and several different classes of doctor were created. For example, those who worked in the country-side might have a shorter training. More importantly, there was an integration of medicine and surgery, and the provision for full-time teachers. This meant that teachers did not have to rely on private practice. Students received state scholarships. In addition to the clinical method, and integral to it, were developments in physiology and pathology. The student and the teacher considered the patient, the signs and symptoms, and the physiology and pathology in coming to a diagnosis.

The classic bedside teaching even today consists of taking a history and carrying out four main tasks

+ Inspection—what can I see?

+ Palpation—what can I feel?

+ Percussion—can I detect differences when I use the body as a drum?

+ Auscultation—what can I hear within the body?

These four tasks became routine in France, and were linked directly to the pathology found in the autopsy room. The development of such clinical methods over the next two centuries is well described by Keele.[4]

Inspection had always been part of clinical examination but was often superficial. Clothes were generally not removed, and the face and the hands were the parts inspected. Palpation was also very limited and, again, did not extend to regions under the garments or to the examination of the pulse. These two aspects alone would have been radical enough on their own when coupled with a pathological interpretation. The method of percussion was first described by Leopold Auenbrugger (1727–1809) in Vienna and published as a short book, *Inventum Novum*. The method was to tap the body using the fingers, or using one finger laid across the part of the body to be examined and then to tap it with another finger, and listen to the sound. Auenbrugger had discovered this while tapping wine barrels, noting how the sounds changed from hollow to full. The procedure was taken up by Corvisart in La Charitè in Paris, who recognised its value. He linked the sounds of percussion to the findings at autopsy and could distinguish in the living patient changes in the lungs, heart and abdomen.

The next major discovery was by Laennec (1781–1826), who invented an instrument for listening into the sounds of the body—the stethoscope. His description of its discovery is one of the great legends of medicine:

> *In 1816 I was consulted by a young woman labouring under general symptoms of diseased heart, and in whose case percussion and the application of the hand were of little avail on account of the degree of fatness...I happened to recollect a simple and well known fact in acoustics, and fancied at the same time, that it might be turned into some use on the present occasion. The fact I allude to is the augmented impression of sound when conveyed through certain solid bodies as when we hear the scratch of a pin at one end of a piece of wood, on applying our ear to the other. Immediately on this suggestion, I rolled a quire of paper into a sort of cylinder and applied one end of it to the region of the heart and the other to my ear, and was not a little surprised and pleased to find that I could thereby perceive the action of the heart in a manner much more clear and distinct than I had been able to do by the immediate application of the ear. From this moment I imagined that the circumstances might furnish means for enabling us to ascertain the character, not only of the action of the heart, but of every species of sound produced by the motion of all the thoracic viscera.*[5]

A new era had begun in understanding lung and heart disease. These four methods, supplemented by the taking of a history, remain the basis of clinical examination to this day. They have, of course, been supplemented by X-rays, scans of various sorts, cardiograms and other tests, but the basis is the same; these new tests simply extend our powers to see, feel and listen. Much more was developed from the process of clinical examination described above, as clinicians recognised that they could use their senses to see inside the body, and the correlation with pathological findings could open new ways of understanding disease.

All these new developments were being experienced by large numbers of students from around the world, who return-ed to their own countries to spread the word, across Europe and America. Clinical teaching had taken on a different meaning. Rigorous history taking (including a family history), inspection, palpation, percussion and auscultation, combined with findings at autopsy, gave the student a new way of thinking about and understanding disease. To this was coupled the practice of measuring and counting events to give a quantitative edge to medical practice, as was the consideration of the natural history of disease, watching how diseases developed and changed.

Until this time, one of the classic maxims of medicine was 'Better something doubtful than nothing'. Pierre Louis (1787–1872) changed this to 'Better nothing, than something doubtful'.[6] He showed that traditional treatments, such as bloodletting, had no real effect, and that it might be better to do nothing than harm the patient. Careful clinical examination and follow-up provided a way of recording the natural history of illness and what happened if the doctor intervened.

The movement passed to Vienna where individuals like Rokitansky and Skoda provided a wider educational prog-ramme than in Paris, and this paved the way for the develop-ments in scientific medicine which dominated the second half of the century.

SCIENTIFIC MEDICINE: THE RISE OF LABORATORY MEDICINE

Medical education in the second half of the 19th century was dominated by Germany and the rise of scientific medicine. The advances were enormous and completely changed the para-digms of health and illness which began the century. Progress in the study of chemistry, physics, bacteriology and immunology resulted in new diagnostic methods (radiology), methods of patient support (anaesthesia and antisepsis) and treatment. By the end of the century, the process of specialisation had also begun. All of these developments had significant effects on medical education. The quotation at the beginning of this chapter from Bernard says it all. It was a period of excitement and change. Before this time science was the province of the amateur; after it became a profession in its own right.

France had developed the clinical method, and by the 1850s the move to German science had begun. However, the French scientific legacy was considerable. François Magendie (1783–1859), for example, founded the *Journal de physiologie (et pathologie) Experimentale* in 1821. Claude Bernard was another, and the publication of *An Introduction to the Study of Experimental Medicine* in 1865 was a landmark, although he did not set up a school in the German sense. The book is worth some further discussion.

Claude Bernard

Bernard's *An Introduction to the Study of Experimental Medicine* formed the basis of much thinking in the middle of the century. He sets out the field and by stating:

> *In order to embrace the medical problem as a whole experi-mental medicine must include three basic parts: physiology, pathology and therapeutics...physiology will teach us to maintain normal conditions of life and to conserve health. Knowledge of diseases and of their determining causes, i.e. pathology will lead us on the one hand, to prevent the development of morbid conditions, and, on the other, to fight their results with medical agents, i.e., to cure the diseases.* [7]

He notes that scientific medicine, like the other sciences, can be established only by experimental means. That is 'by direct and rigorous application of reasoning to the facts furnished us by observation and experiment'.[8] He comments further on observation:

Only within narrow boundaries can man observe the phenomena which surround him; ...to extend this knowledge, he has to increase the power of his organs by means of special appliances; at the same time he has equipped himself with various instruments enabling him to penetrate inside of bodies, to dissociate them and to study their hidden parts.[9]

Here he opens the way for laboratory medicine and the widening range of diagnostic techniques. The way in which medicine will be learned is being re-written and a new vista of education becomes clear. The doctor must think beyond his own senses and extend them both for diagnosis and in order to understand the aetiology and progress of disease. Medical education began to expand to take in these new concepts. As he says:

One must be brought up in laboratories and live in them, to appreciate the full importance of all the details of procedure in investigation, which are so often neglected or despised by the false men of science calling themselves generalisers...A physiological laboratory, therefore, should now be the culminating goal of any scientific physician's studies; but here again I must explain myself to avoid misunderstanding. Hospitals, or rather hospital wards are not physicians' laboratories, as is often believed; as we have said before, these are only his fields for observation;...medicine necessarily begins with clinics, since they determine and define the object of medicine, i.e., the medical problem; but while they are the physician's first study, clinics are not the foundation of scientific medicine; physiology is the foundation of scientific medicine because it must yield the explanation of morbid phenomena by showing their relations to the normal state. We shall never have a science of medicine as long as we separate the explanation of pathological from the explanation of normal, vital phenomena.[10]

The message is clear: the education of the doctor should be scientific if we are to understand the normal and abnormal and learn to treat effectively. These statements had a profound effect on medical education, worldwide.

France

By the end of the century, France had its greatest hero, Louis Pasteur (1822–1895). His researches on applied areas, wine and vinegar for example, led to a series of discoveries which would revolutionise medicine. His work on the 'germ theory' of disease changed the paradigm of health. It is of importance to note that Pasteur was not medically qualified, and thus began one the most interesting aspects of medical research, the role of the scientist. Indeed, it could be said that there is no 'medical research', only research on medical problems, which is open to all who can contribute.

Britain

In Britain, Charles Darwin (1809–1882) was also changing thinking with the publication of *On the Origin of Species* (1859), as were others such as Thomas Huxley, William Prout (1785–1850), Sir Charles Bell (1774–1842) and Marshall Hall (1790–1875), all products of the Edinburgh school. William Sharpey (1802–1880) in London developed physiology, and amongst his students was Joseph Lister whom we will discuss later.

United States of America

Medical science in the United States was also developing, following the return of disciples from Europe and the foundation of the Smithsonian Institute and Johns Hopkins Medical School. William Welch (1850–1934) was typical, and we shall hear more of his educational interests later. He qualified in medicine and then went to Europe, studying physiology with Ludwig and pathology with Cohnheim and Recklinghausen. He returned to New York and set up a pathology laboratory at Bellevue Hospital Medical School and was then offered the chair of pathology at the new Johns Hopkins Medical School, taking up his post in 1885. He returned to Germany to work with Koch and Pettenkofer. A number of those he recruited were graduates of the German system. The developments in America will be discussed in a later chapter, but what flowed from such developments was a radical re-thinking of medical education.

Germany

Germany and German science were at the heart of changes in medical science at the time. The universities had been transformed and specialist scientific institutes developed. These provided the places and people who had time and freedom to innovate. There were two important components of this freedom:

+ *Lernfreiheit*—the freedom to learn.
+ *Lehrfreiheit*—the freedom to teach.

Students could move around, and those who taught could do so unhindered. It is interesting to reflect that in both the development of the clinical method and science, it was both people and the creation of institutions which were important. Part of the ability to teach as they wished was that the scientists trained large numbers of visitors who again returned home to carry on the work; another good example of medical magnets and the dissemination of learning.

German medical scientists involved in this process changed the face of medicine. In 1847, three students, Helmholtz, du Bios-Reymond and Brucke, linked with Carl Ludwig to publish what Bynum[11] has called a kind of manifesto announcing that the aim of physiology was to explain all vital phenomena through the laws of physics and chemistry. This is a remarkably modern statement. Great names such as Virchow moved around the system, in his case transferring from Würzburg to take up the directorship of the newly created Pathological Institute in Berlin, also somehow finding time to be part of the Reichstag. A small window in the Institute looks towards the Reichstag building, and here Virchow could check if it was in session. Koch (1843–1910) was one of the second generation of German research workers. He published regularly, even as a medical student, and his discoveries (e.g. the tubercule bacillus) were of major importance. Koch's postulates— describing the characteristics of microorganisms being the cause of disease—are still taught today. As a result of the developments in Germany, thousands of students came there to work and learn, and returned home to pursue their own careers. This spread of knowledge was to have a profound effect on the subsequent development of medical education in the United States and elsewhere.

The Medical Sciences in the German Universities

The Medical Sciences in the German Universities, written by Theodor Billroth in Vienna in 1876, is one of the most interesting of all the books reviewed in this text. It is erudite, practical and full of humour. Consider the following paragraph found on the first page:

A person must have acquired from books a vast amount of medical knowledge, he may even have memorised from books the technic of its applications; such a person has much knowledge of medicine, and with it all he is no physician. He must see and hear the master's diagnosis, prognosis, and treatment of disease. He must witness the master's skill in action, in order to himself become a physician. The more he knows, the more he will be able to accomplish later. Now the object of our modern endeavour is to make the physician's skill independent of tradition by means of written records to conserve the art of healing for all time, so that it may be independent of the talent of the individual and may be reduced to an absolute science. All knowledge and skill are to be determined and controlled by means of the laws of arithmetic and logic in order to make everything absolute and permanent. How long have we been seeking absolute truth and absolute beauty! "Ye shall be as gods, knowing good and evil."[12]

What a statement, encapsulating all that is good about modern medicine. And then he adds:

I doubt if this goal will ever be reached—at least in the art of healing; certainly not until the art of poetry is wholly resolved into prosody, the art of painting into chromatics and the art of music into acoustics.[13]

It brings one back to the real world. He then offers a very useful summary of the history of medical education to the 19th century. For example, as a professor in Vienna, he makes the link between Leiden and Boerhaave to Vienna via Gerhard van Swieten, and he gives other examples of the work of the Vienna School and sums up progress as follows:

In all subjects the demonstration method of instruction has gradually become preponderant. This began with anatomy, and was then extended to practical medicine, surgery, obstetrics, and then to the natural sciences and physiology. Down to the middle of the 19th century teachers contented themselves with showing and explaining to the students finished preparations, their chief concern being to convey to them the results of research in the most condensed and systematised form possible. But since the fourth decade of this century the German professor has been pretty generally required not only to know the results of the most recent researches, and to teach these to his students, but himself to be an investigator in the branch of science which he teaches...Thus far only the German universities have set themselves this high ideal as their objective; in no other nation is it insisted upon as the most essential trait in the true character of a university...The increased demand on the teachers logically resulted in a higher degree of subdivision and specialisation in the subjects taught; for, assuming that only the investigator can be an excellent teacher, it was necessary to increase the number of teachers.[14]

Billroth emphasised the importance of pathological anatomy in the understanding of disease and considered public health to be important. He also considered the problem of the student. Can he learn too much? Will he be discontented if he practices rural medicine if he has developed an interest in science? Surely physicians do not need to be scholars? He dealt with these and other criticisms of 'scientific' education as follows:

First of all, let me define the position which I have taken toward these criticisms of the modern method of teaching the sciences. The cultured people of all nations must not cease to spread the desire for study and knowledge with all their might, among all classes and in all countries; they must not cease to impose upon themselves and on others increasingly higher intellectual standards; nor must they cease to support the efforts of their governments in this direction...to neglect the education of these leaders, to lower their intellectual and scientific standards, to educate them in such a way that the people will regard them as their own kind—as just so many more artisans, like cobblers, tailors and comb makers—that, in my judgement, would mean the repression of our whole national cultural development, reprehensible in principle and absolutely immoral because it would ruin the nation and make it prey of another long before its natural exhaustion in the course of centuries.[15]

Billroth was unashamedly elitist and nationalist. He also notes that 'Our clinical instruction is purely German in form, and it is characteristically German constantly to find fault with it, to alter and improve it'.[16] He discusses the advantages of a small university and gives the following advice to students:

The smaller universities offer the great advantage that the teacher gets well acquainted with each student and comes to know what he may safely leave to the skill of each individual. Conditions at the larger clinics unfortunately make this impossible. At the beginning of your clinical studies, therefore, avoid the great universities! Visit those only toward the end of your course, and later when you have already begun to practice, return to them from time to time for a few weeks.[17]

He also considers the preparation of the student and is concerned that the scientific spirit is killed outright by the premature development of the medical routine. He gives details of the curriculum for the student, including the hours per subject, and he encourages the student to take secondary subjects, if the hours are arranged 'without time killing intermissions'.[18] His comments on examinations are particularly interesting:

At the examination he falls into the hands of a middle aged practitioner. Now, in view of the rapid flux of medical science, these two will not understand each other at all, or will require a long discussion to reach an understanding. Perhaps the examiner writes his prescriptions in terms of ounces and grains; the candidate knows nothing about that because his instructors, quite properly, have thought it unnecessary to teach it to him. He figures and prescribes in grams.[19]

There is a timeless quality about this sentiment that as knowledge advances, examiners too need to keep up to date.

As will be discussed in a later section, Billroth also writes on the training of teachers. He emphasises the importance of training and records that in 1811 there was a special ordinance: 'An Order for the establishment of training schools for future professors of medicine and related sciences' approved. The good students were to be selected and were to be supervised by a professor. Interestingly, 'They were not to be asked to perform any tasks which might prevent the attainment of their chief purpose, or which are not directly in the line of their official duties'[20]; the forerunner of protected teaching time. The issue is that 'teaching' in this context is not about 'pedagogy' but learning to be a clinical scientist. He advocates the retention of course fees because of the personal contact which it encourages between teacher and student. He is convinced of the importance of the personal influence of great men in forming the next generation of staff. He also notes that:

> There is only one way to train capable university teachers— one way that has been practically tested—and that is to secure for the universities the services of the most distinguished men of science, and to furnish them with the necessary equipment for teaching...We must never forget that a university education aims to train men not only to know their fields, but to be artists in their fields—well rounded men who, scattered to the four winds of heaven, will again become pioneers of culture.[21]

His emphasis here is on originality and creativity. Billroth's book makes for a fascinating and very modern read. It influenced many, and the philosophy behind it was to have international consequences, as we shall see in later chapters.

Other developments in the 19th century

The regular clinical use of the microscope was introduced over this period—from which Virchow was to state that 'omnis cellula a cellula' (all cells, from cells) in his great book *Cellular Pathology*, a record of his lectures at the Institute.[22] Bacteriology became a real science and discoveries were made regularly, identifying the causative organisms behind particular diseases.

Koch has already been mentioned for his pioneering investigations into anthrax, cholera and most particularly tuberculosis, and, of course, for his 'postulates'. It is of passing interest to note that Koch's assistant was called Petri, another name which persists to this day. His announcement of the discovery of the tubercle bacillus was presented to the Berlin Physiological Society on 22nd March, 1882, and it caused major media interest worldwide.

Part of this understanding of infectious disease was the development in understanding of immunology and the biological responses to disease. Numerous vaccines were developed which proved invaluable to the control of infection. For example, crews digging the Panama canal suffered significant attrition due to the effects of yellow fever, and the conquering of this disease was considered 'the first mountain to be climbed'. This was done by the development and provision of an effective vaccine, and was thus instrumental in allowing completion of the canal. Immunotherapy was the answer to many diseases. George Bernard Shaw described these developments in his play *The Doctor's Dilemma*, a caricature of the great British clinician Sir Almroth Wright.[23] As Bynum notes, he was often called 'Sir Almost Right'. Cartoons of the day show patients going to the pharmacy with a jug to pick up immune serum from the horse to cure their illness. Von Behring, a distinguished immunologist, is often shown as the pharmacist.

At the same time, chemists were trying to identify chemicals which could inhibit the growth of pathogenic organisms. Paul Ehrlich, for example, sought to design a magic bullet cure, and after 606 modifications the first active antibacterial was created. The great German pharmaceutical industry began gearing up to produce the active products.

Another important development was the discovery of X-rays by Wilhelm Röntgen (1845–1923) in late 1895. This opened up a whole new prospect for diagnosis and treatment through the work of Henri Becquerel and the Curies.

Antiseptic surgery was pioneered by Lister in Glasgow, Edinburgh and London. The history of its introduction is discussed in a later section of this book. Together with hygiene and cleanliness, antiseptic techniques allowed the surgeon to operate more freely, again setting the base for new surgical developments in the 20th century. Linked to this was the increased use of anaesthesia, again making surgery possible where it had not been before. It is interesting to reflect that it was surgery which benefited most from these developments in science. Several decades were to elapse before powerful drugs were discovered which could assist physicians in helping patients. As will be discussed elsewhere, the introduction of the thermometer and the sphygmomanometer also had an impact on clinical care.

Tropical medicine also benefited from the new research with the identification of organisms and vectors that caused specific diseases, such as in malaria. By the end of the century there were several institutes specifically for the study of tropical disease, including the London School of Hygiene and Tropical Medicine, founded in 1899.[24,25]

By the end of the century, science was dominant as the driving force of medicine and was thus integrated into educational programmes, albeit with more urgency in some centres than others. Patterns of disease began to change, although slowly, and it was not until the 20th century that the fruits of these developments became clear. All of this had to be assimilated into the medical curriculum, and it became more and more crowded. The paradigm of health had been changed to reflect the importance of science and of the understanding of disease.

PUBLIC HEALTH

The 19th century brought very significant developments in the improvement of public health. It was a century of industrialisation, of people moving to cities, of the rise of epidemiology and sanitary reform. There was also a change in philosophical debate, with Benthamite writing on utility and (with others) the need to reform society and deal with issues such as poverty, unemployment and the wellbeing of children. The great Reform Acts opened up the voting franchise until at last women ratepayers were given the vote in local elections in 1907 and full voting rights in 1913.

Johann Peter Frank (1745–1821) was one of those who led the reform in public health process with the publication of *Medical Police* (*System einer vollstandigen medicinischen Polizey*) in six volumes, published between 1779 and 1826. It is a remarkable piece of work and formed the basis of much subsequent health reform undertaken by the state (the police). As the century developed, greater knowledge became available through the sciences of bacteriology and immunology, and the sanitary reforms in Britain pioneered by Chadwick, Farr, and Simon were based much on Frank's work. In R. J. Evans' book *Death in Hamburg*, there is a fascinating account of how one city dealt with cholera. The internal conflict between the city council and the citizens is well described at a time when the infectious causes of disease were being identified.[26]

A similar conflict is dramatised in Henrik Ibsen's (1828–1906) play *The Enemy of the People*, where a local doctor identifies a possible infection in the city baths but is unable to do anything about it as the city council refuses to take any action that might damage trade. In Act Five of the play, the doctor utters the immortal lines that should be known to any-one about embark on a dangerous medical mission: 'You should never have your best trousers on when you turn out to fight for freedom and truth'; a reference to the fact that he had things thrown at him. It becomes so bad that he is forced to leave the city.[27] This is in some ways similar to Karl Popper's famous riposte when challenged by Ludwig Wittgenstein to give an example of a moral rule, he replied: 'Not to threaten visiting lecturers with pokers'—a reference to Wittgenstein's alleged brandishing of a poker at Popper.[28]

This greater understanding of the social aspects of health (social class, overcrowding, employment, poverty and diet) gradually became part of the medical curriculum and will be mentioned again in the next chapter on 20th century developments.

Public health issues in Great Britain were further highlighted in 1854 by the actions of John Snow, a physician in London. During a cholera epidemic in the Soho district, Snow carefully plotted the locations of individual cases and was able to localise the source of infection to a public water pump on Broad Street. He removed the pump handle and thus helped check the spread of the epidemic. Snow's method provided a model for more effective action based in knowledge.[29] Numerous reports were produced (e.g. *Report on the Sanitary condition of the labouring population of Great Britain* (1842) by Chadwick) and this began a movement within which medicine was represented. Epidemiology as a discipline became established and courses and diplomas set up, as further detailed in Fee and Acheson's *A History of education in Public Health: Health that mocks doctor's rules* (1991).[30] The subtitle of this book is taken from a verse by John Greenleaf Whittier:

Health that mocks the doctor's rules
Knowledge never learned in schools.[31]

Thus, even in the 'non-clinical' aspects of medicine, educational programmes were in place and remain so to this day. Epidemiology and statistics are as important to the doctor as the application of the clinical method, something recognised through the ages from Hippocrates to Sydenham. Sir John Simon (1816-1904) wrote: 'The progress which has been made [in preventive medicine] consists essentially in practical applications of Pathological Science'.[32] The changes would not have been possible but for the progress in science. The decline in mortality, however, may not have been due to this.

THE MEDICAL PROFESSION AND REGULATION

One of the most interesting aspects of the 19th century was the development of the medical profession and its organisation. This included the setting up of the British Medical Association in 1856 from the Provincial Medical and Surgical Association, founded in Worcester in 1832. Over the century numerous local, regional and specialist organisations were formed, and a range of journals, such as the *BMJ* (1840) and *The Lancet* (1823), were started. However, the main issue was that of regulation, which challenged the profession and professional organisations such as the medical Royal Colleges to review where they were going. The story is a fascinating one and well told in Charles Newman's *The evolution of medical education in the nineteenth century* (1957).[33] The process concluded in 1858 with the Medical Act, bringing all the players together, with Sir John Simon, the government's chief medical officer, working hard in the background.

At the beginning of the century, the medical profession (at least the formal part of it) was small. In 1800, there were a total of 179 fellows, licentiates and extra-licentiates of the Royal College of Physicians in London; by 1847 this had grown to 683, with 76% being in London.[34] As we have noted earlier in this book, while physicians were university educated, surgeons were not, though the status of surgeons rose throughout the century and culminated in the first medical peerage to Joseph Lister. The hospitals sector continued to expand in London and beyond. There remained a split between the status of hospital staff and the general practitioner, who was seen as the poor relation. The fact that the Medical Act of 1858 (a bill to regulate the qualifications of practitioners in medicine and surgery) might make all doctors equal at the point of graduation was difficult for some to take in. Thus, the story of the setting up of the General Medical Council begins.

The creation of the General Medical Council (GMC)

To read a more full account the reader should consult Newman's book (see above). The first stage in the process was the 'Apothecary's Act for the better regulation of practitioners', which began the gestation of the Council in 1804. By 1806 and after much discussion, an 'outline plan for an intended Bill for the better regulation of Medical Practitioners, Chemists, Druggists and Vendors of medicine' was drawn up giving details of qualifications and educational requirements. It contained information on appointing examiners and divided the country into districts. There was general approval for this, and it was revised further the following year and contained more detailed information: for example, that physicians should be aged 24 and graduates of a university in the United Kingdom. Discussion continued and the author of the bill tried to persuade the College of Physicians to take it on. The president was offended at the way in which this was done and the College found that the bill was objectionable and they would oppose it.

This bill was then taken up by the apothecaries in 1812; they formed an association and hoped that the two Royal Colleges would join. This was the first step toward a GMC. However, the College of Physicians at first refused to help, and then did so by inserting new clauses. Eventually, on 12 July, 1815, the bill was passed and the apothecaries were then able to set up a court of examiners. This allowed the great majority of practitioners in England and Wales to be examined by the Society of Apothecaries and the Royal Colleges, especially the Royal College of Physicians, were by-passed. This was a beginning, but things would continue to change. It is important to remember that these debates were also occurring at a time of considerable change in medical practice (described above)—the introduction of the clinical method, the importance of pathology and the beginnings of a scientific approach.

The process of trying to seek better regulation of medical practice continued, spurred on by a general movement for reform. There were 17 different bodies involved, all of whom had different standards of education and qualification. In addition, and perhaps most importantly, there was no way in which members of the public could distinguish between a qualified and non-qualified doctor. A medical directory had been published by Churchill's since 1845, but it was not complete. There was also the wish that by establishing a register, all doctors would be equal before the law as 'registered medical practitioners'. Herein lay the problem, how could they all be equal, how could apothecaries be of the same quality as a doctor qualified under the Royal College of Physicians? The College resisted the changes.

Enter onto the scene Thomas Wakley, MP, founder of *The Lancet* and dogged reformer with the drive to effect change. Wakley fought almost every one and when rebuffed he tried again. He wanted to set up a London College of Medicine, which would have brought all of the professional bodies together. His passion was reform of the system and the colleges. He became a Member of Parliament in 1835, just after he had begun his reform movement, to which he brought in other Members of Parliament. There was a series of medical bills launched by Wakley and his colleagues. In 1840, it was a 'Bill for the regulation of medical practitioners, and for establishing a college of Medicine and for enabling the Fellows of that College to practise medicine in all or any of its branches and hold any medical appointment in any part of the United Kingdom'. The bill was detailed, describing a 'medical qualification' and providing for the establishment of a council and a register. It did not get anywhere, and a second bill was introduced in 1841. On this occasion, the apothecaries objected and the bill did not get beyond its first reading.

Sir James Graham, Robert Peel's home secretary, began the preparation of a further bill, and after some delay and debate it was introduced in 1844: 'For the better regulation of Medical

Practice in Great Britain'. This bill was very close to the 1858 Act, but on this occasion it was Wakley who opposed it, as did the apothecaries. A new bill was introduced in 1845 which met many of the concerns, and after much more debate it too fell. Wakley and Warburton (a fellow MP) proposed another new bill in 1847, now the seventh of such attempts. Again there were many objections and the opposition was just too great; it was dead by 1850.

A series of bills was then introduced between 1853 and 1858, championed by universities, MPs, members of the House of Lords and the government. Not surprisingly during this process, the public began to wonder what was going on. Did the professional resistance stem from a fear of the scientific approach in medicine? Was it just about stopping progress? By now most people were confused as to what the bill was really about. Much of the debate focused on the composition of any proposed council, the examination system and whether or not there should be separate registers for each country in the UK. Professional divisions remained throughout, and each new version of the bill failed to please everyone. The phrase 'single portal of entry' was beginning to be used as a way of retaining some autonomy for the bodies but providing the beginnings of a solution, Sir John Simon being particularly active behind the scenes. What Simon wanted was a clear definition of a qualified medical practitioner, an accurate register, the application of privileges to those registered, and penalties for those who were not. He put this in a memorandum and by now most of the arguments had been won, except for the issue of representation or nomination to council.

In 1858, the government changed. Lord Palmerston was defeated and Lord Derby became prime minister. Mr. Cowper, who had been progressing this bill, brought it forward again (the sixteenth attempt) under the title of a 'Bill to regulate the qualifications of practitioners in Medicine and Surgery'. The major compromise was to have a combination of representatives and nominated members. The council would not be answerable to Parliament but to the Privy Council. It was Mr. Spencer Walpole, the new home secretary, who devised this and the Medical Council was to make orders to be approved by the Privy Council to establish a register, define qualifications, require examining bodies to cooperate, and to establish examiners. There were to be three branch councils in England and Wales, Scotland and Ireland. There was some dissatisfaction from those who wished a more radical solution, and a further bill (number 17) was drawn up. At the second reading of the Cowper bill (number 16), there was even an attempt to stop the whole process on the basis that medical reform was impractical and that the medical profession should just be left to fight it out. Eventually it went through committee stages, the House of Lords and received Royal Assent on 2nd August, 1858, some 54 years after the process had begun.

The difficult and convoluted history behind the establishment of the GMC demonstrates just how disunited the profession was. The public needed protection from quacks; why didn't it just happen? Certainly the various bodies involved seemed more concerned about their own fate than that of the public. Much was happening across Europe during the fifty or so years of this debate. The French and the Germans had revolutionised the teaching of clinical medicine and the scientific revolution had begun to influence medical education. Changes were already occurring in the UK, and the bill (rather than being seen as a revolutionary process and the start of a new phase of medical education) was only one aspect of that change. It will be interesting in fifty years time to review the current process of re-validation of medical practitioners by the GMC and see if lessons have been learned. That said, the GMC over the last 150 years has provided a vehicle for reform of the profession, a source of information and reassurance to the public, and has always tried to maintain the highest standards of medical practice. The story (and it is a fascinating one) will be continued in the next chapter.

SPECIALIST TRAINING

Specialisation is another part of the professional journey. By the end of the century, many doctors had a special interest, and as we have noted, specialist societies were being set up. It was, of course, resisted by some who thought it demeaning of the profession. Did this mean that some doctors could not do everything? In the long term, specialisation has had a profound effect on medical education, and much of the work in the 20th century has been about how best to train specialists.

Within this specialisation was that of mental health. This began with the establishment of mental hospitals such as Bedlam in London, or 'retreats' such as that set up by Samuel Tuke in York. Clinicians with a special interest emerged, and psychiatry became an established discipline on the medical scene. This formed the background of the work of Sigmund Freud (1856–1939) in Vienna.

STUDENT LIFE

At the beginning of the 19th century, medical students had a reputation for wild fun, drinking and not doing much work. They were generally poor and had to do other things to make ends meet. They may have lived at home to save money and worked with a local practitioner or within a local hospital. A student might earn money as an assistant or by coaching other medical students. Peterson gives the example of John Bland-Sutton, a distinguished surgeon in later life, who earned enough in this way to cover his fees.[35] Doctors had little status, and even when qualified they were not destined to make much money. Peterson also quotes the comments of John Beddoe when he asked Charles Hastings' advice about a medical career. Hastings, the founder of the BMA, responded with an old proverb: 'a physician does not get bread until he has no teeth

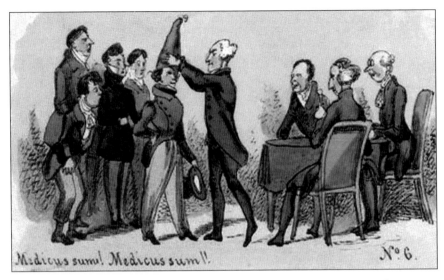

Medicus sum! Medicus sum!!   Nº 6.

This cartoon entitled the 'Graduation' comes from the *Northern Looking Glass* in 1825 and shows students at a graduation ceremony. The title 'Medicus Sum' (I am a doctor) and the dunce's cap reflect the widespread public disquiet about the competence of doctors. By permission of Glasgow University Library, Special Collections.

wherewith to eat it'.[36] Henry Ackland said of the students of St George's: 'Everything wears the air of low men, of low habits as such I have never hitherto come into contact with'.[37] Others tell of battles between groups of students with parts of the human body used as weapons. Attitudes were also different, and at one inaugural exhibition at St George's a senior member of staff could say: 'You are about to begin your medical studies. The sole objects of such studies are two: first to get a name; secondly to make money'.[38] The stories they told were in poor taste, perhaps occasioned by the work in the dissection room. The exception was the university educated physicians who moved in different circles. They were expected to have a liberal education which would bring status and earn respect.

This wild image of the medical student changed across the century; by its end they seemed more serious, perhaps because of the costs. Peterson has summarised what is known. Figures of around £500 to £600 for an apprenticeship are suggested for the best available education in the Victorian period. Apprentice-ships with a leading surgeon at the beginning of the century carried a fee of 500 guineas, and the figure may have been the same even as late as 1884. As is well known, such apprentice-ships and the friendships which developed could last a lifetime. In the London hospitals, fees were £100 for all lectures and hospital practice. With living costs and expenses for books and equipment and examinations, the total would be around £600.[39] Senior staff became role models. S.T. Taylor, a medical student in London in the 1850s, was thrilled when he had a chance to see Sir William Fergusson FRCS perform a difficult operation brilliantly. He records of Sir William:

> *It is said he came to London with only a half crown in his pocket, which is, of course, a gross exaggeration, although in all probability his pockets were not too well lined... [Fergusson] is credited with having an income of £20,000 a year, but of course the exact amount is known only to himself, although there cannot be the least doubt it is a very large one.*[40]

As in the 18th century there were books to help students pass examinations. One such book, *Examinations in Anatomy and Physiology...for the use of students who are about to pass the College of Surgeons or the Medical Transport Board* by Robert Hooper, was published in 1815.[41] It is dedicated to 'Gentlemen Studying medicine and preparing for further examination...as a mark of the author's attention to their interest and welfare'. It is essentially a question and answer book covering everything from anatomy to medicine and surgery.

Some of the notes written by students still survive and give a first-hand account of what was taught and how it was presented. For example, in the Archives of the National Library of Scotland there are hand-written lectures notes on 'Midwifery by Dr Simpson, November 1852' taken by Frederick Cook (MS 3542). This passage describes the rules for the use of chloroform in labour by the great James Young Simpson:

1. Begin it when the patient commences to complain of much pain generally towards the end of 1st stage.

2. Always inculcate perfect quietness around the patient particularly when giving chloroform. If you talk to them you make them often excited.

3. Give it only during a pain and always withdraw it during the intervals.[42]

This advice is direct, taken down from the master. It is clear and would not be forgotten. It is delivered almost like secret knowledge to the waiting disciples.

Other student notebooks written in this period are available for study. Some were associated with a textbook, one of which is 'A syllabus of a course of chemical lectures read at Guy's Hospital'. This book is interesting for several reasons. First, it shows what importance chemistry was playing in medical education in the early 19th century. Second, the book is produced in a printed volume but has blank pages opposite the printed pages throughout for the student to make notes and comments. A copy in the library of the University of Durham was owned by William Barlow and dated October 1811. It has a series of handwritten notes in fine copper plate which record, for example:

Nitrous gas destroys animals in a few seconds

Phosphoric acid is frequently used in medicine

Painter's colic is brought on by lead in paint

Use of bismuth in dyspepsia[43]

It contains notes on the properties of mucus and the chemistry of urinary calculi. The volume is prefaced by an excellent introduction:

In every science taught by lecture, a syllabus has been found to be of advantage to the student. At the same time that it lays before him a comprehensive outline of the syllabus, and points out the several divisions and their arrangement with respect to each other, it defines the meaning and extent of the scientific terms better than more verbal statements would do, and affords a convenient epitome of the rudiments of the science…In preparing this course of lectures, considerable attention has been paid to the order and distribution of the different parts of the subject.[44]

A splendid preface, worth remembering today by aspiring authors of student books.

WOMEN IN MEDICINE

The story of women in medicine is a long and complex one. While there had been famous medical women in the past (for example, Dame Trotula in Salerno), it was still not possible for women to study medicine in Britain in the 19th century. Considering the story of their struggle from the perspective of the 21st century, it is difficult to understand why it took so long. Prejudice still exists even now, but more than 50% of entrants to medicine are women. Literature on the topic and of the period is full of 'battle' allusions, and E.M. Bell's book, *Storming the Citadel: the Rise of the Woman Doctor* says it all.[45] The literature is powerful to read, and while the education and teaching had no special peculiarities (they attended lectures, clinics and dissections), the method by which they obtained such learning was haphazard and subject to sudden change and withdrawal.

The difficulties cannot be underestimated and are well described in Shirley Roberts' book: *Sophia Jex-Blake: a woman pioneer in 19th century medical reform.*[46] There are several names in addition to Jex-Blake associated with the women's movement, and they all knew each other: Elizabeth Garrett (later Garrett Anderson) and Elizabeth Blackwell, the first woman to obtain a medical degree in the USA (she tried 29 medical colleges in the USA before attending Geneva College in New York State).

They were often humiliated because of their superior knowledge, and were excluded from teaching on petitions from the male medical students. They had almost no support from senior medical staff. Decisions for admission made at one meeting were reversed at another. For example, Sophia Jex-Blake was admitted to the Edinburgh Medical School by the Faculty of Medicine, but this was reversed three days later by the Senate after pressure from some medical staff, notably Sir Robert Christison, professor of materia medica. Eventually she was admitted and, with three other students in lodgings in 15 Buccleuch Place, began her studies. Meanwhile, Elizabeth Garrett had passed the MD in Paris with distinction. Jex-Blake continued to pursue the cause, and as a result her study patterns suffered. The opposition remained and even such an illustrious figure as Lord Lister wrote in 1872:

> *Hence it seems clear to me that if women are to be taught to practise medicine, it must be done in entirely separate institutions. Lastly I would remark that even if hospitals be formed for the exclusive education of ladies, I believe it can never be right for young women to study in male wards; and the managers would in my opinion, incur a very grave responsibility if they were ever to introduce such a practice into the Royal Infirmary of Edinburgh.*[47]

In spite of this, progress was made. Jex-Blake got her degree (from Ireland), women's hospitals and clinics were set up. The GMC could not exclude women (though they didn't like it), and Elizabeth Garrett Anderson became a member of the BMA and even addressed its meeting in Edinburgh in 1875.

The GMC resolution is interesting:

> *The Medical Council is of the opinion that the study and Practice of medicine and Surgery instead of offering a field of exertion well suited to women do, on the contrary, present special difficulties which cannot easily be disregarded; but the Council are not prepared to say that women ought to be excluded from medicine.*[48]

After some searching for a suitable hospital in London to link with the London School of Medicine for Women, the Royal Free Hospital was eventually agreeable after some active discussion. It became the school's home (giving access to hospital beds for teaching) and was central to the development of the educational programmes. Elizabeth Garrett Anderson was Dean of the School from 1883 to 1903. It became part of the University of London, and in 1900 the London (Royal Free Hospital) School of Medicine for Women was included in the statutory list of medical schools. By this time, other universities had followed: Manchester University in 1889, Queen Margaret College in Glasgow in 1890, Bristol in 1891 and Durham in 1896.

Sophia Jex-Blake came back to Scotland and set up a clinic for women, and her practice grew. Her pioneering work had paid off, although she herself never adjusted to others taking the lead and resigned from the Royal Free. Even in Scotland her star was eclipsed by the establishment of a rival second medical school for women by Elsie Inglis, another formidable pioneer and one of her colleagues. Over the next 30 years, a number of hospitals for women were created around Britain.

Final victory eventually came with the publication of the Goodenough Report in 1944 (a report we will return to in the next chapter). The Royal Free became incorporated with the hospital, though it had to move, and women were given equal opportunities to have postgraduate education. The report stated:

Without adequate opportunities for obtaining hospital appointments after qualification, medical women cannot qualify themselves properly for general practice, much less can they train for advanced medical work or specialist practice...it seems clear that women doctors are not receiving their fair share of postgraduate appointments, owing to discrimination against them on the grounds of sex.

Such discrimination is unjust to women and, in so far as it may result in the best qualified applicant not securing appointment is contrary to the public interest. Every possible step should be taken to secure that all hospital appointments are filled by open competition, and that the sex of the applicant is not a bar to appointment.[49]

Powerful words indeed, though it took time for this to be implemented fully.

But what was the battle really about? And how can a man even contemplate trying to answer the question? It was probably about two things. First and easiest, it was about equality of women in medicine and being able to fulfil ambition to be a doctor. Second and more complex (but of greater relevance to this book), it was about patients and their right to be treated by a woman doctor if they so wished. The availability of women doctors provided a way by which many women were now able to gain access to someone who they wanted to talk to and get advice about health and illness. For anyone interested in the aim of medicine (of which more later), this is absolutely central. Women achieved that for other women, and gave them choice and a voice in their care.

Medical students in literature

We are all students of medicine, and to that end we must never stop learning. But how are we, the medical students of the past, the present and the future described in literature? The student life is detailed less frequently in books and plays than that of the fully qualified doctor, or of illness and suffering. And yet the subject is interesting. This selection covers the 19th and 20th centuries.

One interesting example of life as a medical student relates to the last topic, that of women in medicine. A novel, *Mona Maclean*, was written in 1892 by Margaret Todd, a medical student and doctor associated with Sophia Jex-Blake and the other women in the late 1900s studying medicine. Its subtitle is *Medical Student* and is written under the pseudonym Graham Travers. It begins in London as the results of the Intermediate

MB are posted, and Mona, a student at University College, has failed again. The scene is typical with crowds of students trying to see who has passed and failed. She is devastated and returns to Scotland and the family, where she spends several months thinking about what to do. She inevitably meets a young man who is also doing medicine but she does not reveal to him her own interest. This part of the story has references to vivisection, dissection and botany. There are comments on the role of women, for example:

"Women" was the reply, delivered with a courteous bow, "Have no power, they have only influence."

Doris flushed, and then said serenely, "We won't dispute it. Influence is in the soul, of which power is the outward form."[50] And again:

"And as a natural consequence, the supply of medical women will exceed the demand in the next ten years in this country. After that, things will level themselves, I suppose; but at present, if a woman is to succeed, she must be better than the average man."

"Whereas at present we are getting mainly the average women, and of course the average woman is inferior to the average man."

"Heretic!"[51]

Here is also a clear statement of why Mona (and presumably Margaret Todd) wanted to study medicine:

"When Mona began her medical career she was actuated partly by intense love of study and scientific work, and partly by a firm and enthusiastic conviction that, while the fitness of women for certain spheres of usefulness is an open question, medical work is the natural right and duty of the sex, apart from all shifting standards and conventional views."[52]

She also gives another reason for studying medicine, one which we will note later in this book in Chapter 12 (The Quest for Competence).

"It is perfectly awful to think how helpless people are who are quite outside of the profession. I think it is worthwhile studying medicine, if only to be able to tell your friends whom to consult—or rather, whom not to consult."[53]

She, of course, returns to London and is greeted by the younger medical students as something of a hero. She helps them with anatomy and their dissections, and there are some interesting conversations between them. She sets out some of her other beliefs.

"It is pleasant is it not, to leave dusty museums now and then and feel Science growing all around one? And what I love about the University of London is that it allows for that kind of thing in its Honours papers."[54]

She passes on the next occasion and gets a first in physiology: 'Mona Maclean, London School of Medicine for Women. Exhibition and Gold Medal'. She eventually marries her admirer and now, both doctors, they set up practice together. They did not set up practice in Harley Street as advised, as they 'were far too enthusiastic to forego the early days of night work, and of practice amongst the poor'.[55] The book ends with a scene which demonstrates the essence of needing women doctors. Ralph, her husband, sees a young girl as a patient. As she enters his consulting room, she bursts into tears. He looks at her carefully and says:

"I think" he said kindly, "you would rather see the doctor who shares my practice." And he rose and opened the door. Mona looked up smiling. "Mona, dear" he said quietly, "here is a case for you."[56]

Patient choice and patient needs being satisfied.

One the most memorable descriptions comes from a brief glimpse of medical students in *Pickwick Papers* by Charles Dickens. The subject of the exchange is Bob Sawyer, the medical student:

"Nothing like dissecting to give one an appetite." Said Mr. Bob Sawyer looking round the table.

Mr. Pickwick slightly shuddered.

"By-the-by, Bob," said Mr. Allen, "have you finished that leg yet?"

"Nearly", replied Sawyer, helping himself to half a fowl as he spoke. "It's very muscular for a child's."

"I've put my name down for an arm at our place," said Mr. Allen. "We're clubbing for a subject, and the list is nearly full, only we can't get hold of any fellow that wants a head. I wish you'd take it."

"No," replied Bob Sawyer, "can't afford expensive luxuries."

"Nonsense!" said Allen.

"Can't indeed," rejoined Bob Sawyer. "I wouldn't mind a brain, but I couldn't stand a whole head."[57]

It is a brilliant evocation of the nonchalance of the student, the bravado and the matter of fact nature of medical life. This tradition has been carried on in modern writers such as Richard Gordon in the *Doctor* books (of which more later) and Colin Douglas, whose first novel, A *Houseman's Tale* (1975), describes many of the experiences and pitfalls that we all went through.

Another rather unusual story in the same vein is called: 'The Life History of a Medical Student. The Awful and Ethical Allegory of Deuteronomy Smith'. The author is anonymous and it is set in Edinburgh, probably in the 1930s. Here is how the examinations are described:

"And it came to pass that at divers times Deuteronomy stood before the elders of the Temples of learning.

And the elders asked him many questions of the bones of men and of beasts, and concerning the herbs of the fields and the metals of the earth whereby the sicknesses of men are healed.

But lo! They were able to ask him nothing that he could not answer, and many wonderful deeds did he perform in their sight.

And because of these things, the elders of the Temple called upon Deuteronomy to appear again before them on a certain day.

And on that day, which was the first day of the eighth month of the year, Deuteronomy and many other young men stood in a great hall.

And they wore gowns adorned with hoods of many colours, and so bright were they that men said that Solomon in all his glory was not arrayed like one of these."[58]

For someone who now sees many graduation days, this is a splendid reminder of its purpose, and pageantry.

But life is not all fun for the medical student. There are considerable stresses and strains and, at times, even boredom. In *Madame Bovary* by Gustave Flaubert, Charles, a medical student, records his feelings:

"The list of lectures which he read in the official timetable set his head in a whirl. They covered anatomy, pathology, physiology, pharmacy, chemistry, botany, clinical medicine and therapeutics, to say nothing of hygiene and materia medica—all words about the etymology of which he knew nothing, words which seemed to him like the portals of sanctuaries in which dwelt the shades of the august. He understood absolutely nothing. No matter how hard he listened, he made but heavy weather of the lectures. Nevertheless he worked, equipped himself with bound notebooks, attended all the courses, and never played truant. He accomplished his little daily task in the manner of a mill horse, which goes round and round in blinkers, doing what he does without knowing the reason for it."[59]

Doesn't sound much fun. In Somerset Maugham's *Of Human Bondage*, a similar picture is painted. Philip is a medical student and he comments on the conjoint examination:

"He was eager to pass it since that ended the drudgery of the curriculum: after it was done the student became an out-patients' clerk and was brought into contact with men and women as well as with textbooks."[60]

"Thank goodness for problem-based learning and the new curricula. Before that he discusses the difficulties and indeed the poverty associated with being a student, and it is not quite like Bob Sawyer's cheerful views of medicine. The difficulty of the examination process is again noted. Of those who have problems he comments:

"They remain year after year, objects of good-humoured scorn to younger men. Some of them crawl through the examination of the Apothecaries Hall: others become non-qualified assistants, a precarious position in which they are at the mercy of their employers: their lot is poverty, drunkenness, and heaven only knows their end. But for the most part medical students are industrious young men of the middle class with a sufficient allowance to live in a respectable fashion."[61]

Students and young doctors also have to face difficult problems and may take time to adjust and learn. A short story by Arthur Conan Doyle, entitled 'His First Operation' shows how it might be done.

It was the first day of the winter session, and the third year's man was walking with the first year's man. Twelve o'clock was just booming out from the Tron Church.

"Let me see," said the third year's man, "you have never seen an operation?"

"Never"

"Then this way please. This is Rutherford's historic bar. A glass of sherry, please, for this gentleman. You are rather sensitive, are you not?"

"My nerves are not very strong I'm afraid".[62]

And so the story continues, with more sherry, a white face, and dreadful expectations. They arrive at the operating theatres where the conversation continues:

"There's going to be a crowd at Archer's," whispered the senior man with suppressed excitement. "It's grand to see him at work. I've seen him jab all around the aorta until it made me jumpy to watch him."[63]

Not perhaps the best preparation for your first operation. He faints of course at the first sight of the patient and wakens lying on the floor, and misses the critical part; the patient didn't stand the chloroform and the operation was cancelled. In a slighter lighter mode, Richard Gordon in *Doctor in the House* describes the medical student's first delivery. The text is interesting but those who remember the film will realise just how touching it was. The scene is set as Simon Sparrow, medical student, arrives at the house:

"Her time is near, doctor," said grandma with satisfaction.

"You have no need to worry any longer, missus," I said brightly...

"Mother," I said earnestly, "How many children have you?"

"Five, Doctor", she groaned. Well that was something. At least one of us knew a bit about it...

"I think it's coming doctor!" she gasped, between pains. I grasped her hand vigorously..."I feel sick", she cried miserably. "So do I", said I. I wondered what on earth I was going to do...Out of my hip pocket I drew a small but valuable volume in a limp red cover, "The Student's Friend in Obstetrical Difficulties." It was written by a hard-headed obstetrician on the staff of a Scottish hospital who was under no illusions about what students would find difficult. It started off with the "Normal Delivery" ...I glanced at the first page, "Sterility" it said...The newspaper that was it...and I scattered over the floor and the bed.

"Is it come yet" she (grandma) said. "Almost" I told her. "I shall need lots more water."

"It's coming, doctor!" ...Suddenly I became aware of a new note in the mother's cry—a higher wailing muffled squeal. I dropped the soap and tore back the bedclothes....

"Do you do a lot of babies, doctor?" asked the mother. "Hundreds," I said, "Every day."

"What's your name doctor, if you don't mind?" she said. I told her. "I'll call 'im after you. I always call them after the doctor or nurse, according."[64]

And the baby is thus called Simon.

In spite of all that is written about the bravado and callousness of the student, they are capable of great compassion and sensitivity, as all who teach them know. They are a wonderful group and it is a privilege to teach them. This is perhaps best brought out in a story by Dr. John Brown, an Edinburgh physician in the mid 19th century, at a time before the use of anaesthetics. The story is called 'Rab and his Friends'. Rab is the dog whose master, James, brings his wife to the Royal Infirmary with a breast lump. The medical students become involved in the care and Ailie, the patient, eventually goes to the operating theatre. The scene is set for the operation and is narrated by the medical student.

"The operating theatre is crowded; much talk and fun, and all the cordiality and stir of youth. The surgeon and his staff of assistants is there. In comes Ailie: one look at her quiets and abates the eager students. That beautiful old woman is too much for them; they sit down and are dumb and gaze at her. These rough boys feel the power of her presence. She walks in quickly, but without haste; dressed in her mutch, her neckerchief, her white dimity shortgown, her black bambazeen petticoat, showing her white worsted stockings and her carpet shoes. Behind her was James, with Rab. James sat down in the distance, and took that huge and noble head between his knees. Rab looked perplexed and dangerous; forever cocking his ear and dropping it fast.

Ailie stepped up on a seat, and laid herself on the table, as her friend the surgeon told her; arranged herself, gave a rapid look at James, shut her eyes, rested herself on me, and took my hand. The operation was at once begun: it was necessarily slow; and chloroform—one of God's best gifts to his suffering children—was then unknown. The surgeon did his work. The pale face showed its pain but was still and silent. Rab's soul was working within him; he saw that something strange was going on—blood flowing from his mistress, and she was suffering; his ragged ear was up, and importunate; he growled and gave now and then a sharp impatient yelp; he would have liked to have done something to that man. But James had him firm, and gave him a glower from time to time, and an imitation of a possible kick; —all the better for James, it kept his mind and his eye off Ailie.

It is over: she is dressed, steps gently and decently down from the table, looks for James; then, turning to the surgeon and students, she curtsies; and in a low clear voice begs their pardon if she has behaved ill. The students—all of us—wept like children; the surgeon helped her up carefully—and, resting on James and me, Ailie went to her room, Rab following."[65]

MEDICAL JOURNALS

Over the 19th century, journals took on an increasingly important role. The number of journals available grew, and in particular the number of specialist journals rose significantly. For example, by the end of the century there were around 120 journals, the majority (50) being of a specialist nature, from a starting base of just a few.[66]

The Lancet (first issue, Sunday 5th October 1823) and the *British Medical Journal* (first issue, Saturday 3rd October 1840) are perhaps the two best known and in particular for their early campaigning style. *The Lancet* especially, through its founding editor Thomas Wakley, played a major part as we have seen in the reform of the medical profession.[67] The *Journal of the American Medical Association* (1883) provided the same function. As journals developed, there was concern that they might confuse the public, or that they would simply be publicity vehicles for doctors seeking new patients or peddling some new type of treatment. During this time, the great medical science journals were being founded: *Journal de physiologie experimentale* (1821), *Archiv fur pathologische Anatomie* (1847), the *Journal of Physiology* (1878), the *Journal of Experimental Medicine* (1896) and many others. Numerous local and regional journals were published over this period. There were a number of public health medicine journals, but one which had a particular influence was *The Builder*, whose editor was George Goodwin. He campaigned for better housing and public health measures, and used a wonderful little rhyme to illustrate his beliefs.

When party broils and wars of creed are rife
When rulers shirk the laws of human life
When duty means the greed for private wealth
You'll likely find a blighted public health.[68]

From an educational perspective what was the value of such journals? First, they provided the doctor with an up-to-date view of new developments. These could be challenged in the correspondence columns and debate encouraged. Second, they provided information on conferences, new books and developments elsewhere in the world. Third, they had a campaigning role, not just in reforming the profession but in highlighting major issues of health, medicine and social welfare. In more recent times, journals have been a source of job vacancies and career opportunities. They also provided an opportunity for the doctor, young or old, to put pen to paper and record the results of a clinical case study, an original piece of observation or the results of an experimental study. In this way there was opportunity for all doctors to contribute to medical literature and to improving health. As we shall see in the 20th century, such practices became the norm and the 'publish or perish' culture developed.

One further aspect, already alluded to, is that the public had access to such journals and thus had the opportunity to see what was going on medicine. The same, of course, is true today, with even greater access via the Internet. This must be seen in a positive way in that it provides the public with information and advice which can then be used to increase awareness and bring a greater degree of choice in consultation.

Most of the characteristics of modern medical journals were developed in the 19th century. Quality has varied over the years, and some journals have come and gone, or been replaced by others. But they still remain an important educational tool for doctors.

The medical society

Many of today's medical societies began in the 18th or 19th centuries as meeting places, dining clubs or travelling clubs,[69,70] and almost all of them had a similar function. In general this included a clinical and scientific educational role, a social function and a responsibility for the welfare of patients in their geographical region. In some, the keeping of a library was an important component of the society. The ethos of this kind of society is best summed up in a series of quotations, the first of which is taken from Sir William Osler's essay on 'The Educational Value of the Medical Society':

"The first, and in some respects the most important, function is...to lay a foundation for that unity and friendship which is essential to the dignity and usefulness of the profession...The well-conducted medical society should represent a clearing house, in which every physician of the district would receive his intellectual rating, and in which he could find out his professional assets and liabilities. We doctors do not "take stock" often enough and are very apt to carry on our shelves stale out-of-date goods. The society helps a man to keep "up to the times" and enables him to refurnish his mental shop with the latest wares...The presentation of case histories may be very instructive, but this is often a cause of much weariness and dissatisfaction...In no way can a society better help in the education of its members than in maintaining for them a good library...[for the member for whom] the rolling years have brought ever-increasing demands on his time, the evening hours find him worn out yet not able to rest, much less snatch a little diversion or instruction in the company of his fellows whom he loves so well...he is the one above all others who needs the refreshment of mind and recreation that is to be had in a well-conducted society."[71]

The second is from Sir Heanage Ogilvie in an address to a newly formed medical society:

"The functions of a medical society are social and educational, and of these the first is undoubtedly the most important, because it leads naturally to the second...Unity and friendship among the doctors of a district is most easily brought about by the pleasant and free intercourse which a well conducted dinner meeting of a medical society provides."[72]

Underlying these social and educational functions, there was a firm commitment to the needs of patients, well expressed in the aims of the Massachusetts Medical Society, founded in 1781:

"To do all things as may be necessary and appropriate to advance medical knowledge, to develop and maintain the highest professional and ethical standards of medical practice and health care...for the health and welfare of the citizens of the commonwealth."[73]

Many societies have essentially stuck to this model and survived. But will it be sufficient for the future? Will the societies which began many years ago continue? Fortunately, there are some pointers as to which factors make for a successful society, and two articles in particular make interesting reading: 'The decline and fall of the scientific society'[74] and 'The evolution of medical societies in Britain—Have they a future'.[75, 76, 77] In summary, the following factors seem to be important:

+ A general approach is required. The medical society cannot compete with the specialist approach. It should make up in breadth what it cannot do in depth. Topics which cross boundaries and raise general issues are to be encouraged, as well as general reviews of recent advances.

+ A social function is important. The ability to meet colleagues and their partners in a relaxed, but stimulating atmosphere is the essence of a good society. However, this must not be the only part of the society. An educational input is also essential. A 'medico-convivial' society has superficial attractions, but would be unlikely to meet with all tastes.

- The admission criteria must be appropriate: groups of doctors must not be excluded but membership must also be seen to be a privilege. The general medical society should appeal to all groups of doctors.

- The organisation should be seen to be efficient and responsive to changes in medical practice and knowledge.

- The society should maintain and foster links with other medical societies and groups.

- Above all, it seems to be the balance which is most important if the medical society is to find a place in medical education.

In the paper entitled, 'Dr. Welch's influence on medical education', the concept of the 'Heritage of Excellence' is raised as an important part of medical education.[78] That heritage is still with us, just. What will the future hold?

CONCLUSIONS

The 19th century was a watershed in medical education. The development of the clinical method and the increasing use of scientific principles and the results of experimental research changed the way doctors worked. Journals began to replace books as the way to keep up to date, specialties developed, new societies appeared, and there was a much greater link between the patient and the laboratory. The increase in knowledge and understanding of disease gradually became manifest in better treatments and care. The paradigm of health had been shifted towards a scientifically based model: and the change in approach of Cullen at the beginning of the century to Koch at the end could not have been greater.

All this had to be incorporated into a medical curriculum which became increasingly crowded, though with less emphasis on lectures and more on practical work and demonstrations. Bedside clinical teaching had been revolutionised in France and was now accepted as the preferred mode of learning.

Regulation had taken up a very considerable amount of time, and the eventual form of the GMC allowed for further development. But the process diverted much energy and clearly exposed professional differences. However, the medical profession was now poised to reap the benefits of the new science in the next century.

All of this was not just about filling minds with facts but changing the thinking of doctors. Perhaps not surprisingly, this was not always successful, and resistance to change (demonstrated throughout this book) required leadership and a clear vision of what needed to be done. The next chapter illustrates how some of these changes were accomplished in the United States of America.

REFERENCES

1. Bernard C. An introduction to the study of experimental medicine (1865). New York: Macmillan and Co; 1927; 146.
2. Newman C. The evolution of medical education in the nineteenth century. Oxford: Oxford University Press; 1957; 12.
3. Ibid, 48.
4. Keele K D. The evolution of clinical methods in medicine. Being the FitzPatrick Lectures at the Royal College of Physicians 1960–61. London: Pitman Medical Publishing Co; 1963.
5. Laennec R T H. A treatise on the diseases of the chest (1821). Translated by J Forbes. London: T & C Underwood; 1961; 284–5.
6. Bynum W F. Science and the practice of medicine in the nineteenth century. Cambridge: Cambridge University Press; 1994; 44.
7. Bernard, 1.
8. Bernard, 2.
9. Bernard, 5.
10. Bernard, 14.
11. Bynum, 98.
12. Billroth, T. The medical sciences in the German universities (1876). Translation with an introduction by William Welch. New York: Macmillan and Co; 1924; 1–2.
13. Ibid, 2.
14. Ibid, 27.

15. Ibid, 45.
16. Ibid, 68.
17. Ibid, 77.
18. Ibid, 95.
19. Ibid, 118.
20. Ibid, 208.
21. Ibid, 224, 252.
22. Virchow R. Cellular pathology. 2nd edn. London: Churchill; 1860.
23. Shaw G B. The doctor's dilemma. London: Penguin Books; 1946.
24. Manson-Bahr P. History of the School of Tropical Medicine in London. London H K Lewis; 1956.
25. Walker M E M. Pioneers of public health. The story of some benefactors of the human race. Edinburgh: Oliver and Boyd; 1930.
26. Evans R J. Death in Hamburg: society and politics in the cholera years. London: Penguin Books; 1990.
27. Ibsen H. The enemy of the people. (The World's Classics) Oxford: Oxford University Press; 87.
28. Edmonds D, Eidinow J. Wittgenstein's poker: the story of a ten-minute argument between two great philosophers. London: Faber; 2001; 2.
29. Simon J. English sanitary institutions. 2nd edn. London: John Murray; 1897.
30. Fee E, Acheson R M. A history of education in public health: health that mocks doctors' rules. Oxford: Oxford University Press; 1991.
31. Ibid, Preface.
32. Bynum, 225.
33. Newman.
34. Poynter F N L, ed.. The evolution of medical education in Britain. London: Pitman Medical; 1966; 51–2.
35. Peterson M J. The medical profession in mid-Victorian London. Berkeley/London: University of California Press; 1978; 43.
36. Ibid, 48.
37. Newman, 41
38. Newman, 43
39. Peterson, 68–9
40. Peterson, 158–9
41. Hooper R. Examinations in anatomy, physiology, practice of physic, surgery, material medical, chemistry and pharmacy. New York: Collins; 1815.

42. Archives of the National Library for Scotland. Hand-written lectures notes on 'Midwifery by Dr Simpson, November 1852'. Taken by Frederick Cook. MS 3542.

43. Babington W, Marcet A, Allen W. A syllabus of a course of chemical lectures read at Guy's Hospital. London; 1811.

44. Ibid.

45. Bell E M. Storming the citadel: the rise of the woman doctor. London: Constable; 1953.

46. Roberts S. Sophia Jex-Blake: a woman pioneer in 19th century medical reform. London: Routledge; 1993.

47. Ibid, 134.

48. Ibid, 98.

49. Report of the Inter-departmental Committee on Medical Schools. (Goodenough report) London: HMSO; 1944; 100.

50. Travers G. Mona Maclean, Medical Student. Edinburgh: Blackwood; 1892; 322.

51. Ibid, 393–4.

52. Ibid, 355.

53. Ibid, 453.

54. Ibid, 395.

55. Ibid, 511.

56. Ibid, 511.

57. Dickens C. The Pickwick Papers. Continental Edition. Oxford: Oxford University Press; vol II, p. 4.

58. Smith D. The Awful and Ethical Allegory of Deuteronomy Smith, or The Life History of a Medical Student. By a Student of Medicine. Edinburgh: E&S Livingstone; 1891; 64.

59. Flaubert G. Madame Bovary. (The World's Classics) Oxford: Oxford University Press; 8.

60. Maugham S. Of Human Bondage. London: Pan Books; 1975 edition; 320.

61. Ibid, 265.

62. Doyle A. C. His First Operation. In: Round the red lamp. London: Metheuen; 1912; 12.

63. Ibid, 13.

64. Gordon R. Doctor in the House. London: Longmans; 1961; 106–8.

65. Brown J. Rab and his Friends. Everyman Library. London: J M Dent; 1907; 33.

66. Bynum W F, Lock S, Porter R. Medical journals and medical knowledge: historical essays. London; Routledge; 1992; 30–31.

67. Sprigge S S. The life and times of Thomas Wakley (1879). New York: R.E.Krieger Publishing Co; 1974.

68. The Builder 1875; 780.

69. Shaw A B. The oldest medical societies in Great Britain. Med Hist 1968; 12: 232-44

70. Poynter F N L. British medical societies. The Practitioner 1968; 201: 238–45.

71. Osler W. On the educational value of the medical society. Aequanimitas (London 1904).

72. Ogilvie H. The place of medical societies in the doctor's life. Lancet 1946; I:525–6.

73. Relman A S. Two hundred years young: The Massachusetts Medical Society. N Engl J Med 1981; 305: 1088–9.

74. Hanlon C R. The decline and fall of the scientific society. Surgery 1959; 46: 1–8.

75. Ractliffe D S. The evolution of medical societies in Britain— Have they a future? Bristol Medico-Chirurgical Journal 1979; January/April: 3–14.

76. Power D'A. British medical societies. London: Medical Press and Circular; 1939.

77. Jenkinson J. Scottish medical societies. 1731–1939. Edinburgh: Edinburgh University Press; 1993.

78. Gregg A. Dr. Welch's influence on medical education. Bulletin of the Johns Hopkins Hospital 1950; 87: 28–36.

7

Bridging the centuries: America leads the way

Education of the public and the organisation of modern society are placing new responsibilities upon medicine. Medical knowledge has been put into general circulation. It is now widely appreciated that health is a vital factor in every phase of life—in the home, the school, the office, the factory and on the farm. It is the greatest asset of the individual and the nation. The happiness and the prosperity of a people are largely dependent upon mental and physical vigor. The efforts to make knowledge regarding the conservation and promotion of health widely effective in the population, and to train physicians, nurse, dentists, public health officers, laboratory technicians and other personnel required in a satisfactory program of medical care are essential features of modern community life.[1]

Final Report of the Commission on Medical Education, 1932

AMERICAN MEDICAL EDUCATION

The 20–30 years each side of the beginning of the 20th century were particularly important for medical education in America and the rest of the world. As has been noted, changes in medicine and medical education occur within a social and political context.[2] America entered this period in Civil War (1861–65), and with peace established, the country expanded and developed rapidly. People from all over the world came to live and work in America, some freely and others forced to do so for a variety of reasons. The history of American medicine during the period covered in this chapter has been well documented by Welch (1915–6), Flexner (1910), Norwood, (1944 and 1970), Shryock (1966, 1947), Field (1970) and Ludmerer (1985) (see Further reading).

Medical schools had been set up in 18th century America, usually by graduates from Europe. The first two schools were established by Edinburgh graduates: William Shippen and John Morgan founded the first medical college in Philadelphia in 1765, and King's College New York (Columbia University) followed in 1767. Morgan summarised some of his thoughts on the ideal college in an address delivered at a public commencement held at the College of Philadelphia on May 30–31, 1765. Entitled 'A discourse upon the institution of medical schools in America', it was written while Morgan toured Europe, mainly in Paris. The discourse contains some interesting and negative comments about his co-founder Dr. Shippen. In a comment reminiscent of Hippocrates' first aphorism he says:

> *Medicine is a science as important in its object, as it is difficult in the acquisition. It is very extensive in its research and presupposes the knowledge of many other sciences. The cultivation of it requires no small ability, and demands of those who engage in the arduous pursuit an enlarged and benevolent mind.[3]*

Later he comments:

> *...it is necessary that a plan be marked out for directing students, and that they should be taught a regular course of every distinct branch of medicine; the infant state, and the want of professed teachers, have hitherto clogged medical pursuits in America with innumerable obstacles.[4]*

All this however was about to change.

On June 21, 1768, America's first commencement was held in Philadelphia and 10 young medical students were granted degrees, including Benjamin Rush. The Medical College in Harvard opened in 1783, Dartmouth in 1798 and Yale in 1817. Training was generally by apprenticeship and, for example, Rush was bound to John Redman for a six-year term. He learned by watching the master attend patients and by reading medical books in the library. Students acted as servants, caring for horses, sweeping the office and collecting fees. Rush, in his five years as a student, was absent no more than eleven days, and was out of the house only three evenings. Redman served an extensive clientele, with two apprentices. Rush prepared and compounded medicines, visited the sick, and read at intervals all the books he could. Rush borrowed other books, and read Boerhaave's lectures on physiology. It was a very good training.

Rush was particularly interested in the use of the lancet and calomel. According to Cullen, the body and disease could be compared to a house with 100 different rooms, each room with a different lock. Rush said: 'I am capable of entering every apartment of my house with the assistance of a single key—bloodletting'.[5]

Americans went to Leiden and then Edinburgh and trained under Cullen and Monro. They visited Paris and met the Hunter brothers, Cheselden and Smellie in London. Their thirst for knowledge carried them to Europe's leading physicians and surgeons.

But in spite of other schools being formed, there was a general feeling that standards were deteriorating, and the character of students was questioned. Daniel Drake, in a pamphlet written in 1847, urged students to 'forego the pleasures and amusements of the city. The eye that is dancing with pleasure or dull from its excess sees but imperfectly the aspects of disease in the clinical wards'.[6]

The cost of being a medical student in America was similar to that in Europe. There was a matriculation fee, and fees were paid to the professor, upon which a class ticket was granted. This printed admission card provided access to courses, and the cost varied but was around $15 per ticket on average.

The beginning of reform: 1825–1846

Poor teaching and facilities became evident, and the first convention to deal with this was held in Northampton in June, 1827. There was a thorough discussion of what constituted a good medical education, and proposals made, for example, on necessary prerequisites, including a knowledge of Latin, geometry and natural philosophy. By the early 1830s, Northampton was seen to be a failure and little reform resulted. The big problem was quackery and the unlicensed practitioner (as in the UK).

In 1846, at a national medical convention, N. S. Davis proposed a series of solutions, including the establishment of a national committee. This subsequently became the American Medical Association (AMA) in 1847. As usual, there was much subsequent debate and resolutions, but little action. Again, there was considerable discussion on preliminary education—good education and natural philosophy, mathematics, Latin and Greek as a prerequisite to entering medicine.

American medical reform was influenced by the European example. Paris had replaced Edinburgh as the centre of medical education, and the 1849 committee recommended the French emphasis on clinical teaching. More committees were set up, along with different ways of organising the meetings. Subgroups were to report to the AMA and it was agreed that AMA standards should be rigorously enforced—but there was little action as the AMA had limited power. The Civil War stopped all discussion at a time when things might have changed.

The situation deteriorates further: 1860–1890.

During the last three decades of the 19th century, the scientific revolution in medicine was underway in Germany. Pathology and bacteriology were developing; the importance of prevention had been recognised and mortality rates began to fall. However, in spite of the fact that advocates of medical reform in America had worked for almost 50 years, the situation in the colleges had grown worse. Schools continued to proliferate, diploma mills had developed in response to the inadequacies of the licensing laws, and inferior students were still being admitted to the colleges and turned into physicians.

Sporadic improvements

From its founding in 1859 to 1870, the Chicago Medical College stood alone in opposition to destructive competition, striving to maintain a high standard. When Charles Eliot became President of Harvard University, the medical college was essentially a proprietary school with a curriculum of four months of lectures during each of two years. Students were required to attend eight months of apprenticeship at the Massachusetts General Hospital. Examinations required up to nine students to be examined at one time.

Eliot became convinced of the need to change. He proposed a three-year course with a graded curriculum, and a faculty with fixed salaries. This split the faculty into two factions, with Henry J. Bigelow (professor of surgery) being the leader of the opposition. Eliot finally told the faculty that further debate was useless and carried out the changes in 1871. This was approved by the Harvard Corporation which was lay dominated. Medical colleges in Pennsylvania, Syracuse and Michigan all followed Harvard's lead.

The American Medical Association (AMA) was formed in May 1847 in Philadelphia. Work was done on the requirements for a medical degree, on premedical education, a code of ethics, and on licensing. A drive began to increase licensing in Illinois, and in 1881 the AMA board established a committee to investigate which colleges were in good standing. They found more evidence of diploma mills operating, and this was highlighted by journalists.

The purpose of the AMA is noted in Morris Fishbein's, *A History of the American Medical Association*:

> *For cultivating and advancing medical knowledge; for elevating the standard of medical education; for promoting the usefulness, honor and interests of the medical profession; for enlightening and directing public opinion in regard to the duties, responsibilities, and requirements of medical men; for exciting and encouraging emulation and concert of action in the profession; and for facilitating and fostering friendly intercourse between those engaged in it.*[7]

As we have discussed, the *Journal of the American Medical Association* was first published on the 14th of July, 1883. At around the same time, the American Academy of Medicine was established, as was the American Medical College Association.

The Johns Hopkins development

Johns Hopkins was a banker, and in 1873 he established a board of trustees to construct a hospital which would compare with anything in Europe. In 1876, a university medical school was established and Daniel Coit Gilman was appointed president. The esteemed surgeon John Shaw Billings was appointed dean, and this helped to attract an excellent young faculty: William Henry Welch (Pathology), William Osler (Medicine), William S Halstead (Surgery) Howard Kelly (Obstetrics) and Franklin B Mall (Anatomy). Together, they transformed the hospital from an auxiliary part of the medical college to an integral part of medical education. The change was from reading medicine to practising it, and the laboratory became as another aspect of medical education. The significance of this development is that within two decades more than 60 medical colleges had appointed three or more professors who held Hopkins degrees. The Hopkins experience demonstrated that a superior medical college could be developed in America, and its establishment was one of the most significant in American medicine.

The Association of American Medical Colleges

Johns Hopkins University played a major role in bringing about a renewal of the effort to improve American medical education. In 1890, a series of meetings was held in Baltimore to discuss the need for educational reform, and there was a national meeting to discuss 'medical education in this country and measures for its improvement'. Linked to the AMA, the Council on Medical Education was set up in 1906 and this was to play a major role in 20th century improvements in medical education. It identified low spots in medical teaching and attacked poor standards in preliminary education. By 1909, some 50 schools would require premedical college work by applicants. Before this, in 1900, Johns Hopkins was the only institution with such requirements.

The Flexner Report and its aftermath

In 1910, Carnegie Foundation president Henry S. Pritchett asked to inspect the results of the AMA survey of medical education. Pritchett then recommended that the Carnegie Foundation undertake examinations of medical, legal, engineering and theological education. Pritchett had read Abraham Flexner's *The American College*, a criticism of the elective and lecture system. He asked if Flexner would review medicine. At first, Flexner thought that he had confused him with his brother Simon, who was director of the Rockefeller Institute for Medical Research. However, he agreed and a new chapter in the history of medical education was begun.

Flexner know little about medical education; however, he familiarised himself with the subject and visited numerous institutions, especially Johns Hopkins. Ultimately, he developed a view of the ideal college embodying in a novel way the best features of medical education in England, France and Germany. He inspected the nation's colleges: entrance qualifications, faculty sizes (to determine if extensive enough to prepare students for the scientific practice of medicine), college finances, laboratories and hospital facilities.

Programmes and facilities for every college were described in his report, and he made specific proposals for a national system of medical education. He advocated the reduction of medical colleges from 155 to 31 regional institutions. When Carnegie published the report, the press completed the work and within a few years half the colleges had disappeared. Flexner's role did not cease, and he made contact with philanthropists and used his influence to secure grants to re-structure some of the more promising schools.

The Flexner Report: Medical education in the United States and Canada. A Report to the Carnegie Foundation for the Advancement of Teaching, 1910

The introduction to the report, by Henry S. Pritchett, makes interesting reading in itself. He looked to Johns Hopkins as the model but recognised that the changes advocated in the report could not be enacted immediately, all across the country. He raises the issue of 'educational patriotism':

> *By educational patriotism I mean this: a university has a mission greater than the formation of a large student body or the attainment of educational completeness, namely the duty of loyalty to the standards of common honesty, of intellectual sincerity, of scientific accuracy. A university with*

educational patriotism will not take up the work of medical education unless it can discharge its duty by it; or if, in the days of ignorance once winked at, a university became entangled in a medical school alliance, it will frankly and courageously deal with a situation which is no longer tenable. It will either demand of its medical school university ideals and give it university support, or else it will drop the effort to do what it can only do badly.[8]

Pritchett is also very clear about the need for the report. To summarise:

+ In the last 25 years there has been enormous over-production of uneducated and ill-trained medical practitioners.

+ This over-production is due in the main to the existence of commercial schools sustained by advertising methods to attract unprepared youth.

+ Until recently, the medical school has been profitable, but now with the need for laboratories it has become expensive.

+ The existence of poor schools has been justified by the need for poor boys to attend.

+ A hospital under complete control of the medical school is as necessary to a medical school as a laboratory.[9]

What a splendid statement with which to start the report. The report begins with a review of the history of American medical education, some of which has been discussed above. Flexner notes that between 1810 and 1840, some 26 new schools were established, and between 1840 and 1876 another 47 more. As an example, there were 39 in Illinois and 14 in the city of Chicago.[10]

The following chapter is entitled 'The proper basis of medical education' and is certainly worth a re-read in the 21st century. Flexner notes that knowledge is growing and new techniques and methods have appeared and can be put into action. However, he states:

Provided, of course, the physician is himself competent to use the instrumentalities that have been developed. There is just now the rub. Society reaps at this moment but a small fraction of the advantage which current knowledge has the power to confer. That sick man is relatively rare for whom actually all is done that is this day humanly feasible—as feasible in the hamlet as in the large city, in the public hospital as well as in the private sanatorium. We have indeed in America medical practitioners not inferior to the best elsewhere; but there is probably no other country in the world in which there is so great a distance and so fatal a difference between the best, the average and the worst.[11]

As Flexner puts it clearly, here is the rub. How do we ensure that doctors remain up to date and practise at the highest standards? He concludes this chapter by indicating that the minimum entry standards in medicine are a two-year college course in which the sciences are featured. He is concerned with the entry to medicine of those who may not have the means, but argues that it should be possible if 'he lays his plans, be prudent, and stick to his purpose'.[12]

There follows a chapter on laboratory branches of medicine as part of the course of study. He quite clearly sees medicine as part of science and notes:

On the pedagogic side, modern medicine, like all scientific teaching, is characterised by activity. The student no longer merely watches, listens and memorises; he does...an education in medicine nowadays involves both learning and learning how; the student cannot effectively know, unless he knows how.[13]

This is problem-based learning, student-centred and action-based. He makes further comments on the value of the lecture:

The lecture indeed continues of limited use. It may be employed in the beginning of the subject to orientate the student, to indicate relations, to forecast a line of study in its practical bearings; from time to time, too, a lecture may profitably sum up, interpret, and relate results experimentally ascertained. Textbooks, atlases, charts occupy a similar position. They are not in the first place a substitute for sense experience, but they may well guide and fill out the student's laboratory findings.[14]

In another passage he takes this further:

...the student brings his own faculties into play at close range—gathering his own data, making his own construction, proposing his own course, and taking the consequences when the instructor who had worked through exactly the same process calls him to account: the instructor, no longer the fountain pouring forth a full stream of knowledge, nor a showman exhibiting marvellous sights, but by turns an aid or antagonist in a strenuous contest with disease.[15]

Flexner argues strongly for the adjacent working of the clinic and the laboratory, and for using the literature to gain experience. The doctor will thus get into the habit of using journals to keep up to date.

He then gets to the meat of the report and the 'reconstruction'.[16] He notes wisely that 'the solution deals only with the present and the near future...in the course of the next 30 years needs will develop of which we here take no account'. He recognises that reports on medical education have a limited shelf life and will be overtaken by events and the environment. He then sets out the principles which form the basis of the report—summarised here:

1. The medical school is properly a university department.
2. They should be in a city and not in an 'out of the way' location.
3. There should be only one in each town.
4. Students will tend to study in their own states, therefore facilities should be made available for them to do this.

He notes that these principles have been disregarded in America. He then proceeds to look at each state and makes suggestions as to how many medical schools and where they should be. He also covers the basis issues for state boards, preliminary educational requirements, the facilities of the medical schools and the examinations for licensure. He has a separate section on the education of women which emphasises the choice available to them and their role in medicine:

Woman has so apparent a function in certain medical specialties and seemingly so assured a place in general medicine under some obvious limitations that the struggle for wider educational opportunities for the sex was predestined to be an early success in medicine. It is singular to observe the use to which victory has been put. [17]

Flexner then gives details of the number of students and schools available. He has a similar view on the education of the negro, which from the 21st century is difficult to read. For example: 'The practice of the negro doctor will be limited to his own race'. But looking back to what Flexner himself wrote about reports and their inevitable short lifespan, perhaps he might be excused. It is what others note as making decisions in a particular environment, at a particular time, in a particular political situation.

The report finishes with a note on every medical school in the USA and Canada. He is highly critical of some:

The foregoing account makes it clear that really satisfactory medical education is not now to be had in Alabama. [18]

Wisconsin presents a simple problem. The two Milwaukee schools are without a redeeming feature. [19]

In the matter of medical schools, Canada reproduces the United states on a greatly reduced scale. Western University (London) is as bad as anything to be found on this side of the line…McGill and Toronto are excellent. [20]

And so it goes on. No wonder people stopped and action began to be taken. To those who write reports, the Flexner

Report of 1910 is one to look at. The problem is analysed, principles set and clear guidance is given. Finally, it is interesting to note that the Carnegie Foundation approved the setting up of the report at its meeting in November 1908. It was signed off by Pritchett in April 1910, some 150 medical schools having been visited and data gathered from each.

Full-time teachers were created and this enabled Halstead, Janeway and Howland at Johns Hopkins to be full-time professors. For the first time, medical education and medical research became full-time occupations for every member of the faculty of an American institution, though there was a need to provide higher salaries.

In 1924, Flexner evaluated the changes. Since 1910, half the colleges had disappeared. There was a general improvement of equipment and facilities, and everywhere laboratory subjects were taught by full-time specially trained professors. There had been a great reform in the medical curriculum, with a four-year graded course separating preclinical from clinical.

Finally, Flexner notes in his autobiography the influence of Johns Hopkins:

> *Having finished my preliminary reading, I went to Baltimore —how fortunate for me that I was a Hopkins graduate!— where I talked at length with Drs Welch, Halstead, Mall, Abel, and Howell, and with a few others who know what a medical school ought to be, for they had created one...I thus became intimately acquainted with a small but ideal medical school, embodying in a novel way, adapted to American conditions, the best features of medical education in England, France and Germany. Without this pattern in the back of my mind, I could have accomplished little.*[21]

Medical Education: A comparative study, 1925

Flexner followed up his 1910 report with a fascinating comparative one in which he visited medical schools across Europe and reflected on them. As before, he takes an historical perspective on medical education and also notes some important educational issues:

> *The practitioner of medicine therefore uses—or should use—the same type of intelligence that is used in the solution of a problem. It makes not the slightest difference whether the problem is entirely new, or merely new to him. In a very real sense every case is unique, so that there never comes a time when the watchful intelligence, observing and interpreting, absolutely necessary in investigation, becomes superfluous or irrelevant in medical practice.*[22]

Two aspects of this quotation—problem solving and the ability to deal with new issues—remain relevant to medical practice and will be discussed later. He reiterates the importance of a scientific education and that medical education 'must be conceived as primarily the effort to train students in the intellectual technique of inductive science'.[23] He agrees that Billroth's book *Lehren und Lernen der medicinischen Wissenschaften* ranks with Claude Bernard's great book on experimental method, both of which were discussed in the previous chapter.

The bulk of the book covers the clinics, laboratories and hospitals he visited during his travels. They are fascinating. He describes Chief Medical Officer Sir George Newman, chief medical officer in England, as one of the doyens of medical education, and we shall review his work in the next chapter. He also gave evidence to the Haldane Commission on University Education, which will also be discussed in a later chapter. It is the detail which is impressive. He describes the work in individual universities, and notes strengths and weaknesses. Anyone seeking to find out how things were going in their medical school in the first two decades of the 20th century might look here first.

Final Report of the Commission on Medical Education. Association of American Medical Colleges (1932)

This report brings together much of the thinking about medical education at the time. It emphasises, as noted in the opening quotation of this chapter, that medicine is practised in a social context; it is part of the community and serves the community. It notes the changes which are occurring, and will occur, in medical care, and the problems of making good care available to the whole population. The report reflects on the uneven burden of illness and that:

> *Medical knowledge is the property of society and the principles involved in providing the application of that knowledge to serve different elements in the population have been demonstrated.*[24]

This report includes a discussion of health care in rural areas. It also covers the supply and distribution of physicians, the need for specialists and the importance of postgraduate education. The internship is seen to be an important part of the process. Not surprisingly, there is a section on licensure, as well as preventative medicine, premedical education and the medical course as a whole. It finishes with a section entitled, 'The Challenge to Leadership' and makes the forcible point that:

> *The hope of democracy is in trained leadership. The medical profession is the trustee of the essential knowledge and has the personnel necessary to solve a large national problem. Possessing that knowledge it is in a position to make a vital contribution to public welfare. Medicine will occupy its proper place in society to that extent that it provides leadership and properly trained personnel for the program of medical service, which should be built upon thoughtfully conceived plans of medical and postgraduate education,*

proper organisation of the profession, and the advocacy of unselfish and courageous public and professional policies.[25]

Not a bad way to finish a report. A rallying call to medical leaders which is timeless.

THE OUTCOME

The end result of the Flexner reports was significant change, and much has been written on the subject (e.g. *Beyond Flexner: medical education in the twentieth century* by Barzansky and Gevitz, 1992). This book notes that there have been many commentaries on the Flexner Report, having been analysed from many dimensions, and such discussions themselves have been criticised.[26] The contrast between Osler and Flexner has also been used as a vehicle to contrast the 'art' and the 'science' of medicine. Concerns have been expressed about Flexner's views on women and the opportunities for black people. However, his conclusion, based on considerable evidence in the report, was that medical education in America was really poor and needed to be changed. Much like the reform of the medical profession in Britain, a great deal was already underway, and the report was a step in the process, not the beginning.

The impact of the rise of European medical education, most notably in Germany, ensured that there were already a good number of well-educated physicians available to change the American medical school. The huge impact of Johns Hopkins in the reform process cannot be overestimated, as noted above in Flexner's own words. In addition, medical organisations—the AMA and the AAMC—were beginning to have an impact at the turn of the century after several decades of internal debate.

So why is the report still seen as a classic if it was all happening anyway? As Hudson points out, it is perhaps because not everyone has read it, and it is constantly 'misunderstood'.[27] The report called for major social change and was highly influential. His recommendations—cutting the number of ill-trained physicians and poor medical schools, recognising the importance of premedical education, the role of science, the importance of engaging in research, the need for medical schools to have access to hospital beds and the importance of licensing of doctors—were not new in themselves, but provided an impetus to speed up the process. In Hudson's words: 'Flexner's contribution was not so much revolutionary as catalytic to an already evolving process'.[28] It enabled the release of money for the purposes of medical education.

Flexner's closeness to the Hopkins model has sometimes been equated to his support for the 'lockstep' model of education. He is against rigidity and groups of fixed classes moving in fixed order. Flexner notes:

> *Anything more alien to the spirit of scientific or modern medicine or to university life could hardly be contrived. We have seen that it is impossible to set aside any definite set of facts or skills as constituting the "best" training for medicine. Medicine is scientific, if at all, mainly because of attitude and technique.*[29]

There has also been the concern that Flexner sacrificed the 'art' of medicine for the 'science'. Again, this is overplayed and Flexner wished only that the approach was based on science and evidence. He believed that the 'art' was also important. In his book, *Learning to Heal*, Ludmerer says: 'Contrary to popular perception, neither Abraham Flexner nor the American Medical Association participated in the creation of modern American medical education' as things were already moving, but 'profoundly influenced the final form the system took'.[30] Perhaps that is the mark of the successful report, one which builds on the present changes, but influences the rate and direction significantly. As will be seen in the next chapter, large numbers of reports have been written on medical education and only a few have had a significant impact. Perhaps Flexner discovered the secret: to go with current changes but to shape the vision and give direction.

CONCLUSIONS

This chapter had the subtitle, 'America leads the way'. From the late 19th century, with the establishment of Johns Hopkins and subsequent reforms including the Flexner Report, America was in the forefront of change in medical education. As we shall see in the next chapter this impetus was maintained in the 1950s and 1960s with new ways of thinking about medical education which had global impact.

REFERENCES

1. Association of American Medical Colleges (AAMC). Medical Education. Final Report of the Commission on Medical Education. New York; 1932; 380.
2. Hodges B. The many and conflicting histories of medical education in Canada and the USA: an introduction to the paradigm wars. Med Educ 2005; 39: 613-21.
3. Morgan J. A discourse upon the institution of medical schools in America. With a preface containing, amongst other things, the Author's apology for attempting to introduce the regular mode of practising physic in Philadelphia. Philadelphia; 1765; 2.
4. Ibid, 19.
5. Kaufmann M. American medical education: the formative years 1765–1910. Westport, Connecticut: Greenwood Press; 1976; 58.
6. Kaufmann, 47.
7. Fishbein M. A history of the American Medical Association. Philadelphia: Sanders; 1947; 30.
8. Flexner A. Medical education in the United States and Canada: a report to the Carnegie Foundation for the advancement of teaching. New York: The Foundation; 1910; xiii.
9. Ibid, x–xi.
10. Ibid, 6.
11. Ibid, 22.
12. Ibid, 43.
13. Ibid, 58.
14. Ibid, 61.
15. Ibid, 93.
16. Ibid, 143.

17. Ibid, 178.
18. Ibid, 186.
19. Ibid, 319.
20. Ibid, 325.
21. Flexner A. I remember: the autobiography of A. Flexner. New York; Simon and Schuster; 1940; 115.
22. Flexner A. Medical education: a comparative study. New York: Macmillan; 1925; 8,
23. Ibid, 13.
24. AAMC, 386.
25. Ibid, 400.
26. Barzansky B, Gevitz N, eds. Beyond Flexner: medical education in the twentieth century. New York: Greenwood Press; 1992.
27. Hudson R P. Abraham Flexner in historical perspective. In: Barzansky B, Gevitz N, eds. Beyond Flexner: medical education in the twentieth century. New York: Greenwood press, 1992; 7.
28. Ibid, 13.
29. Flexner 1925, 137.
30. Ludmerer K M. Learning to heal: the development of American medical education. New York: Basic Books; 1985; 7.

8

The educational revolution: the 20th century

On the pedagogic side, modern medicine, like all scientific teaching, is characterised by activity. The student no longer merely watches, listens and memorises; he does...an education in medicine nowadays involves both learning and learning how; the student cannot effectively know, unless he knows how.[1]

Abraham Flexner in The Flexner Report, 1910

INTRODUCTION

Perhaps surprisingly, the 20th century (extending into the 21st century) is by far the most interesting in the whole history of medical education. So much has changed, both in the knowledge base of medicine but also in the way in which learning occurs. The pace of change has quickened and shows no sign of slowing down. This is reflected in two ways: first, the enormous changes in the knowledge base; second, in the number developments in education and learning which have occurred. The number of 'reports' has increased, and there have been a succession of initiatives, not all of which have been evaluated. In addition, there is now greater concern about public issues in medicine and in the involvement of patients. While biomedical science remains at the heart of the learning process, there is increasing interest in the arts, the humanities and social sciences in the education of the doctor. One aspect which was raised at the beginning of this book and should be pointed out again is that for most of the 20th century, doctors were referred to as 'he' and the word 'men' is most frequently used. This it not a reflection on the views or values of the present author, but reflects opinion at the time.

The 20th century has been one of enormous change in knowledge and technology. This explosion in knowledge has shaped some of the changes in medical education and continues to do so. For example, at the beginning of the century, a 4- to 5-year programme equipped the doctor to go immediately into practice, and to do so in almost any branch. This is no longer the case. In addition, there was a need for more and more doctors, and as the numbers of students increased, new medical schools were established, giving the founders opportunities to change and begin again.

Society has also changed and there are now different expectations of what medicine can and should do. There is also a different relationship between the patient and the doctor. In the UK, the National Health Service (created in 1947) had a major impact on medical education, and in other countries the healthcare system also affects the way in which medical education is delivered.

Medical education in the 20th century (and early years of the 21st) has been dominated by a series of major reports and radical changes in the way in which learning is delivered. This has been a worldwide phenomenon, though in this chapter the impact on the education of doctors in the UK will be emphasised. This is not to exclude other significant changes elsewhere but reflects the particular interest of the author. Such reports are often seen as dull and boring, and associated with a bureaucratic process which stifles imagination and innovation. They are generally not like this. The reports below show just how well thought through the issues have been; they are lively and informative.

One of the most interesting aspects of this historical review is the assessment of which reports were effective (as determined by the implementation of their recommendations in one form or another) and which were not. Equally interesting is the composition of the committees who wrote the reports: a list of the great and the good in medicine.

Note that the last 15 years (1990–2006) will be treated only superficially in Chapter 9. Some of the most recent reports will be noted and described, but little can be said now of the long-term impact of these reports. That will be for others in the future to assess.

The beginnings of change

The process of change really began at the end of the 19th century and beginning of the 20th century in the United States, and this aspect of medical education has been dealt with in Chapter 7. The impact of this period has been considerable, and the process of change in American medical education continued in the 1950s and 1960s, with equally important outcomes in the UK. This will be discussed later in this chapter.

THE REPORTS ON MEDICAL EDUCATION IN THE UK

This part of the chapter will summarise the most frequently quoted reports on medical education in the UK over the 20th century. This might seem somewhat repetitive and boring, but these reports set out the key issues and changes in medical education over the period. A further reason for giving details of such reports is that some of them are now difficult to find. They provide a fascinating glimpse into the thinking behind the educational process. It is difficult to be critical of them at this distance, and from the excerpts the reader will make up his or her own mind about them. For example, in the 1881 GMC report there is a statement that students should be 'tested' on each subject studied. There is no explanation of this, nor any particular detail on the level of competence that should be reached. But that is how it was. We must remember that our reports, or our contribution to them, will be viewed in a similar way in the future. It is inevitable that the choice of reports reviewed is somewhat selective; there is much still to be learned from them and the author apologises if the reader's 'favourite' report has been missed.

The General Medical Council's Report on Education and Examination (1881)[2]

This report sets the scene for the 20th century by laying out requirements for medical schools in the UK. While there were changes to the report (notably in the 1920s and 1930s), it remained as the basic document until 1947, though modified through other general GMC reports.

It begins with entrance qualifications and provides a clear description of the university preliminary examinations and the subjects to be included: English (with grammar and composition), history, geography, Latin, mathematics, elementary mechanics, and one of a range of optional subjects, including Greek, logic, botany or elementary chemistry.

The report recommends that 21 shall be the earliest age at which the candidate can obtain a licence to practise. The course of professional study shall occupy at least 4 years. There follows a list of subjects 'without a knowledge of which no candidate shall obtain a qualification enabling him to be registered'. (Note that all references are to men.) These included chemistry, anatomy, physiology, materia medica and pharmacy, medicine, surgery, midwifery and forensic medicine. The subjects are separated into two divisions, essentially pre-clinical and clinical. The Council 'will view with approbation any encouragement…to prosecute the Study of the Natural Sciences before they engage in studies of a strictly professional character'.[3]

As far as the professional examination is concerned, each of the candidates should be 'tested' in all of the subjects mentioned.[4]

In the 1881–2 Medical Acts Commission Report it is noted:

It would be a mistake to introduce absolute uniformity into medical education. One great merit of the present system, so far as teaching is concerned, lies in the elasticity which is produced by the variety and the number of educating Bodies. Being anxious not in any way to diminish the interest which the teaching Bodies now take in medical education, or to lessen their responsibility in that respect, we desire to leave to them as much initiative as possible. In certain matters of general importance, such as the duration of study and the age at which a student should be permitted to practice, common regulations ought, we think, to be laid down; but we wish to record our opinion that nothing should be done to weaken the individuality of the Universities and Corporations, or to check emulation between the teaching institutions of the country.[5]

This report then shows how the 20th century began, and as we will see what a long way it has come.

Subsequent reports were published in 1890, 1909, 1922 (when the medical curriculum extended to five years, exclusive of physics and chemistry), 1936 and the most detailed one in 1947. The 1947 report will be discussed in more detail in this chapter.

Sir George Newman. *Notes on Medical Education* (1918)[6]

Almost a century ago, Sir George Newman, a most distinguished predecessor of the author as chief medical officer to the government, was a prolific writer on medically related subjects. He was well read in the humanities, as is reflected in his own writing. He had a particular interest in medical education and, indeed, is singled out in the Flexner Report for special mention.

This short report, addressed to the president of the Board of Education, is wide ranging and full of interest. For example, he makes a fascinating reference to medical students in English literature, including Dickens, Trollope and Eliot. He begins by setting out the changing conditions of medical practice and most importantly lists the official duties of the medical practitioner, including certifications of births and deaths, inspecting houses for disinfection, diagnosis of mental health issues, dealing with dangerous and offensive trades, and so on.

He cites the words of pioneering British biologist Thomas Henry Huxley ('Darwin's bulldog') at the formal opening of The Johns Hopkins University in 1876. Professor Huxley declared that the medical practitioner must be able on the one hand to prevent disease by his knowledge of hygiene, and on the other to divine its nature and to alleviate or cure it. In order to achieve these great ends, the practitioner must first understand health; he must have:

> *...a thorough and practical knowledge of the conditions of health, of the causes which tend to the establishment of disease, of the meaning of symptoms, and the uses of medicines and operative appliances; next he must understand the nature of disease, the structure of the human body and its manifold actions implying a knowledge of anatomy, physiology, chemistry and therapeutics.*[7]

It is interesting to compare this written in 1876 with the GMC guidance in 1881.

Newman then sets out the knowledge required: a scientific knowledge of the nature of disease, the signs and symptoms of disease, the treatment of disease, prognosis and what the signs of death portend (a reference to autopsy work). Most importantly, he follows this with the statement: 'If this be the type of medical practitioner the times require, the question arises, what kind of education will produce such a practitioner?'[8]

He argues for a university education, but that the doctor must have something more than learning: 'He must also be a skilled craftsman, and knowing his way among men, he must be, in a general sense a humanist'.[9] The whole section on the pursuit of learning in medicine is worth reading and is very contemporary. For example:

> '...the service of the public requires a well informed and skilful doctor, but also an educated man, and before the professional training, and also as part of it there must be a general equipment, adding not only to the pleasure and usefulness of life but also the standard and character of the medical training built on it.[10]

He quotes his namesake Cardinal Henry Newman: 'If then a practical end must be assigned to a University course, I say it is that of training good members of society'.[11] He then follows with Sydenham: 'The chief deficiency of medicine is not want of efficacious medicine. Whosoever considers the matter thoroughly will find that the principal defect on the part of physic proceeds not from a scarcity of medicines to answer particular intentions, but from want of knowing the intentions to be answered'.

In dealing with 'instruction' he makes several points. First, a university is a place where students work in constant association with other students and in close contact with their teachers. The second concerns the quality and status of the teachers. They should possess not only high academic qualifications in learning and skill in the craft, but also undoubted pre-eminence as teachers. He makes no comments on how a 'good teacher' is to be identified, nor makes any statements on the training in this aspect of the work. Third, that all training should be carried out under favourable conditions—with staff, laboratories, time, remuneration, etc. Lastly, university teaching is ultimately synthetic and works towards universal ends. It is not a mere cramming place or 'grind shop'.

> *In short, the teacher in a university is the pivot of the method. He must be learned in his subject, skilled in craft, competent in administration, experienced in research, and catholic in mind. He should reach his post not by favour, by merit of age or seniority, by social convention, but chiefly because he is a teacher and a leader of men.*[12]

What a splendid summary of medicine and medical education. Nowadays, one might only add the ability to keep up to date by continuing professional development and by the regular publication of clinical outcomes. The importance of inter-professional working and teamwork would also be emphasised, as would the relevance of management.

There then follows a section on the curriculum which covers the subjects to be included. More interestingly is a long paragraph on 'The relation of examination to teaching'. The point is made, from the Royal Commission on University Education in London (1913), that: 'Examinations are a subsidiary function, which can never take the place of education and may very easily injure it'.[13] As Huxley said in 1874: 'Examination, like fire, is a good servant, but bad master'.[14] Newman is quite critical of many examinations which 'nullify education and bring all the pernicious influences and evils of the cramming system'.[15] As we know only too well, examinations should follow the process of education, not lead it. What is required, Newman says, is a new spirit in teaching, and ideals which can not be imposed from outside but by growth from within. He emphasises the cultivation of the laboratory method and the scientific spirit in teaching, as well as an understanding of the social life and conditions of the patient.

As chief medical officer, he had a particular interest in the teaching of preventive medicine. The objectives are to:

+ Prevent disease arising or spreading.
+ Reduce the death rate.

- ✦ Prolong the span of man's life.

- ✦ Increase the physical capacity and powers of resistance of the individual and the community.[16]

What should be taught are the causes and conditions of disease in relation to social and communal conditions, the study of beginnings of disease, the relation of disease to environment and external conditions, sanitary administration and the application of the scientific method.

Finally, there is a section on the place of research in medical schools. It is a splendid and reflective section on the past, present and future. He argues for a more intimate association between teaching and research on the one hand, and laboratory research and clinical research on the other. He again quotes the Royal Commission on University Education in London: '…it is a necessary condition of the work of university teachers that they should be systematically engaged in original work'.[17] This includes an exhortation to continue to study medicine after graduation. He argues for arrangements for postgraduate training and facilities for all practitioners to bring their knowledge and practice up to date.

All in all, it is a splendid publication, full of good sense and very modern. The language is perhaps a little different, and the pace of change in medical knowledge has been more rapid than could have been conceived at the time. The principles, however, seem very sound and form the basis of some of the conclusions in the final section in this book.

Postgraduate medical training in the 1920s

While browsing, a pamphlet on this subject was noted, dated 1920.[18] The pamphlet describes the position in Glasgow and indicates that pre-first-world-war postgraduate medical education (PGME) was imperfectly organised, though a scheme was being developed. After the war, the topic was taken up and a committee of the university, chaired by the principal, Sir Donald MacAlister (who was also the president of the GMC at the time), reviewed the issues again. It noted that medical centres in Germany and Austria regularly attracted large numbers of medical men from all over the world. The Americans and the French were organising their resources for postgraduate work, as was London. A postgraduate council had been set up under the direction of Sir William Osler. A Postgraduate Medical Association had been formed, as had a Fellowship of Medicine (founded in 1918). These two organisation merged in 1919.

The Glasgow committee decided that it should not be left behind 'with its abundance of clinical opportunities'. A postgraduate medical association was set up by the university. Its membership included teachers from the university and the main teaching hospitals, but significantly not from the Faculty of Physicians and Surgeons of Glasgow. It would set up practitioner courses, weekly clinical demonstrations, advanced and comprehensive courses on such topics as obstetrics and child welfare, school inspection and hygiene, tuberculosis and venereal diseases. Other topics were suggested for the future. Facilities would be available for research work and degrees such as the DSc and the PhD. Young specialists might be attracted to 'work with our leading men'. It was decided that the question of finance would greatly influence the success of the venture and that fees should be charged. The government would be asked to assist. Here then is a small taster of what was happening across the country to improve postgraduate education.

Report of the Interdepartmental Committee on Medical Schools: The Goodenough Report (1944)[19]

This report to the Ministry of Health and the Department of Health for Scotland had wide ranging implications. It was set up '...to enquire into the organisation of Medical Schools, particularly in regard to facilities for teaching and research, and to make recommendations' and began its work in 1942. As in previous reports, the gender used is male.

It is interesting to note the thoroughness of the work. It met 50 times, and in 34 meetings oral evidence was heard. Two of the meetings, each lasting several days, were held in Scotland. At the start of the report, several useful definitions are provided, and the first section offers general comments on the 'Relation of Medical Education to a National Health Service'. Here one of the most relevant statements on the importance of medical education is set out:

> *Properly planned and carefully conducted medical education is the foundation of a comprehensive health service. If such a service is to have continuing vitality it must be founded on highly developed and vigorous systems of general and professional education for members of the medical and allied professions, and it must evoke the enthusiastic and intelligent cooperation of the general public.[20]*

This is such an important statement, and perhaps the only modern change would be to replace 'medical' with 'professional' to reflect the changing patterns of care and the wide range of staff involved in the delivery of patient care. The emphasis on public involvement is also critical.

The aims of medical education are described as guiding:

> *...medical students to such development of mind and character as will enable them when qualified to give maximum service to the community. It must help a student to acquire a scientific foundation for his professional work, a proper outlook on the promotion of mental and bodily health, an adequate knowledge of disease, a sympathetic understanding of people and their environment, a sound judgement and the ability to observe accurately, reason logically, and assess the claims of new knowledge.[21]*

There is a very important section on the selection of medical students which proposes:

+ that before he begins his medical training a student must have received a good general education at least up to the recognised standard of entry to a university

+ that selection should not be based on examination results alone

+ that prospective students should be interviewed before acceptance and weight should be attached to the con-clusions found at such interviews and to confidential reports on an applicant's previous career

+ that selection machinery must be supplemented by arrange-ments to weed out as early in the course as possible (particularly in the first year) those students who prove unsuitable.[22]

The report notes the methods employed in the USA and Canada for selection and asks that they receive close study.

The main recommendation which was rapidly taken up and implemented was on a compulsory pre-registration year. There was, it is noted, enthusiastic support for the proposal that every student, after final examinations, should be required to serve as a junior house officer for a period of 12 months in one or more approved hospitals before being admitted to the Medical Register and allowed to enter independent practice. Here is the beginning of postgraduate training, and one of the themes of subsequent reports was the extension of this principle in all aspects of medicine.

Research is seen as fundamental with the statement 'a community that wishes to support scientific research must first find and train the men who have the ability and impulse for scientific enquiry. It must create the most favourable conditions for their work and give them the tools they need'.[23] In an age of tensions between providing for the delivery of a quality service to patients, and changing and improving practice by research, these words remain as powerful as ever.

The section on teaching the teachers is also of interest. The characteristics of the good teacher are first described: wide and sound knowledge of the subject, skills in clinical medicine, a keen interest in students, their development and ideas, and an ability to inspire and guide them. It is suggested that help and guidance and the acquisition of skills in the art of teaching would be useful, and that in the past too little attention has been paid to the training of teachers of medical students. Apart from illustrating some of the difficulties of being a teacher of medicine, no positive suggestions are made as to how to take this forward.

The report also makes recommendations on the content of the curriculum, its overcrowding and the length of the course, along with a number of other recommendations.

Within the report are important implications for women in medicine (noted earlier, in Chapter 6). In particular, the importance of women having access to postgraduate education was recognised.

There is an important section on the involvement of the general public in medical education. For example, it notes that all of us, rich or poor, may need medical help at some time and, therefore, the public should be willing partners in the further-ance of medical education and research. There is a comment, but with limited supporting evidence, which is central to cur-rent debate: 'There is convincing evidence that the care and treatment of the sick reaches the highest standards when it is associated with the conduct of teaching and research, and when every step in the treatment must be fully and openly dis-cussed'.[24] The report cites the evidence presented by the County Councils Association which says that 'the presence of a medical school improves the medical facilities for the inhabitants of the district in which it is situated'.[25] The debate continues.

Finally, there is a section on postgraduate education covering the issues of facilities required and the need for refresher courses in various specialities, especially general practice. The authors saw it as 'lacking in adequacy and completeness'. In relation to specialist training, the report notes that the trainee 'should be regarded throughout as primarily a trainee…and must have adequate time for the critical scrutiny of whatever he is doing and for reading, reflection and research'.[26] There follows discussion of the establishment of a postgraduate organisation, with the main emphasis being on London. There is no formal discussion of 'creating a specialist register', though there are allusions to the length of time and experience required to become a specialist, as defined by the medical Royal Colleges. As has been noted earlier, there is specific mention of the need for women to have the same opportunities as men in postgraduate education, the final issue of equality.

The report is an excellent summary of medical education in the 1940s, and a series of its recommendations were instigated, bringing significant changes in the education of doctors.

Recommendations as to the Medical Curriculum. General Medical Council (1947)

These recommendations of the GMC are a direct response to the Goodenough Report. But this document could not be more different from Goodenough. Read from a 21st century perspective it seems to be introspective and at times even petulant. It begins almost with a defence. The GMC is not allowed to interfere with the conduct of examinations, and the object of the Council 'is and always has been' to give practical assistance to licensing bodies and medical schools. But, it goes on, 'there is nothing in the Act, even if it desired, to prescribe a uniform curriculum…upon all students'.[27]

The document then goes through the various recommendations of the Goodenough Report in detail. Some it agrees with, others it most definitely does not. It makes the preliminary point that the GMC was just about to revise their guidance when the Goodenough Commission came along, and did some of it on its behalf, though this accelerated the process. It refers to the recommendation that the GMC should, without delay, carry out 'a drastic overhaul of the medical curriculum'. In summary, it does not quite achieve this.

The document refers to the Council being asked by the minister of health in 1944 to undertake a revision of all recommendations, and that the Council had also been in touch with medical school and licensing bodies about this. These bodies made it clear that recommendations should not be used as an instrument by 'means of which the Council would seek to dictate the selection of any teachers of any subjects in the Curriculum or the methods by which any such subject should be taught'.[28] This is clearly a major drawback to the GMC, as their power to reform the curriculum was thus very limited. There is even an apologia in the introduction, hoping that they will not be laid open to 'misconstruction' on this point if they offer certain observations. They sent a delegation to 'The New World' to see what was going on in Canada and the United States.

The document first tackles the crowding of the curriculum referred to in Goodenough. The most they can do is to ensure that there is nothing in the recommendations to encourage the licensing bodies and schools to retain anything which is unnecessary or premature for students to learn. As far as the length of the curriculum is concerned they cannot agree with the report that the total length of the course of training leading to the final examination should not exceed four and a half years. Though it does make the very contemporary point that the longer the course, the more of a burden it will impose on students of 'limited means'. One of the major planks of the Goodenough Report is thus not taken forward.[29]

As far as the general and pre-medical background was concerned, the Council left the recommendation as adopted in 1937, with no change. There are interesting comments on specific subjects. For example, in relation to statistics: 'the Council think it preferable not to include in the new recommendations as to the period during which, or the relation with other subjects in which it should be taught'.[30] In regard to social medicine, it was decided not to include any new recommendation as to instruction during the pre-clinical studies, and that there should be no change during the clinical period. It was surgery which caused the most powerful response:

The Council agree that it would not be desirable, even if it were practicable, to attempt to include, in the instruction of students in Surgery, instruction expressly intended to equip them to undertake major operative surgery. But they cannot agree with the Committee that the possibility that any student will, as soon as he is entitled to practise on the public, be called upon to undertake minor operative Surgery is so remote that instruction in this subject can be safely omitted from the instruction given during the period of Clinical Studies.[31]

Psychiatry was different and the Council was supportive of including it as a separate subject. There is a fascinating discussion on sex hygiene. The Council notes:

If, for example, Bodies and Schools should become convinced of the importance of providing instruction in the subject of Sex Hygiene, on the ground that questions and problems about the relationship between the sexes are often referred to general practitioners, it may be advisable that such instruction should be given as part of instruction in Social Medicine.[32]

There is a feeling reading this document that the Council were annoyed that Goodenough had reported first, and that they might have liked to have changed things but were not able to do so.

The National Health Service (1947)

The creation of the NHS in 1947 had a profound effect on the development of medical education. For the first time there was a national service within which the learning of medical students and postgraduates could be planned. Each NHS hospital and the consultants who were employed had a responsibility to provide teaching. The earlier quotation from the Goodenough Report emphasises the importance of education to the NHS. However, it was in postgraduate education that the NHS proved to be particularly useful, especially after the development of regional postgraduate centres and Deans who were able to coordinate the training of the young doctor and provide throughout the region the facilities and experience required. Planned programmes were developed which covered the main teaching hospitals and the district general hospitals whose staff were delighted to be involved. Where national specialities were developed, postgraduates from any region were able to go for further experience. The ability to coordinate and use local, regional and national resources was indeed a major effect of the creation of the NHS, and it might be a useful exercise to compare such a system with other systems worldwide. As will be discussed later, the last 15 years have seen significant changes in the NHS, and the impact of those changes is still being assessed.

Dealing with a national system also allowed for the development of speciality interests and the creation of national centres of excellence for dealing with particular conditions or procedures, for example, in cardiac surgery, transplantation, specialist genetic services, children's services and mental health. Such national services not only allowed the development of skills and expertise but provided an important training function and allowed the gradual expansion of the service as the skill base expanded. Such developments were just as relevant to other groups of health professionals.

The training of a doctor: Report of the Medical Education Committee of the British Medical Association (1948)

The report of this committee, chaired by Henry Cohen, came at just the right time and stimulated a great deal of discussion, some of which will be mentioned below. It begins with a brief historical background and refers to the many discussions on medical education in Britain and America which were current at the time. It sets out some principles, including the importance of life-long learning, the difficulty in selecting students, the importance of adding new subjects to the curriculum but without making it too overcrowded, the real concerns about the problems of memorising large amounts of information rather than principles, and the isolation of some departments and the need for integration. The aim of the medical curriculum is discussed and it is agreed that:

> ...the aim of medical education is not to impart to the student a mass of factual information in each branch of medicine, but to equip him with sound basic principles, including the scientific outlook and method, a knowledge of the fundamentals of the medical sciences, competence in, and understanding of, certain indispensable techniques, and an intellectual resourcefulness and initiative in the handling of unusual unexpected situations. Sound habits and methods of study are the foundation of continued self education. Time must be available for healthy exercise and recreation and for independent reading and leisurely reflection.[33]

The comment on resourcefulness in unexpected circumstances is interesting and does not come up often in the many papers and reports on the aims of medicine. The committee goes on then to note that it does NOT accept 'in its full implication the oft reiterated view that the aim of the curriculum should be to produce a competent general practitioner'.[34]

Chapter 13 on the selection of medical students reviews the historical background and notes that as the number of applicants now exceeds places, and that there are no restrictions for social and economic reasons, something must be done. They agree that there are two obligations imposed on those who control choice of medical students. First, they must seek to secure those who will benefit from higher education, with a natural ability for medicine. Second, the community has a right to expect that the money it expends will receive the greatest benefit possible. They review all of the current issues associated with selection. They end up by suggesting that the best way is to interview by a committee to encourage a wide range of views, perhaps with a preliminary sifting related to intelligence testing. The key recommendation is that the committee review decisions at the end of the first and second years to see if they should continue, and allow members of the committee to compare their earlier assessment of the candidate with their performance.[35]

The review then goes into extensive detail on the curriculum and includes an important chapter on 'The Integration of Medicine' in which the case is made against compartmentalisation. Methods of teaching are described and there is a quotation from Professor Noah Morris: 'What is the ability to teach? Surely the best teacher is the individual who infects his or her students with the best habits of thoughts, the best technique and the best habits of life'.[36] The authors note that too often the ability to teach is not regarded by appointing bodies as a primary qualification in a teacher of medicine. They note that the 'chief should treat the student as a disciple and not merely as an attendant'. The chapter finishes by noting that preparation for teaching is lacking in universities, and comments: 'Few are born teachers; most would benefit from such a course. Efforts should be made to remedy this defect by providing suitable courses in association with university departments of education.'[37]

This is an impressive document in contrast to the GMC report of 1947, and it paved the way for further action.

THE PROFESSION RESPONDS

Following the GMC report of 1947, and on the basis of discussions at the time, the profession responded with a spate of articles in the *British Medical Journal* and *The Lancet*. One of the first of these was a leader in *The Lancet*, 'Ways of learning'.[38] This is an important article in that it records the opinions of students and staff on a variety of questions. Is the student's burden heavier that it used to be? Are the only facts which stick in the memory those which are learned by toil? Are films a valuable teaching method or a soporific? Have subsequent teachers improved on the methods of Socrates?

It is the responses which are interesting, and these come from staff and students.[39] There are positive responses to experience in social medicine and, indeed, to the role of film in education. It should be noted that these 'methods of imparting information are of the soporific type…and that nothing replaces adequate teaching at the bedside'. The responses support the importance of the student handling the case from the beginning, taking his own notes and seeing the case through to discharge.

As far as the burden of learning is concerned, one respondent notes that: 'I am always slightly sceptical about the alleged great need for lightening the student's burden. In my experience the good and indeed the average student takes the present burden in his stride without suffering any obvious detriment. The weak brothers are generally the most vocal in their protests, and their evidence is suspect'. Other quotes include:

I am afraid that I am rather disposed to take the view with some misgivings the so called modern methods of teaching. In fact my own method is probably the oldest of all, namely the Socratic method!

The most important of all teaching is that done at the bedside. The crowded state of our schools and the pressures of war time work has tended to make the classes so large that the intimate bedside teaching of former years has not been possible.

A systematic lecture course in all the main subjects has considerable value in spite of arguments to the contrary.

Recently in a class of twenty students only two knew how to perform the simple test for occult blood in the stools. The average student is becoming robot-minded. He sees specimens sent for laboratory examination, and radiograms taken and expects to get a diagnosis ground out from a clinical sausage machine.

The problem of the medical school now and always will be to find good teachers.

These are wonderful vignettes of medical education 60 years ago. Perhaps they should be repeated now.

Further examples can be found in the September 1949 issue of the *BMJ* in an article on 'Reform in medical education'[40] by W. Melville Arnott (William Withering professor of medicine, University of Birmingham), followed by one on the teaching of physiology by G.W. Pickering (professor of medicine, University of London).[41] Here are two very distinguished professors of medicine committing themselves in print to changing medical education.

Arnott, for example, notes the historical background and begins with a comment on the scientific method in medicine. There is then an interesting section on 'Faults of educational practice'. Then a useful comment on the selection of teachers, the characteristics of which are laid out in detail but with no comment on their preparation as teachers. The selection of student, he notes, 'is a highly controversial field'. The final sentence in this section is of interest: 'Students who show an outstandingly poor performance during the earlier years of the course should be discouraged from continuing. Britain is no longer wealthy in terms of either manpower or of treasure, and she can no longer afford the luxury of square pegs in round holes'. The possibility of integration of the curriculum is noted, and there is a comment on the place of surgery (from a professor of medicine). He notes that: 'However in my opinion the time has come for a real rapprochement between surgery and medicine. The community of work and interest is far greater than the divergence. The physician need not be a surgeon, but the surgeon needs to be a physician'. Lightening the burden on students is raised, as is the introduction of teaching in social medicine. He finishes by quoting Sir Thomas Lewis in his evidence to the Goodenough Committee when he said that medical teaching should:

> ...aim at sending the student forth with a well trained mind, familiar with and critical of sources of information, possessed of a sound knowledge and experience of all common disease and manifestation of disease—whether common or rare—that is clearly understood. Thus a substantial foundation will be laid upon which by building as he has been taught, his mind can become well stocked.[42]

Pickering highlights the distinction between education and instruction. He notes that in medicine, until recently, the instruction method has been the one used because of the historical background in medicine, the crowding of the curriculum and the small size of university staffs; all very familiar. Under the heading 'Techniques of education' he includes the lecture, the tutorial and the practical class. He urges that we do not forget the student, and while he considers the performance of the student during the year (continuous assessment) he doubts that we are in a position to do away with examinations.

In the 1950 volumes of the *BMJ* there is a series of articles on teaching and learning. First is an interesting article by J.A. Lauwerys, professor of comparative education in the University of London.[43] He discusses methods of teaching including a fascinating account of 'The Project'. This is one of the first references to problem-based or topic-based learning, and he refers to the French concept of a 'centre d'intérêt', where a topic is considered in an integrated problem-based way. He ends his paper with a section on the training of teachers, left to the last as being the most puzzling and difficult challenge of all.

He poses the question as to whether university teachers would profit from special training in methods of teaching and of education. He offers a few suggestions. The young teacher should have an experienced teacher attend his lectures and comment on them. Heads of departments should have staff meetings on educational issues and perhaps some weekend meetings on education. He notes that in his view it would be unwise to go further than this.

In the same issue of the *BMJ* there are papers on the 'Art of lecturing', 'Methods and men in the teaching of clinical medicine' by none other than Sir Henry Cohen. There is an interesting one on 'Some mechanical aids to instruction', which includes a discussion on the use of the blackboard, models, the epidiascope, lantern slides, motion pictures, tape and wire recorders and the new possibility of television. Finally, there is a fascinating article by a London medical student.[44] He asks three questions

+ What are we training for?
+ Do first things come first?
+ Where does the fault lie?

He is critical of many aspects of the process, including clinical attachments which he notes may have carried some responsibility in the past but are now a gigantic fraud. The ward visit is at its best superb—at its worst unbearable. A full dress systematic lecture is of little value. Routine bread and butter information which can be found in standard text books provides poor material for a 60 minute discourse. He fully supports the tutorial system. He does not believe we need full-time clinical teachers as many part-time consultants are excellent, and as long as there is a surfeit of registrars (doctors in training), there is little need to do more. He finishes with a note on the art of medicine:

Medicine is a great liberal profession not a trade, and one would have thought that some effort would be made to bring this home to medical students…the selection of students for character rather than brains would be a step in the right direction, but it is equally important that emphasis is placed throughout the course on those aspects of medicine which make it an art as well as a science.[45]

Listening to students and patients has real value.

The articles in *The Lancet* are just as interesting. For example, R. S. Aitken, Regius professor of medicine in the University of Aberdeen writes in 1945 on 'The teaching of medicine'.[46] He says that the aim of the teachers is three-fold: 'to help the student acquire some knowledge of human disease; to train him to think, so that he can apply knowledge to the cure and pre-vention of disease; and to initiate him into that intimate pers-onal relationship between doctor and patient which is peculiar to and indispensable to good medicine'. His next paragraph uses a wonderful set of phrases: 'The bare bones of knowledge are appallingly numerous, and they cannot like sagas be learned by rote'. He notes the Goodenough Report and emphasises the importance of psychological and social medicine.

The second article in this series is by W. H. Oglive, surgeon to Guy's Hospital, who writes on 'The education of the surgeon'.[47] He begins with a section on 'Finding the surgeon':

What is this man, the surgeon that we are educating? Is he born or made?…a first class surgeon must be a first class man, but a first class man will not necessarily make a first class surgeon. A preliminary selection is therefore advisable …in the English Fellowship this selection is performed by the primary examination.

Having found our man, how are we to make him a good surgeon? What is a good surgeon? I will have the temerity to quote myself: In judging a surgeon five aspects of his work at least must be considered. Knowledge of anatomy, physiol-ogy, pathology, surgical history, contemporary literature and the work of other surgeons; wisdom, that is clinical sense and sound judgement based on accumulated experience; originality, the power to build scattered observations into something new; ability to instruct by word of mouth and pen; and technical operative skill.

His comments on the acquisition of wisdom are fascinating:

Wisdom is acquired as far as it can be acquired by clinical study and discussion, by seeking out wise men, watching their methods, and listening to their comments. The teacher should never, figuratively at any rate, mount the platform. The six feet that separate the rostrum from the front bench are seldom spanned, but the barrier between experience and immaturity melts before personal contact. The relationship to be sought is not that between master and pupil but between master craftsman and apprentice.

Finally, his comments on the appointment to a senior surgical post:

The senior posts in the teaching hospital staff should not be subjected to change, but men need not be appointed to them until they are about 45. If the weaned registrars instead of being shaken off at the end of their appointment are placed at one of the hospitals in the group, invited to all conferences and discussions, given their share in a rota on clinical lectures and asked to assist in the teaching of such subjects as applied anatomy, if they are given a change of posting from time to time and allowed fallow periods for travel and study, a body of men will grow up around the parent school from whom the selection of senior teachers can be made with a knowledge of what they are rather than what they may be, and each will develop into the best type of surgeon that his natural gifts allow.

The Royal College of Physicians

Around this time the Royal College of Physicians was particularly active. The Gousltonian Lectures by Ellis (see later) were perhaps a stimulus. They produced two reports on the curriculum. The first of these was directed to the GMC who were considering changes to the curriculum. It covers the general areas described above but makes some interesting points. For example:

+ 'Compared to their forerunners many students now start medicine with less cultivated minds, and those who develop late or specialise late may not be able to start at all.'

+ 'Qualification no longer entitles the doctor to practise medicine, surgery and midwifery wherever he wishes and without supervision.'

+ The authors also note the importance of changes in practice, specialisation and in the patterns of disease.[48]

They conclude by noting that:

...the reforms needed to effect these changes can be determined only by experiment in medical schools, for which the current Recommendations of the General Medical Council allow little scope. If the Council saw fit to substitute for these detailed recommendations a broad statement of educational objectives they would give a valuable lead to the schools which would be encouraged to study their problems afresh. It is suggested that extended use of the General Medical Council powers of inspection, both of medical schools and examinations, would enable them to meet their statuary obligations without issuing instructions except on matters of "general importance" as defined by the Medical Acts Commission of 1881.

The second report of 1956[49] reiterates much of the 1955 report. As we shall see, the recommendations were taken up in the final report of the GMC in 1957.

AN AMERICAN INTERLUDE

In the 1940s and 1950s, there began a series of profound changes in medical education which came to have worldwide significance. The impact was considerable and is still ongoing. It is difficult to interpret the changes in the UK without a description of the process which occurred and its influence. Something special happened, and this is beautifully described in George Miller's book, *Educating Medical Teachers* (1980). He begins by making the obvious point that we do not prepare well for major life events like marriage and parenthood, and notes that: 'The task of medical teaching is accepted deliberately and dispassionately, yet the preparation for that influential role is equally frail'.[50]

The most exciting part of the process begins in Western Reserve University (now Case Western Reserve). This was the place which more than any other demonstrated the power of curriculum innovation.[51] Joseph Wearn was appointed dean in 1945 and inherited a school which was facing problems, its survival threatened. He set about the task of change and showed enormous enthusiasm and vision. He changed the organisation of the faculty into a place where all of the medical teachers were expected to be part of establishing and implementing educational policy. His own background supported the spirit of enquiry and the need for evidence, and his belief that the programmes should be student focused. This was the beginning of a revolution. It is a remarkable story and one with profound implications across the world. It was noted that similar approaches were being used at Harvard Medical School, Stanford, Albert Einstein College of Medicine and other institutions in the USA, England and Australia. A footnote to the article refers to changes at the University of Durham (Newcastle upon Tyne), and the author of the present volume has checked the changes in the course introduced in 1962 and they bear a strong resemblance to those in Western Reserve.[51]

The story of the revolution continues in Buffalo, New York, associated with other developments in Western Reserve,

Cornell and Colorado. Miller quotes Ward Darley, executive director of the Association of Medical Colleges: 'The first organised effort to study and evaluate the broad spectrum of teaching and learning processes in medicine was developed as the Project in Medical Education at the University of Buffalo in 1951'.[52] This was the culmination of many years of debate and discussion in the USA, which has been discussed earlier in this chapter. In Europe, the same issues were being considered but little done to change things. The mood at this time is well summed up by Slobody, professor of paediatrics at New York Medical College in 1950:

1. effective medical teaching has not been developed to its fullest extent

2. the principles of education have the same relationship to medical teaching as basic sciences have to clinical medicine

3. the proper application of the principles of education will improve medical training

4. medical colleges should make the basic principles of education an intergral part of the curriculum. Graduate courses leading to a master's degree in medical education should be available to prospective teachers.[53]

As always, it was people who changed things together with funding from a sympathetic and far-seeing Commonwealth Fund. Lester Evans, a paediatrician and an executive director of the fund and Edward Bridge, the dean, were the prime movers, and the concept of teachers and tutors meeting regularly became seminars in medical education. Encouragement from the dean was critical and the first year of the programme seemed to be a success. It was developed further in 1951–2. While other places had used a wide range of clinical experiences (for example in Case Western), the uniqueness of the Buffalo approach was in the seminars for tutors. Student participation in educational planning was encouraged. Interestingly, the next development was to bring into the programme a sociologist and anthropologist, Nathaniel Cantor, to lead the educational development, a move which was later described as 'An adventure in pedagogy'.[54] There was, of course, dissent and not everyone agreed that this was the right approach. Experiments were tried elsewhere but often were not successful because of the inability of the 'educationalist' to interact with the medical teachers. Activity and evaluation continued at Buffalo with positive outcomes such as:

+ heightened awareness of the general purposes of education

+ increasing awareness in appreciation of the role of basic scientists by clinical participants and vice versa

+ increased awareness of the complexity of formal education

+ recognition that knowledge of a subject is an essential but insufficient criterion for the preparation and identification of a good teacher.

These were very important conclusions in the 1950s. There were more issues in the development of medical teachers and a summer school was instituted. Links was made on a worldwide basis, and institutions positively continued to learn from each other.

The next stage was to export the concepts to other medical centres, or as Miller puts it 'initial colonisation'. Once again the Commonwealth Fund was asked to provide the crucial resource to enable this to happen but on this occasion they declined. However, they agreed that they could fund a consultant in another medical school and then see what happens. The Medical College of Virginia in Richmond was chosen for this purpose. The experiment worked well and demonstrated the viability of the concept—that of having an educational consultant in residence. The importance of student learning, as well as staff development, became increasingly recognised. As always, senior support for the initiative in the institution was crucial. The second outpost was Stanford University, and others followed.

The links to changes in the UK are many and some will be picked up later in this chapter. For example, the Royal College of Physicians Report on Medical Education was forthright: 'In the past ten years no country has produced so many wise Reports on the improvements on medical education, and no country has done so little about it'.[55] A key figure in the changes to be described was John Ellis (later Sir John), then a physician at the London Hospital and sub-dean of the London Hospital Medical School. With a Rockefeller Grant, he toured the leading centres in the USA and reported this in a Goulstonian Lecture to the Royal College of Physicians, and subsequently published. He notes in his conclusions that a way forward would be to: 'establish a means whereby it can be studied. Research is needed in three things—in learning, in teaching, and in the pattern of medical practice'.[56]

He wanted a national council or institute of medical education. His report influenced the 1957 GMC report, as we shall see, and resulted in the establishment of the Association for the Study of Medical Education (ASME) in 1956 and the establishment of the *British Journal of Medical Education* (now *Medical Education*)—once again, the power of an individual to change things and make things happen. These threads will be picked up later in the chapter.

Over the next ten years, the projects around learning and teaching in medicine grew and interesting maps of the dissemination of the new thinking have been produced.[57] A very large number of medical education and development units were set up across the USA and worldwide. New methods of teaching and evaluation flourished, and simulation techniques and problem-based learning were introduced. The World Health Organization became involved and produced a series of initiatives around preparation for teaching, and in particular in developing countries. Fellowship programmes were established to allow staff to visit and exchange experiences. They saw three levels of expertise: educational specialists, educational leaders and educational practitioners.

New medical schools were set up across the world and had the great advantage of being able to begin from scratch and set the curriculum and learning methods without the encumbrances of the past. There is a subsequent section which describes this in more detail but they included Ben Gurion University in the Negev Desert in Israel, the MacMaster Faculty of Medicine in Canada, The Maastricht school in the Netherlands, Xochimilcho Faculty in Mexico City and the University of Newcastle in Australia.

Before returning to the story in the UK it is worth returning to an almost final comment in Miller's book: '…what needs most to be acquired in medical school is not a vast body of knowledge, much of which will be outmoded by graduation, but a set of attitudes and values that will persist throughout a professional career'.[58]

He makes a plea at the end that medical schools should value their teachers and award them appropriately.

FIRST WORLD CONFERENCE ON MEDICAL EDUCATION, LONDON (1953)[59]

The first World Conference on Medical Education came at an important time. Things were beginning to change and the great and the good in medical education met for a week to discuss issues around four main themes.

1. Requirements for entry into medical schools

2. Aims and content of the medical curriculum

3. Techniques and methods of medical education.

4. Preventative and social medicine

In all, over 90 papers were given and the resultant volume is substantial and records the thinking on medical education in the middle of the 20th century. It would not be appropriate to summarise the whole volume but one or two points will be raised.

First, the challenges to medical education: Sir Lionel Whitby, Regius professor of physic at Cambridge and the conference president, set these out. They included the accumulation of medical knowledge, the kind of student who should enter medical school, the role of the teacher, and the curriculum itself. He also makes the point that social medicine is the main contact with the laity, as it covers that part of medicine which can be readily understood, and the execution of it, particularly the financial aspects lies, in their hands.

There is a very interesting chapter on the history of medical education which sets the scene for much subsequent discussion. In addition, there is a very useful introductory chapter entitled 'What is education?', which illustrates some of the philosophical background issues.

The section on the entry requirements to medical schools makes the familiar point that too many students apply and therefore, the need for selection. Academic qualifications are the obvious way, but there is a useful discussion on wider aspects of the individual's character and personality. It notes the obvious, but rather wasteful method of admitting everybody and failing a substantial number in the first or second years. It also makes the important point that entrants need more than a science background, and a knowledge and interest in the arts would be of value. This is refuted in several other sections of the volume. Finally, it notes that no method of selection is perfect!

There is a single chapter on 'Teaching the teachers'.[60] In it, the author argues for better preparation for teaching. This view is contradicted in several other chapters. For example, in a section on the aims of the medical curriculum, one very distinguished and senior academic contrasts teaching in schools and teaching in university. He states:

> ...whereas the former consists essentially of the presentation of a limited body of data to children and adolescents, the

proper task of the latter is surely to escort the student to the railhead, as it were, of knowledge and then leave him adequately equipped for further exploration. While the pedagogic facility is certainly an advantage, I maintain that it is a quite subsidiary qualification and not even essential in education at a university level.[61]

This debate continues and will be discussed again in subsequent sections.

Having a whole section on preventative and social medicine is a novel aspect of this conference. We have seen how the Goodenough Report emphasised its place, and the GMC's lukewarm response. Here is a full section which covers epidemiology, genetics, psychiatry, social environment, the home setting in medical education, occupational health, infant and child care, housing and nutrition. All in all a very impressive collection of speakers and papers.

In summary, this volume sets out where things were and the challenges to be faced, though it is interesting to note that there is no discussion on postgraduate or specialist medical education. At the start of the 21st century, many of the questions remain, debate about many of them is still fierce and solutions still elusive.

CHANGES IN MEDICAL EDUCATION

Sir John Ellis

The two articles cited earlier in *The Lancet* of 1956 were of particular importance. They followed a visit to the USA by Sir John Ellis and were delivered as the Goulstonian lectures before the Royal College of Physicians in 1956.[62] They were a major input into the 1957 GMC report. The purpose was to review the changes in medical education and to consider what further developments might be required.

Ellis begins with a consideration of the 'block' system by which medical education was divided into two blocks, essentially preclinical and clinical. His critique is that this does not deliver the curriculum in an integrated way, and he regards the second MB examination (the break between the two blocks) as one of the failures in the adaptation of medical education to changing circumstances. He refers to previous reports (all listed in this chapter) which have suggested change but which have not been taken up. In particular he refers to the introduction of the National Health Service (NHS) which has had mixed effects. There was a wish to ensure that teaching was continued and expanded but this had proved difficult financially. He also notes that as the NHS itself has expanded there has been a rise in specialisation which has had a compounding effect on teaching. As specialisation has developed, 'the student finds it more and more difficult to gain a sense of proportion' and has less responsibility.

Ellis also comments, with many others, that entrants to medicine have become more specialised, most only doing science subjects for entry. He argues for a balanced education. He produces a caricature of the student journey through medicine with frustration and lack of learning, and cramming facts for examination. It is a production line with no time to think. The educational potential of the pre-registration year recommended by Goodenough is applauded, though this could become another barrier. However, Ellis notes that the system is outworn and needs real change.

His visit to America stimulated his thinking, and he was impressed with the intense nature of the thinking on medical education, and with the number of fulltime appointments in the system. He recognises that the first objective is to define the aim of medical education. He quotes from Dr. Ham, who wrote the article on the Case Western experiment: 'The curriculum is the course through which the student travels; it is a definition of limitations as well as opportunities'. The building blocks are:

1. A statement of the aim—what we are trying to achieve in the period of undergraduate training.

2. A formulation of educational objectives—what kind of discipline we must teach to achieve it.

3. An analysis of the process of learning which the student should employ to master this discipline, together with the techniques of instruction.

4. The framing of an educational plan in which these processes and techniques are arranged at the most suitable stages of the student's development.

5. Implementation of this plan by translating the theoretical ideal into a feasible curriculum.

Ellis makes the point that it is now clear that the aim of medical education must be to give the student a foundation upon which he can later build a training for any branch of medicine. He gives three objectives:

1. To cultivate in the student the power of accurate observation.

2. To develop the power of logical thought.

3. To acquire empirical knowledge. Only with experience will the student develop clinical judgement.

His plan to achieve this in the curriculum is sequenced as follows:

1. The study of the normal.

2. The study of the causes and effects of variation from the normal.

3. A short introductory course in clinical method.

4. A period of practice of clinical method—a clerkship.

5. A stage of consolidation—designed to combine the study of special pathology and the systematic study of clinical medicine.

6. A stage of more experience mainly in the wards, by attachment to firms.

7. A stage of special outpatient teaching and of midwifery and paediatrics.

8. A stage of practice under supervision, both in the outpatient department and outside hospital.

9. A stage of responsible practice under supervision, i.e. the pre-registration appointments.

I suspect many courses were subsequently designed to this model.

It is of interest that in arguing for this plan, Ellis considers the alternative—that at Case Western—with the introduction of clinical teaching from the start. He does not think that 'this helps the student to acquire any better basis in clinical method and I think it may result in one not so good'. He does find merit in some aspects—the tutorial system, interdepartmental teaching and the ability to put an educational plan into effect—but overall he considers his plan superior.

The key issue is the method of reform, and Ellis argues that this is the role of the medical school through a curriculum planning committee. There is a need for freedom to experiment, and he argues that the GMC should give this freedom. The link with the NHS and the Department of Health are also of vital importance. He leaves to the end a critical reform:

The third step in the reform of medical education is, therefore, to establish a means whereby it can itself be studied. Research is essential in three things—in learning, in teaching, and in the pattern of medial practice. On the first two depends the future improvements in medical education On the last depends the nature of the work the students are eventually going to do. All three are the vital concern of the university medical schools. Their investigation requires a focus from which stimulation as well as correlation can come. A body capable of providing this focus must be found in the

> *form of either a national council or an institute of medical education. Here is the supreme opportunity for collaboration between the Royal Colleges and the medical faculties of the universities—a collaboration at the educational level which would inevitably form a basis for wider cooperation in all fields of medical practice.*[63]

From this the Association for the Study of Medical Education was formed.

General Medical Council: *Recommendations as to the Medical Curriculum* (1957)[64]

This report was quite different from the 1947 one. It is not apologetic, and its recommendations began a wave of change in medical schools. It makes the important point on page two that it was not until 1950 that the Council had the power to appoint visitors of medical schools to report as to 'the sufficiency of the instruction given to students'. This was a crucial concern of the 1947 report where they really had no power to intervene. It was clear that the Ellis Report on medical education, noted earlier, had an important influence on the recommendations.

It is interesting to note that the President's Address to the GMC on 26th November, 1946, contains details of the GMC visit to North America. It was paid for by the Nuffield Foundation and the Rockefeller Foundation, and included visits to New York, Cornell, Columbia, Chicago, Michigan, Toronto, McGill, Harvard and Johns Hopkins. This was at a time, as we have noted, of considerable excitement in medical education in North America. They acquired valuable information as to the requirements for medical practice, and the content and layout of the curriculum.

Following the 1947 report they carried out a great deal of work and in this had the full cooperation of medical schools. They recognised that one of the criticisms of the 1947 report was that its recommendations were too precise and detailed and did not allow scope for innovation and initiative. They recognised the congestion in the curriculum and the burden on students memorising factual information. The primary purpose of these recommendations was to reduce congestion.

For example, the minimum length of the whole period of training is specified but without guidelines on the time allotted to specific subjects, and no attempt is made to indicate precisely the scope of instruction in particular subjects. Visitations to medical schools were to be changed, with small groups visiting and looking at the curriculum as a whole.

Two key recommendations for professional education were: 'It is desirable that interdepartmental teaching should be encouraged throughout the whole period of professional study', and that 'the memorising and reproduction of factual data should not be allowed to interfere with the primary need for fostering the critical study of principles and the development of independent thought'.[65]

Many medical schools, including the new ones set up in the 1960s, took these recommendations to heart. For the new schools these will be discussed separately. In the case of the author of this book, he began his medical course in Glasgow in 1959, during which time the faculty and senate were actively discussing a new curriculum based on the GMC recommendations. This was completed in 1964, and having left medicine for two years to complete a science degree, the author returned to a new 'integrated curriculum'. This brought together in the clinical years a range of subjects, from basic to clinical, in a topic-based approach. The graduating class of 1967 did not realise at the time that they had been part of a much wider movement of reform and change.

Preventive medicine was discussed in the recommendations and was to be linked to local authorities and social welfare services.

The 1957 GMC report was short, only 15 pages, yet it had a real impact and illustrated what could be achieved when all worked together and Council took the lead.

Reports on universities

In the midst of these reports on medical education, two very important reports on university education appeared and were the subject of scrutiny. The first of these was the Hale Report on teaching in universities, and this is dealt with in detail in Chapter 14. The second was on higher education itself—the Robbins Report.

Higher Education Report: the Robbins Report (1963)[66]

This report set the direction for higher education for a generation. Its main conclusions were to create a number of new universities in the UK, to increase the status of institutions of advanced science and technology, and to suggest upgrading colleges and polytechnics to universities. In the process it covers a wide range of issues, some of which are relevant to the themes in this book.

The report begins with a redefinition of the aims of higher education. They include 'the instruction in skills suitable to play a part in the general division of labour'. The report makes no apology for this being first, not because they think it most important but because it is sometimes ignored and under-valued. Second, it makes the point that what is taught should be taught in such a way as to promote:

> *...the general powers of the mind. The aim should be to produce not mere specialists but rather cultivated men and women. And it is the distinguishing character of a healthy higher education that even when it is concerned with practical techniques it imparts them on a plane of generality that makes possible their application to many problems...[67]*

There follows a very important section on the selection of students, and the methods employed. It uses a now familiar mantra: 'In this field perfection is unattainable'. The authors comment favourably on the use of the school report, and then note that in the USA, universities like Harvard use additional tests (especially the Scholastic Aptitude Test) and recommend further work on this. These would not be to replace academic examinations but to supplement them.

The report comes out very positively in favour of integrating teaching and research: 'we are in total disagreement with the extreme view that would remove research altogether from universities and concentrate it in research institutes...It is the essence of Higher Education that it introduces students to a world of intellectual responsibility and intellectual discovery in which they are to play their part'.[68]

The authors then consider methods of teaching, and they describe the range available. However, their most interesting comments are on whether or not every university teacher should have a period of instruction in teaching techniques before he takes up his duties. Following a survey of teachers themselves (the majority of whom thought it desirable), they recommend that 'all newly appointed junior teachers should have organised opportunity to acquaint themselves with the techniques both of lecturing and of conducting small group discussions'.[69] This is an important conclusion, and as we shall see later it was acted on, albeit slowly and in a piecemeal fashion.

The recommendations in this report were profound and had a wide impact across the sector, including in medical education.

Royal Commission on Medical Education: the Todd Report (1965–68)[70]

This was one of the most significant reports in the history of medical education, though its recommendations were hardly acted upon at the time. However, now almost 40 years later and through a range of other reports, the Todd recommendations have almost all been enacted. This illustrates one of the most interesting aspects of the history of medical education—the up-take time for new ideas. We have seen in the 19th century the machinations around the establishment of the General Medical Council, and in the Todd Report we see the concept of specialist registration being advocated, being ignored and then through a series of other mechanisms being eventually introduced. These subsequent reports will be discussed shortly. It is interesting to note that the author of this book recently came across a letter, received in 1966, from ASME and NFER asking students to fill in a questionnaire for the Commission, giving the student view of medical education.

The report begins by setting the scene in the UK from an historical perspective, and in paragraph 4 makes the following statement:

> *We have had to accept, for our purposes, the virtual absence of systematic factual information about the practical processes of medical teaching in Britain and their effectiveness; we have recommended that provision be made for proper study of the aims and methods of medical teachers, as part of a substantial research effort in medical education in coming years.* [71]

This was a significant indictment of the lack of research and investigation of medical education in the UK. The report then covers a wide range of issues. It makes the important point that:

> *...the aim of the undergraduate course should be to produce not a finished doctor but a broadly educated man who can become a doctor by further training. We are convinced that undergraduate medical education should be firmly in the hands of a university and that a university degree course should be a requirement for the entry of British students to the medical profession.* [72]

From a postgraduate perspective, the report notes the establishment in 1967 of a Central Committee for Postgraduate Medical Education and welcomes it. In this context it sets out a proposed plan for postgraduate education. It should comprise: an intern year, general professional training, further professional training, and continuing education and training. These were radical suggestions at the time: a planned programme leading to a consultant post with a continuing process of education. The process would create 'junior specialists and then specialists' when they might be considered for a consultant appointment. A new grade of 'hospital specialist' would be established.

The authors noted also that some witnesses suggested that continuing professional education should be compulsory for all doctors in the NHS. They note that 'even if we thought such compulsion desirable in principle (which we do not) we could not define criteria which covered all forms of continuing education'.

From an administrative point of view, they recommended that there should be a central body known as the 'Central Council for Postgraduate Medical Training in Great Britain' responsible for the general oversight of postgraduate education and training. It would work through regional organisations and supervise arrangements for education.

Crucially, they recommended that the GMC should assume a function in postgraduate education similar to that it discharges in undergraduate education. 'The Council should specify in broad terms, and constantly keep under review, the professional training, experience and qualifications necessary to achieve recognised competence to exercise independent clinical judgement in a specialty and should keep a register of those who have been judged to have reached the required standard'.[73] It would do this in association with the appropriate professional bodies. This aspect caused much discussion and it was to be 30 years before a specialty register was established.

The undergraduate medical course was considered in detail. It notes that the basic attraction of medicine for the young is the opportunity it offers him of serving humanity in any one of many ways, for example, by helping the sick or infirm, in advancing medical science by research, or by improving the organisation of medical care. The fundamental problem is to devise a course which achieves these aspirations. The authors emphasise that the course should be primarily educational. The aim of medical education should be:

1. To produce, on graduation, a person with a knowledge of the medical and behavioural sciences sufficient for him to understand the scientific basis of his profession and to permit him to go forward as medicine develops.

2. To provide a general introduction to clinical method and patient care in the main branches of medicine and surgery, together with an introduction to social and preventive medicine. It should be taught in a way which will inculcate a desire to continue learning.[74]

The report then covers the structure of the curriculum and the length of the course in more detail.

Interestingly, it refers to the work in Western Reserve University on integrated medical courses, and the work done in several UK medical schools. Small-group teaching and clinical clerking are noted and there is special mention of elective periods of study. It recognises that this is not a new proposal, but mentions that it is often placed close to examinations, diminishing its value.

The section on the selection of medical students begins with the sentence: 'We have found dissatisfaction in many quarters with the basis on which applicants are selected for admission to the undergraduate medical course'. Not much has changed then. It further comments: 'There will always be differences of view on such matters and we think there can be no possibility of reaching even a broad measure of agreement until a means has been found of relating the characteristics of the candidate to his eventual professional performance'.[75] They recommend more research.

There follows a significant discussion on the need for more medical places, recommending that existing schools increase their number of students and that several new medical schools be created. These new schools had an opportunity to put into practice the lessons from the past, and in a subsequent section this will be considered in more detail.

The Todd Report runs to over 400 pages. It took 3 years to complete, and the Commission held over 100 meetings and obtained evidence from a wide group of individuals and organisations. The Commission was composed of some of the most distinguished medical leaders of the middle of the 20th century, including Sir John Ellis who drafted much of the report. Yet its recommendations were only implemented in a limited way. Now, at the beginning of the 21st century, some 35 years later, most have been enacted.

New medical schools and changes in the old

The 1960s and 1970s saw the development of several new medical schools and modifications in existing ones. For example, the University of Newcastle (1963) and the University of Dundee (1967) were established and separated from the parent universities of Durham and St Andrews.

Existing medical schools refashioned their curricula in the light of the GMC report of 1957 and during the discussions of the Todd Report. Some of these changes flowed directly from the changes occurring in North America. For example, the curricula in Glasgow and Newcastle (Durham) medical schools changed significantly. In Glasgow, a curriculum committee was set up after the 1957 GMC report and over the next few years refashioned the course. Sir Charles Illingworth, professor of surgery, convened the group and the outcome was an integrated curriculum with topic teaching, phrases which will recur several times in this section. The curriculum was introduced in 1961 and the faculty papers make reference to the changes in medical education occurring in the UK and in North America. Sir Andrew Watt Kay took over from Sir Charles Illingworth in 1964 and, as we will see, chaired the advisory group in Leicester and gave advice to Nottingham. Therefore, these changes had an impact on the development of several new medical schools in the UK.

One of the new schools was at the University of Southampton, where the foundation dean was Professor Donald Acheson (later Sir Donald). His background in epidemiology and community medicine gave this school a community flavour in its first successful years.

A second school was set up at the University of Leicester, chaired by Sir Andrew Watt Kay, a member of the Todd Report and professor of surgery at Glasgow. The new curriculum (personal communication, Professor Ken Wood) was to be flexible and based on an integration between the basic sciences and clinical medicine. It would be 'topic' based, very much like the Glasgow course. The first intake was to be in 1975.

A third new medical school was to be in Nottingham. The composition of the advisory group was simply a list of the great and good in medicine in the UK. The final report of the group was produced in 1965 and the first intake was to be in 1970. The curriculum would encourage curiosity in the learner and avoid the defects of curricula elsewhere by taking steps to avoid overcrowding of information, lack of integration between subjects, and too many examinations. An interdepartmental committee would be drafted to plan the curriculum, and 'the droit de seigneur' by which a professor claims and is conceded a permanent quota of a student's time was not to be tolerated. The curriculum would be topic-based and flexible. The advisory group took advice from a wide range of institutions, including Aberdeen, Glasgow, Newcastle, Harvard, Rochester, Stanford and Western Reserve, Duke and Auckland.

The relationship between these new medical schools and existing ones worldwide was thus clearly established, and the new curricula were based on the concepts of integration, topic teaching and flexibility.

Report on the Responsibilities of the Consultant Grade (1969)[76]

This report produced by Sir George Godber, the then chief medical officer (CMO) at the Department of Health, is an interesting one. Sir George was one of the most respected

CMOs, with very significant standing and long experience. The document, which was in part a response to the Todd Report, criticised the lack of planning in postgraduate training and the difficulties with career planning when each consultant was supported by a sizable group of junior staff. This could result in the exploitation of junior doctors, who were virtually un-appointed consultants or were forced to transfer to a junior level in another specialty. The author of the present text, who was a surgical trainee in 1969, remembers this period well: few job opportunities, time expired and very experienced senior registrars with little hope of promotion. Sir George's solution was to propose specialist registration and a proper career structure. In evidence given later to the Short Report on medical education in 1981, he noted that the report failed totally in its purpose. However, it did open up a dialogue between the Department of Health and the professional bodies.

Report on the Committee of Inquiry into the Regulation of the Medical Profession: The Merrison Report (1975)[77]

The genesis of this report is in itself interesting. The commission was set up after a long dispute within the medical profession about how it should be regulated. The dispute had come to a head with the introduction by the GMC of an annual fee for the retention of a doctor's name on the medical register, rather than a once-only fee. This was felt unjust. To precipitate a crisis, they refused to pay the fee and the GMC threaten to remove them from the Register. At this point the secretary of state for social services intervened and the commission was set up, averting the crisis.

The review begins by considering the basis of the power of the GMC and its stewardship of the Register. Registration is founded on a standard of competence, and the GMC needed to specify this and take action to ensure that this was the case. Thus, the GMC must recognise a certain standard of education and define the course of undergraduate medical instruction required to attain that standard. The report recognises that such an organisation as the GMC must be independent of the providers of health services and ought not to be a creature of government.

The commission's broad conclusion was to reform the GMC and to change its composition and structure. It also proposed new areas of **responsibility**, and in particular to include a role in postgraduate education. This was a new role but in line with thinking in the Todd and Godber reports. Thus, the GMC was to be given powers over all aspects of medical education: basic, general and specialist. It was to oversee the 'coordination of all stages of medical education'. This was a very significant change. It also recommended that the GMC should be involved in educational research, and perhaps undertake studies of such subjects as methods of assessment of the student.

Specialist education was to complete the education of the doctor, providing the skills and knowledge of particular disciplines. The details (because they vary from specialty to specialty) needed to be determined by the specialty itself. General practice was also considered in a similar way.

The commission notes that:

> ...our establishment as a Commission may be said to have resulted partly from suspicion of the GMC's plans for the organisation of specialist education following the report of the Royal Commission on Medical Education. It soon became clear to us that a large part of the difficulty that had arisen over the GMC's plans for the organisation of specialist education arose because of widespread misunderstanding of the relationship between education and registration.[78]

The registering body must control standards, but other bodies may (as in undergraduate education) also be involved in its delivery.

Not content with this radical view, the commission also looked at re-licensing, a subject which, it notes, reflects a 'growing interest in this country in schemes of tying continued registration to periodic test of competence'. Although they were impressed with evidence from abroad, they did not feel able to recommend the introduction of any scheme of relicensure. That would have to wait for another two decades.

The Merrison Report was of great significance to the medical profession. It changed the structure and organisation of the GMC and sent out important messages on specialist education. These were followed up over the next few decades.

Competence to Practice: the report of a Committee of Enquiry set up for the medical profession in the United Kingdom: The Alment Report (1976)[79]

This committee, chaired by E. A. J. Alment, was set up by the British Medical Association and the medical Royal Colleges to be widely representative of the medical profession. Its remit was to review 'the present methods of ensuring the maintenance of standards of continuing competence to practise and of clinical care of patients and to make recommendations'. Its significance is that the report was published so shortly after the Merrison Report and is, to some extent, a commentary on it.

The report defines a competent doctor as 'one who brings to bear upon his medical work a reasonable level of knowledge and understanding of the nature of his task, and exercises appropriate skill in the practice of his profession'.[80] The committee agrees that basic medical education should be generic to all doctors, with no specialisation at this stage.

However, the report then makes a very fundamental point which differs significantly from Merrison, Todd and Godber. It states that

> ...if the objective of medical education is to teach the sciences basic to medicine, together with a comprehensive understanding of clinical method and the development of clinical judgement to it, then recognition of a doctor's competence to practise medicine after he has completed such education satisfactorily should be a once and for all matter, lost

only through deterioration of mind or body by age or illness. These views we share, and we believe they are also upheld by the universities. This concept of education is fundamental to the relationship between education and the licence to practise.[81]

The committee also make an interesting further comment on Merrison, finding the term 'highest level of clinical responsibility' inconsistent with Merrison's view of specialist education as a continuing process. 'The doctor may have reached a stage beyond which he is no longer required by any statuory other regulation to refer to another on the clinical decisions that he takes, but educationally he will continue to learn from his own experiences and from that of his colleagues'.

Standards of clinical training will be drawn up by specialty based committees, the joint higher training committees. It makes the point that although the doctor is not subject to further formal examinations, his progress is reported to the committee. Further it notes that: 'In the United Kingdom, however, appointment to a consultant post is not necessarily the consequence of having reached specialist status in the educational sense'. Relicensure is dealt with quickly: 'There is as yet no evidence to justify relicensure, not because there is no evidence that doctors fail in their competence in certain respects and that this can be detected, but rather because a system of licensing for all could not be based on measurements satisfactory enough to justify it'.[82]

This report thus gives a good picture of professional views some years after the Todd Report and shortly after Merrison. There seemed little appetite for change.

Medical Education: Fourth Report from the Social Services Committee: The Short Report (1981)[83]

This report was drawn up to consider the number of doctors required and the career structure in hospitals. The problem was a now familiar one. How many doctors do we need and what should the career structure be? The problems of poor working conditions of junior doctors, short-term contracts and poor career prospects were all raised. The report begins with an analysis of medical workforce planning numbers, and then has a most useful section on history and background, from Goodenough to Merrison, and all in between. It reviews background documents on planning reviews from all quarters. It covers service requirements and makes a fundamental point in considering that a much higher proportion of patient care than at present should be provided by fully trained medical staff. From this it followed that there should be an increase in consultants and a decrease in the number of junior doctors, but the report does not advocate a subconsultant grade. It also does not call for an increase in medical student numbers, but does recommend that medical schools should consider more mature students for entry.

More significantly, the committee strongly advocated that specialist training in all fields should take the form of planned programmes which include experience in both teaching and non-teaching hospitals. The GMC was again to be the coordinating point for postgraduate medical education. The report makes no formal comment on specialist registration but records that Todd, Merrison and Godber had all recommended it. However, it states: 'the Royal Colleges who held responsibility for approving postgraduate clinical training programmes have not adopted this suggestion'.[84]

It is over twenty years since this report was written. Again, much has changed but the process has been slow with much compromise on the way.

EXTERNAL PERCEPTIONS OF MEDICINE

Over the period 1950 to 1980, several very influential books appeared which had a profound effect on the profession and as a consequence on medical education. They were all based on the concept that medicine had gone wrong, that it was not serving the public and that unless it changed it would lose all influence. These books were of considerable importance, and having re-read then, it is not difficult to see why. At the time there was annoyance and concern by the profession and, indeed, by the author of this volume, who was indignant that others could write in this way. How dare they! What did they know about medicine! As it happens, quite a lot. But what made these works so effective was the ability of the writers to see the medical profession through different eyes.

The first worth mention is *Mirage of Health* by Rene Dubos, published in 1959. It set out the arguments that health was one component of human happiness, and that the search for perfect health for every one was likely to be futile. He makes the important comment that 'it is not the function of medicine to become identified with political action'.[85] Medical training does not impart that kind of wisdom. This view might be questioned and will be picked up later in this book. In his conclusions he writes:

> *Men naturally desire health and happiness. For some of them, perhaps for all, these words have implications that transcend ordinary biological concepts. The kind of health that men desire is not necessarily a state in which they experience physical vigour and a sense of well being, not even one giving them long life. It is instead the condition best suited to reach goals that each individual formulates for himself.*[86]

The issue of quality of life clearly is defined. He describes others' views of health. For example, Aristotle said: 'The nature of man is not what he is born as, but what he is born for'. Katherine Mansfield wrote as she was dying: 'Work is more important than life', and 'By health I mean the power to live a full, adult, living, breathing life in close contact with what I love—the earth and the wonders thereof—the sea, the sun. I want to be all that I am capable of becoming'.[87]

Dubos clearly feels that medicine can contribute only a part of such a sentiment, and cannot by itself remove all pain and suffering. There are other dimensions which are important, including the spiritual one.

The second book is *Medical Nemesis: The Expropriation of Health*, written by Ivan Illich in 1975. The book has as its opening sentence: 'The medical establishment has become a major threat to health'.[88] He describes the process of medicalisation of life, a process by which the doctor has taken control of health and by which a physician-based healthcare system has grown beyond its bounds. In a chapter entitled 'The epidemic of modern medicine', he describes the expanding proportion of new disease burden which is in itself the result of medical intervention, and that medicine has not changed life expectancy. Doctors' effectiveness is in fact an illusion. He continues with a discussion on useless medical treatment, doctor inflicted injuries and defenceless patients. He uses the term 'nemesis' to represent the divine vengeance visited on mortals who infringe the prerogatives of the gods. Nemesis is the inevitable punishment for inhuman attempts to be a hero rather than a human being. The book is uncomfortable reading, and at the time represented an important view. It might be useful to go through his list of examples, now 30 years on, and see if things have changed.

The third book is by Thomas McKeown and was published in 1979. *The Role of Medicine: Drama, Mirage or Nemesis?* picks up the themes of the other two books and provides much substance to support them. The book is full of charts and figures, and is all the more powerful as the author was a distinguished epidemiologist. As with the other books, he concludes that 'the contribution of clinical medicine to the prevention of death and increase in expectation of life in the past three centuries was smaller that that of other influences'.[89] He questions the role of medicine, but of particular interest (to this book) is the chapter on medical education. In it he begins by stating that the aims of medical education should be broader than they are at present. His case for wider aims is based on several factors:

+ Other influences on health—social, behavioural environmental, nutritional, etc.

+ An extended concept of health care. Diagnosis and treatment should not be the only function. This neglects other aspects of care, such as the mentally ill and those with chronic disease. The interests should extend to non-personal aspects of health, and if so medical education will have to change.

+ Selection of medical students. He makes the point that there is no reason to doubt that applicants are motivated and that they have high intellectual abilities. However, they enter medicine with predominant notions of diagnosis and treatment that most patients are cured, and that health depends on medical intervention. He makes a key point when he writes:

I do not think that the difficulty of training doctors to meet the needs of society arises because the wrong people are chosen... The failures to enlarge the concept of the medical task are usually due to subsequent training, to what they see and hear during years in a medical school and teaching hospital. The important influences are the medical curriculum and the image of medicine projected at the teaching hospital.[90]

This is such an important statement and reflects views going back centuries of the hidden agenda in medicine and the need to change the nature of the teacher as much as the teaching.

The fourth book is *The Unmasking of Medicine*, by Ian Kennedy and published in 1981 following his Reith Lectures. This is a powerful book, critical of medicine and its structures. His aim 'is to expose and then examine the real face of medicine'.[91] He makes it clear at the outset that one of his targets is the power of the doctors and the profession. He describes the social institution which has grown up around doctors, and how the treatment of illness is for doctors and them alone since only they have the competence. He goes further: 'to embrace a notion of health which calls for positive political action and the creation of appropriate economic conditions is to concede that "health" is fundamentally a political term. Most doctors are unwilling to do this'. He is scathing about the values of modern medicine: 'The earlier Hippocratic tradition of concern for the whole person in his environment…has been ousted by the post Renaissance view that illness is a mechanical failure'.[92] He also notes that: '…by thinking in terms of disease, we have been led to believe that diagnosis leads to cure. This, sadly, is far from accurate. There is little to be gained by labelling if not much can be done once the label has been arrived at'.[93] He makes it clear that modern medicine has taken the wrong path. It is too scientific in its teaching and practice, and 'it may not produce what is so often needed: someone who can care'.[94] It is hospital-based rather than considering preventative measures.

Taking and making decisions, Kennedy argues, are not just medical tasks. Many of them, he contends, are not technical, but ethical and moral. Such decisions are not the province of one group (doctors) but of society as a whole. Doctors are not uniquely competent to make ethical decisions. Such big decisions as who lives or dies are too big for doctors to decide on. He argues for more learning by doctors on ethical analysis. In his view (in 1981), the GMC is concerned largely with etiquette rather than competence. He makes the point that 'the medical profession can never be expected to become the champion of the consumer's cause. When such measures as self audit are met with hostile rejection, it is clear that other approaches from the consumer are called for. The profession is not going to help'.[95] In his conclusion he suggests a new relationship between doctor and patient, and that the power of the doctor is to be challenged, and the balance of power redressed.

This is a powerful book—even reading it again after 25 years. Much has changed, and much written at the time has challenged doctors to think about how medicine should be practised. The relationship between patient and doctor is a fundamental one, and one which will be discussed later in this book.

These four books, and others such as Henry Miller's *Medicine and Society*, acted as a backdrop to the changes being made in medical education. Miller's book has a section on medical teaching and he refers to the 'crisis in medical education'.[96] Written in 1973, it notes the changes in the previous 25 years, and the conflict between learning the science and cultivating the personal and human qualities required of the doctor. He notes the changes in the USA and, in particular, those at Western Reserve and the need to think beyond the teaching hospital into learning medicine in the community.

From the perspective of the 21st century, 20–40 years later, has much changed? Has the curriculum been modified? Has medicine learnt its lessons? There has been much change, some of it to be described later in this book. But much more has still to be done, and in the themes developed from the historical survey some pointers to the future will be set out in Chapter 10.

THE EDINBURGH DECLARATION 1988[97]

This was drawn up at the World Conference on Medical Education in Edinburgh in 1988. It contains twelve points which reflect many of the current issues, but a few particularly interesting ones. For example:

+ Ensure the curriculum content reflects national health priorities.

+ Train teachers as educators, not solely as experts in content.

+ Complement instruction about management of patients with increased emphasis on promotion of health and prevention of disease.

It finishes with a flourish:

By this declaration we pledge ourselves and call on others to join us in a sustained and organised programme to alter the character of medical education so that it truly meets the defined needs of the society in which it is situated. We also pledge ourselves to create the organisational framework required for these solemn words to be translated into sustained and effective action. The stage is set; the time for action is upon us.

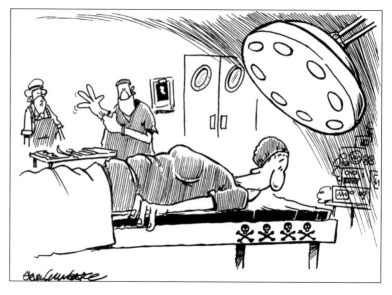

A cartoon in response to the publication of mortality statistics in Scotland. The patient is given a visible reminder of the competencies of the doctor written on the operating table. By permission of Stephen Camley, published in the *Glasgow Herald*.

CHANGES IN THE EDUCATIONAL PROCESS

Over the period 1950–90 there were major changes in the learning process. These included the use of different methods of teaching, such as problem-based learning, simulated patients, special study modules, etc. These are dealt with in more detail in Chapter 10.

Ethical issues

Ethical issues have been part of medical practice since the time of Hippocrates and now the emphasis is even greater; there was a notable report on the subject in 1988, the Pond Report. It begins with the obvious point:

> *It is often claimed that medical ethics cannot be taught. Competence and compassion, it is argued, are acquired by experience or "osmosis", while the moral views of individuals differ and ultimately are a personal matter.*[98]

It then raises the question as to whether or not this is true, and asks if there is a place in medical education for ethics as a subject. The report then sets out how such a subject might be part of the medical curriculum. It defines the two meanings of medical ethics. The first relates to standards of professional competence and conduct. The second refers to the study of ethical or moral problems raised by medical practice. It is this second meaning which began to receive more prominence, and included not only patient issues but those related to public health. One key part of the learning was to allow:

> *...greater awareness and understanding, on the part of doctors, of their own and others' moral thinking, and thus have an important part to play in facilitating better communication, not only between doctors and patients, and doctors and other health professionals, but also amongst doctors themselves.*[99]

Of particular interest for this volume was that they reviewed existing practice in medical schools in the UK by writing to all the deans. The replies showed significant variation, and that overall the total number of timetabled hours was not large.

Ethics teaching was encouraged, particularly in obstetrics, general practice and community medicine, and in a few schools short ethics courses had been introduced. Very few medical teachers appear to have had any specific training in medical ethics.

The report made a number of recommendations. In summary:

+ medical ethics teaching should be taught at regular intervals throughout the course

+ clinical teaching should normally begin from clinical examples and small group discussion should be emphasised

+ interested teachers should be encouraged to undertake further study

+ multidisciplinary teaching should be encouraged

+ care should be taken to ensure that teaching was not being undertaken by persons who held particular views and promote a personal agenda

+ examinations should reflect an interest in ethics

+ elective courses should be arranged for interested students.[100]

Following the Pond Report, the GMC paper *Tomorrow's Doctors* published in 1993[101] made an explicit statement on the role of ethics and noted that teaching in this subject should be developed: 'Ethical and legal issues relevant to the practice of medicine' together with 'our awareness of the moral and ethical responsibilities involved in individual patient care and the provision of care to populations of patients'.

In 1998 the UK consensus statement was published and set out a core curriculum.[102] The core content included informed consent and refusal of treatment, the clinical relationship, confidentiality, medical research, human reproduction, the new genetics, children, mental disorders and disabilities, life, death, dying and killing, vulnerability of doctors, resource allocation and rights.

This has recently been evaluated[103] and indicates that while progress has been made there is a need for further investigation of the subject across the curriculum, with improved methods of learning and assessment. There is a particular issue about teaching of the theoretical base. The most important issue is the need for capacity, capability and leadership in facilitating learning.

Such recommendations have been a valuable spur to improving the learning experience of students. Since that report there have been numerous papers on the methods and resources available for the teaching of medical ethics (see Bibliography). It has also been suggested that there might be value in taking an ethics history as part of the consultation process.[104]

Arts and humanities

In a similar and related way to ethics, there has been an increasing interest in the arts and humanities in health and medicine. While this is not a new issue, the interest derives from a feeling that scientific eyes may not be the only way to look at health and illness. So why might we be interested?

First, the use of the arts and humanities allows us to consider people as whole individuals, whole communities, and in particular, issues around quality of life. The range is con-siderable. It includes literature, philosophy, music, the visual arts, theatre, arts in the community, and many other subjects.

The philosophical interest has, of course, been very long standing and includes ethical issues and the dilemmas faced by doctors. However, it is broader than this, and an interest in philosophy or the humanities allows us to analyse problems, to consider arguments, and to be clear about how we feel, how we know and how we might act.[105] An exposure to the humanities also allows us to understand how others might feel, and helps us to see problems from their perspectives. Up until the last 50 years or so, it would have been expected that most people coming into medicine would have had an arts degree or some background in philosophy, logic and rhetoric. As this is no longer the case, there has been an increasing discussion on how such a background might assist in improving patient care.

The major themes in relation to the arts and health are concerned with their possible value in professional education, in therapy and in community well-being. The evidence is slowly building up that the arts do change these aspects of the doctor's work, but more needs to be accumulated. Over the last few years there has been a spate of conferences, papers, seminars and debates on such subjects, and centres for the study of arts and humanities in health and medicine are developing across the world (see Bibliography).

For example, there is increasing interest in the use of literature in medical education. This can range from short stories, poetry, novels, whether or not they have a direct link to clinical practice. Indeed, studies with students have shown that they prefer 'serious' literature rather than those only related to doctors and clinical practice.[106] For example, books such as *Trainspotting* by Irvine Welsh, or Roddy Doyle's *The Woman Who Walked into Doors*, *Saturday* by Ian McEwan, all illustrate a range of health problems, including domestic violence and neurological disorder, which are dealt with from the point of view of the writer, rather than the physician. This alternative perspective gives added power, and such books have the potential to make the student or the doctor think differently about how they work, and how they act. The portrayal of illness is another aspect of such novels, particularly chronic disease and in some instances psychiatric illness. Such works add a different dimension to medical education.

For this reason, the collection of a library by individual doctors has always been part of medical education. While medical books tend to dominate such collections, most of the great libraries of physicians in the past have covered a very wide range of subjects and indicated a degree of learning and erudition well beyond medicine. The use of books is critical, as the following two quotations suggest:

To study the phenomena of disease without books is to sail an uncharted sea. While to study books without patients is never to go to sea at all. [107]

Sir William Osler

Medicine is my lawful wife but literature is my mistress. When I am bored with one I spend a night with the other. [108]

Anton Chekhov

The arts are increasingly seen as part of professional and, in particular, medical education. Courses, seminars and discussions occur with increasing frequency, and the bright, intelligent, fact-filled medical student finds such events a wonderful release—to think of life, quality of life and clinical issues in a different way. They stimulate imagination, curiosity and creativity; all things which are central to the role and aim of the doctor, and of medicine.

O'Donnell has suggested in a provocative article that doctors act as performance artists in that they have to take on many different parts in the course of a professional career. [109] The commonest of these is the 'bedside manner', which can be switched on at will. He argues against simple checklists of 'communication skills', and that most doctors find these obvious and would like to move beyond them to a greater understanding of themselves through the arts and humanities.

Increasingly, as hospitals are being built and developed (or redeveloped), the place of art has grown in importance. A wide range of new buildings incorporate sculpture, paintings and the visual arts, and events such as poetry readings, music and theatre take place within the hospital setting. They add a different dimension for those in hospital who may be suffering from a variety of illnesses and who can see music and art as a further facet to their lives. These projects are now being evaluated across the world, and there is the beginning of an evidence base which suggests that they make the environment more comfortable, more human, and thus enriched.

Art therapy is also playing an increasing role. This may range from painting and music, to movement and dance. Each of these can contribute to quality of life of the individual patient and provide a release from pain and sickness, and allow, in spite of physical illness, a creative spirit to take over. The importance of being able to continue to think and create is an extraordinarily powerful one in the midst of illness.

In a similar way there is increasing use of art in the community. Public sculpture, displays, theatre and music all add to the concept of a community, and they help to create that community and build it into something richer and more cohesive. Such projects can range from large public sculptures through to lantern displays and other art and craft-related activities.

Humour also plays a substantial part in improving the quality of life.[110] This may be through films, videos, books or cartoons, all of which have known effects on blood pressure, hormone release, immunity and a general feeling of well being. Perhaps we should use humour more frequently in clinical practice.

Changes in the diagnostic process have also had effects an patients. In Thomas Mann's *Magic Mountain* there is an important reflection by one of the main characters (Hans Castrop) when he sees his X-rays.

Hans Castrop saw exactly what he should have expected to see, but which no man was ever intended to see and which he himself had never presumed he would be able to see: he saw his own grave. Under that light, he saw the process of corruption anticipated, saw the flesh in which he moved decomposed, expunged, dissolved into airy nothingness— and inside was the delicately turned skeleton of his right hand and around the last joint of the ring finger, dangling black and loose, the signet ring his grandfather had bequeathed him… With the eyes of this Tienappel forebear…he beheld a familiar part of his body, and for the first time in his life he understood that he would die.[111]

The arts are also particularly important for a number of specific groups, including the disabled and those with mental health problems. The roles of dance, theatre and drama, and painting, either by the patient or by those caring for them, illustrate and illuminate difficulties in everyday living, and help others to understand and deal with them.

Emphasis has been made on the importance of quality of life. The following quotation from Oliver Wendell Holmes in *The Professor at the Breakfast Table* expresses this very clearly:

The longer I live the more I am satisfied of two things. First, that the truest lives are those that are cut rose-diamond fashion, with many facets. Second, that society in one way or another is always trying to grind us down to a single flat surface.[112]

This quotation from a distinguished American physician illustrates an important point: patients are not flat surfaces associated with single physical diseases. They are whole people with feelings, thoughts and anxieties. The arts may give us an additional way into helping to improve the quality of life of those we look after.

POSTGRADUATE AND SPECIALIST EDUCATION

Postgraduate and specialist education has always been part of the training process, and in general the medical Royal Colleges and the universities have provided such programmes through the award of specialist diplomas and degrees. This has been supplemented by short courses and opportunities for continuing professional development. However, until relatively recently, this was not a formal programme and there were no national mechanisms for approval of specialty training.

The first important initiative was the introduction of the mandatory pre-registration year recommended in the Goodenough Report of 1944, and implemented in 1951. The second initiative occurred in 1961 at a conference called in Christchurch College in Oxford and organised by the Nuffield Provincial Hospitals Trust.[113] It was an astonishing success, occurring as it did in the midst of changes in the NHS and some professional unrest. Those who attended (again, a list of the great and the good) returned home and set about developing postgraduate centres and an organisation to deliver programmes of education for those in training. By the late 1960s, most were established and John Lister writing in the BMJ could report on the number of centres, regional organisations, tutors and programmes up and running.[114] There were of course problems, money and people being the main ones, but it was an amazing success.[115] In 1986 there were several celebrations and publications to celebrate the 25th anniversary of the Christchurch initiative, including a special commemorative issue of postgraduate journal Update. In this issue, Lister again updates the progress and details the hospital, general practitioner and regional organisations.[116] When the author of this present volume became postgraduate dean in the West of Scotland in 1984, he inherited an organisation which covered all specialties and with a regular annual review of all those in training. These were subsequently reflected in the report Hospital Doctors: Training for the Future (which will be discussed later). The Christchurch conference started a movement—the postgraduate centre movement—which has grown and become more sophisticated with the years.

Over the 30-year period (1970–2000) the specialist bodies, including general practice, worked at establishing educational programmes and assessing quality in medical practice. Practice visits and specialty visits began to assure the quality of the educational experience, and there was significant debate on the content and methods of assessment. This influenced appointments at senior level in all specialties and raised the quality of the applications. Specialist societies sprang up, reflecting the increase in specialisation, and provided mechanisms for exchange of information and experience. The more general societies (usually local ones) may have suffered as a result, and the increased pressure on staff made attendance in the evenings at such events less attractive.

From the 1950s to the 1990s there was debate on the formal structure of postgraduate and specialist education and the possibility of re-accreditation or revalidation. It took, however, until the mid-1990s for the issue of specialist education to be tackled, and the first few years of the 21st century before revalidation became a possibility. These are both discussed later.

Associated with this is the concept of apprenticeship, a longstanding learning process of working with a master. Recent educational developments, a formal curriculum, planned programmes in specialist education and more objective methods of assessment have tended to downplay such a personal form of learning. While it can be a hit and miss process (the master and the learner may not hit it off) and may lack the range of subjects which are required (the professional practice of the master may have a limited range), there remains some merit in the one-to-one interaction. Both secret and tacit knowledge may be passed on, and there is an opportunity to work and learn and be mentored by one person. A bond can develop allowing the sharing of experience and skill. In other words, it should be part of the process rather than the only method of learning and gaining experience. If managed appropriately, planned rotations to build up experience can be combined with an apprenticeship model.[117]

Increasingly, research is seen as a relevant part of postgraduate education. The publication of papers and books, and the presentation of work at seminars and meetings are considered 'good' training for the aspiring specialist. Appearance in citation lists are compared and are sometimes seen as more important than clinical experience. The truth, of course, is a bit of both. The ability to design an experiment, test an hypothesis and critically appraise the literature are important skills. They encourage a life-long, in-depth interest in a particular subject, which may be followed through for the remainder of the career. The spirit of curiosity and the wish to change things is part of being a doctor. It should not be seen as just one more hurdle before getting a specialist post.

THE DEVELOPMENT OF THE MEDICAL COLLEGES AND FACULTIES

Following the establishment of the older colleges there has been a steady development of new colleges and faculties, catering for a range of specialties. Such organisations have generally been established for several purposes: to maintain standards, to develop educational programmes and to assure the public of quality of care in the particular specialty. The have provided a focal point for educational development. The box below lists the dates of establishment.

Royal Colleges and Faculties: dates of establishment

Royal College of Surgeons of Edinburgh, 1505
Royal College of Physicians of London, 1518
Royal College of Physicians and Surgeons Glasgow, 1599
Royal College of Physicians of Ireland, 1654
Royal College of Physicians of Edinburgh, 1681
Royal College of Surgeons in Ireland, 1784
Royal College of Surgeons of England, 1800
Royal College of Obstetricians and Gynaecologists, 1930
Faculty of Dental Surgery, 1947
Royal College of General Practitioners, 1952
Royal College of Pathologists (College 1963), 1970

Royal College of Psychiatrists (Society 1841), 1971
Royal College of Radiologists (Faculty 1939), 1975
Faculty of Public Health Medicine, 1978
Faculty of Occupational Medicine, 1978
Royal College of Anaesthetists (Faculty 1948), 1992
Royal College of Ophthalmologists (Society 1880), 1988
Royal College of Paediatrics and Child Health, 1996

These colleges and faculties provide a huge range of educational programmes and keep members up to date with specialty developments through meetings and journals. The majority were not there 100 years ago, an example of the pace of change. They gather and meet regularly as the Academy of Medical Royal Colleges to discuss matters of mutual interest. In 1998 the Academy of Medical Sciences was established to give national and international leadership in the medical sciences and to promote the application of research to the practice of medicine and to the advancement of human health and welfare. In addition, they aim to promote excellence in research and training, enhance public understanding of the medical sciences and their impact on society, and to assess and advise on issues of medical science which are of public concern.

These two organisations representing the educational and research arms of medical practice provide a powerful resource for improving the care of patients and the public. It is interesting to note that there is no Academy of Medical Educators in this list; perhaps there should be.

THE RISE AND RISE OF GENERAL PRACTICE

For centuries, general practice (sometimes in the guise of the apothecary) had a bad press. They were the lowly paid, poorly educated and very hard working. By the 1950s there was considerable concern and demoralisation, just the right time to set up a college. In 1952, a small group of GPs got together and set up a steering group chaired by Sir Henry Willink. It had its first meeting in February 1952, with 7 GPs and 5 consultants. At the 8th and final meeting in November of the same year, a college was legally constituted and a foundation council formed. Regional faculties were set up and the first full council was elected with William Pickles as president, George Abercrombie as chairman and John Hunt as honorary secretary. Pickles was a GP based in Yorkshire and had written a fascinating book on epidemiology based in practice, an example of curiosity, data analysis and practical application. Pickles notes in his introductory chapter that the object of the book was to stimulate other country doctors to keep records of epidemic disease. He ends the chapter with: 'We country practitioners are in a position to supply facts from our observation of nature, and it is, I feel most strongly, our plain duty to make use of this unique opportunity'.[118] Pickles was one who recognised the opportunity of practiced-based research and its value to patients and the public.

The college began to influence vocational training by setting standards for a practice to be accredited as a training practice, and over the years it gradually but effectively raised and expanded these standards. Through working parties and reports, the work of the college had a major impact on learning, but just as importantly on the quality of care provided to patients. GPs are now the generalists, the general physicians, with a well-functioning education programme and rising standards.

MEDICAL ASSOCIATIONS AND JOURNALS

A subject can be said to come of age when associations, societies and journals are formed to cater for those with special interests in that subject, thus developing a research and literature base. In the subject of medical education these are essentially 20th century creations. While general journals published articles in this area and medical societies discussed educational issues (and still do), it was only in 1926 that the *Bulletin of the Association of American Medical Colleges* was produced, followed over 40 years later with the *British Journal of Medical Education* in 1966. This section will consider these developments briefly, and there is a whole history in telling their story.

The journals

A quick search on the Internet produces an interesting list of journals publishing articles in medical and biological education (see box below). Of course, the mainstream journals and clinical specialty journals continue to have a strong interest in this area, and that will undoubtedly continue.

Journals of medical education	
Academic Medicine	Journal of Continuing Education for Health Professionals
Advances in Health Sciences Education: theory and practice	Journal of Medical Internet Research
BMC Medical Education	Journal of the International Association of Medical Science Educators
Education for Health	Medical Education and its related journal Clinical Teacher
Journal of Audiovisual Media in Medicine	Medical Education OnLine, Medical Teacher
Journal of Biocommunication	Teaching and Learning in Medicine

A few of these journals will now be discussed in more detail.

Academic Medicine

This began as the *Bulletin of the American Association* in 1926 and became a journal in 1929. It was then published as the *Journal of Medical Education* in 1951, before becoming *Academic Medicine* in 1989. It has a long and interesting history.[119] Publication was initially quarterly, and by 1927 the number of pages had increased from 40 to 96. Its circulation was 3,000, and in addition to America it was distributed in Europe, Africa and the Far East. It maintained, at this time, statistics on medical student admissions, including how many students actually completed their courses.

The mission statement adopted in 1989 was:

To be a leading influence in academic medicine by taking vigorous action to promote responsible, productive debate of important issues within the academic medicine community and the health care and policy communities; to be the primary forum for dissemination and discussion of vital research, information, and ideas concerning the education of physicians, the institutions conducting that training, and administrators, faculty, and the staff involved; and to help all involved in academic medicine to understand better the broad issues of medical education and to improve their contributions to the field.[120]

Over the next decade, the journal changed considerably in editorial and management terms, and in 2005 the editor (Dr. Michael E. Whitcomb) and the editorial board decided that the journal should move further in the direction of addressing the key concerns of the academic medical community. The outcome of this is recorded in a note from the editor published in 2005, in which he describes the discussions of the editorial board on what the primary focus of the journal's content should be for the future.[121] It was described as having two audiences: the medical education research community and those in leadership roles in medical institutions. The debate was about whether this could and should continue. The board stated its strong opinion 'that *Academic Medicine* should now strive to be the journal that those holding leadership positions in medical schools and teaching hospitals turn to first for information that will help them address the major challenges facing their institutions and academic medicine as a whole'.[122] To do this it should continue to publish research reports and articles, particularly those with new, innovative or more effective approaches to educational initiatives. It also encouraged the publication of multi-institutional studies, reviews and a greater number of articles dealing with leadership issues.

These are important and significant developments in a journal with a long and distinguished history.

The *Journal of Medical Education* (now *Medical Education*)

This journal was established in 1966 (and will be celebrating its 40th anniversary in 2006 with a special edition on the history of medical education). It has had five editors to date; John Ellis 1966–75, Henry Walton from 1976, and jointly with Graham Buckley from 1996 and John Blyth until 2005. The current editor is John McLachlan. The early issues are interesting to look through. An editorial in the first issue debates the need for a new journal, and pays its respects to the *Journal of Medical Education*. Its purpose was to enhance communication across the community. The point is made that 'Medical education is now one of the subjects of medicine, albeit still a very diffuse and empirical one. Already it has a profuse literature, but as it is increasingly submitted to objective study more information is obtained which should reach a wider audience'.[123] The topics in 1966–7 look very familiar even today:

+ Student selection
+ The doctor's job
+ Looking ahead to the computer
+ Aspects of learning

- The use of videotape recording
- Individual study and educational technology
- Role of genetics in medical education
- Marking multiple choice examinations
- Projectors
- The role of the university in the future
- Factors influencing the development of the curriculum
- Teaching medical ethics
- On evaluating the success of teaching
- Attitudes of patients to clinical teaching
- The measurement of medical student attitudes
- Testing clinical competence
- An integrated final year examination.

These are just a few of the topics in the first year of publication. They were written by a wide range of authors and were of an international nature. In recent years, a number of new developments have enhanced the journal's role. For example, the section on 'Really good stuff' opens the door for shorter publications and information from other sources. Collection of the 'Most popular articles' and 'Most read papers' are useful. In 2004, it launched the *Clinical Teacher* which is aimed at the 'active, practising clinician' and to provide a 'digest of current research, practice and thinking in medical education…includes reviews of the literature related to clinical teaching….the latest thinking about modern teaching'.[124]

Medical Teacher

Medical Teacher, published in the UK, is one of the leading international journals for educators in the health sciences. It is aimed at the practising medical teacher and includes accounts and assessments of methods of teaching and learning, assessment and curriculum planning.

The journal was first launched in 1979 by Update Publications with Anne Patterson as editor. There was dwindling financial support of *Medical Teacher* in the form of advertising revenue and the journal was sold to Carfax Publishing in 1984 and re-launched under the editorship of Professor Ronald Harden. The Taylor and Francis Group acquired the journal in 1999 and it has expanded under their ownership to eight issues a year and a readership in over 70 countries worldwide. The journal has been adopted as the journal of the Association for Medical Education in Europe (AMEE) and the Canadian Association of Medical Education (CAME).

Over the years the journal has featured how education and medical education in particular is an evolving and progressive process as new approaches are tried, tested and developed or discarded. A series of articles in the anniversary issues in 2004 highlighted that while many of the details of techniques in medical education have seen significant change, in many ways the principles have remained the same.

Since it was first published the journal has recognised the changing problems that healthcare workers have in their day-to-day practice as teachers. It has highlighted the move to a scholarship in education and advancement of medical education as a discipline with its own field of knowledge and skills.

Association for the Study of Medical Education (ASME)

This association began following the 1957 GMC report and the meeting called by the Royal College of Physicians of London to consider setting up an organisation to allow free communication on medical education. Its first president was Sir Russell Brain PRCP (later Lord Brain), with Sir John Ellis as secretary. It has never had an executive function in medical education but provides a forum for all concerned to meet and present papers on educational issues. Its role is expanding and includes many non-medical members. ASME now has 1248 members and 89 corporate members.

The early history of ASME is well summarised in an article in the first issue of the *British Journal of Medical Education* in 1966.[125] Its purpose was to provide 'all those who carry such responsibilities (for medical education) with a medium of communication and such services as they may need'. The founders wanted to ensure that they created an association in which 'every organisation connected with medical education could share and to which any doctor or teacher of any age and in any medical discipline or any branch of medical practice could contribute if he were concerned in or for medical education'. The original purposes were to exchange information, organise meetings, maintain a bureau where information could be collected, stored and made available, to encourage and promote research in medical education and do anything else required to promote the interests of medical education. In the last section of the paper, it is noted that:

> *It is abundantly clear that attitudes to medical education are quite different now from 10 years ago. Change is expected, wanted, and indeed under way. It is generally realised that postgraduate training is as important as undergraduate education. The necessity of continuing education is accepted. It is obvious that many different bodies are, and must remain, involved and that, so far as the professional bodies are concerned, specialisation is likely lead to an increase in their number.*

In this editorial there is little direct reference to 'non-medically qualified people' with an interest in medical education, or education in related disciplines such as nursing, pharmacy and others, though it is implicit. Certainly at the present time, many members and those attending conferences come from a wide range of backgrounds. The current mission statement notes: 'The Association seeks to improve the quality of medical education by bringing together individuals and organisations with interests and responsibilities in medical and health care education'. There has been debate about changing the title of the association to reflect this.

Other associations

There are of course many national associations for medical education: a European Association and a World Federation for Medical Education (WFME). For example, the WFME was founded in 1972 and is a global organisation concerned with the education and training of medical students and medical doctors at all levels. It comprises six Regional Associations for Medical Education and has been particularly concerned about global standards in medical training and has published several reports on this subject.

WOMEN IN MEDICINE

Following the publication of the Goodenough Report, the playing field was levelled for women in both undergraduate and postgraduate education. While the official view was that equality had been established, many women still found it difficult to achieve the career progression of their male colleagues. For example, there are many more men than women taking up a surgical career, and while this may be due to many reasons, one is likely to have been that males were preferred by other males when jobs became vacant. By the late 20th century and into the 21st century, the number of women medical students now exceeds men in many schools, and figures of 70% women are not unusual. We await the impact of this on clinical practice and the choice of specialty.

CONCLUSIONS

It should be obvious that this chapter has merely skimmed the surface of the vast historical resource available to study medical education in the 20th century. What has been attempted has been an overview, concentrating on major developments in teaching and learning. The external environment (increase in knowledge, the changing organisation of health care and the increasing importance of patient and public involvement) have determined much of the agenda. The last 15 years have passed at an increasing pace, and this period will be discussed briefly in the next chapter. The main themes which were set out at the beginning of this book are now well established.

+ What is the aim and role of medicine?

+ The quest for competence.

+ How do we select medical students and specialists?

+ What kind of curriculum is required to deliver these aims?

+ Can we think beyond learning to research and development, innovation and improving the quality of care provided?

These topics will be developed further in Chapter 10.

REFERENCES

1. Flexner A. Medical education in the United States and Canada: a report to the Carnegie Foundation for the advancement of teaching. New York: The Foundation; 1910; 58.
2. General Medical Council. Recommendations on education and examination. London: Spottiswood and Co; 1881.
3. Ibid, 13.
4. Ibid. 13.
5. 1881–2 Medical Acts Commission Report. Report C-3259-I; para 37.
6. Newman G. Some notes on medical education in England: a memorandum presented to the president of the board. London: HMSO; 1918.

7. Ibid, 15.

9. Ibid, 18.

10. Ibid, 19.

11. Ibid, 20.

12. Ibid, 24.

13. Ibid, 24.

14. Ibid, 27.

15. Ibid, 27.

16. Ibid, 91.

17. Ibid, 110.

18. Glasgow pamphlet. University of Glasgow; 1920.

19. Inter-Departmental Committee on Medical Schools. Report of the Inter-Departmental Committee on Medical Schools (Goodenough Report). London: HMSO; 1944.

20. Ibid, 9.

21. Ibid, 39.

22. Ibid, 106–107.

23. Ibid, 234.

24. Ibid, 42.

25. Ibid, 42.

26. Ibid, 213.

27. General Medical Council. Recommendations as to the medical curriculum. London: HMSO; 1947; 6.

28. Ibid, 10.

29. Ibid, 13.

30. Ibid, 20.

31. Ibid, 26.

32. Ibid, 42.

33. Medical Education Committee of the British Medical Association. The training of a doctor: report of the Medical Education Committee of the British Medical Association. London; 1948; 9.

34. Ibid, 9.

35. Ibid, 10–13.

36. Ibid, 60–68.

37. Ibid.

38. Ways of learning. Lancet 1945; 2: 239–40.

39. Ibid, 256–7.

40. Arnott W M. Reform in medical education. BMJ 1949; 2: 487–502.

41. Pickering G W. Teaching of physiology. BMJ 1949, 2: 502–505.

42. Arnott.

43. Lauwerys J A. Methods of education. BMJ 1950; 2: 471–74.

44. Some comments on medical education in Britain. A London medical student. BMJ 1950; 2:496–8.

45. Ibid, 498

46. Aitken R S. The teaching of medicine. Lancet 1945; 2: 225–31.

47. Oglive W H. The education of the surgeon. Lancet 1945; 2: 229–31.

48. The curriculum: views of The Royal College of Physicians. Lancet 1955; 2: 132–4.

49. Second report of medical education. Lancet 1956; 1: 437–8.

50. Miller G E. Educating medical teachers. Cambridge: Harvard University Press; 1980.

51. Ham T H. Medical education at Western Reserve University: a progress report for the sixteen years, 1946–62. N Engl J Med; 267: 868–874 & 916–923.

52. Miller, 5.

53. Slobody L B. How to improve teaching in medical colleges. J Assoc Am Med Coll 1950; 25: 45–49.

54. Miller G E. An adventure in pedagogy. JAMA 1956; 162: 1448–50.

55. The curriculum: views of The Royal College of Physicians. Lancet 1955; 2: 132–4.

56. Ellis J R. Changes in medical education. Lancet 1956; I: 813–18, 867–72.

57. Miller, 180-82.

58. Miller, 210.

59. First world conference on medical education, London, 1953. Oxford: Oxford University Press; 1954.

60. Ibid, 539–44.

61. Ibid, 280.

62. Ellis 1956.

63. Ibid, 872.

64. General Medical Council. Recommendations as to the Medical Curriculum. London: GMC; 1957.

65. Ibid, 10.

66. Committee on Higher Education. Higher Education: Report of the Committee appointed by the Prime Minister under the chairmanship of Lord Robbins, 1961-1963. London: HMSO; 1963.

67. Ibid, 6.

68. Ibid, 181.
69. Ibid, 189.
70. Royal Commission on Medical Education. Royal Commission on Medical Education, 1965-1985. Report, etc. [Chairman, The Rt. Hon. the Lord Todd]. London; 1968.
71. Ibid, 20.
72. Ibid, 23.
73. Ibid, 81.
74. Ibid, 86.
75. Ibid, 121.
76. Department of Health and Social Security. Report of the Working Party on the Responsibilities of the Consultant Grade. (The Godber Report) London: HMSO; 1969.
77. Department of Health and Social Security. Report of the Committee of Inquiry into the Regulation of the Medical Profession [Chairman: A W Merrison] London: HMSO; 1975.
78. Ibid, 140.
79. Committee of Enquiry into Competence to Practise. Competence to practise: the report of a Committee of Enquiry set up for the medical profession in the United Kingdom. [Chairman: E A J Alment] London: The Committee; 1976.
80. Ibid, 1.
81. Ibid, 9.
82. Ibid, 43.
83. Social Services Committee. Fourth Report from the Social Services Committee. Medical education, with special reference to the number of doctors and the career structure in hospitals (The Short Report). London: HMSO; 1981.
84. Ibid, ivii.
85. Dubos R J. Mirage of health: utopias, progress, and biological change. New York: Harper & Bros; 1959.
86. Ibid, 228.
87. Ibid, 229–30.
88. Illich I. Medical nemesis: the expropriation of health. London: Calder & Boyers; 1975; 11.
89. McKeown T. The role of medicine: drama, mirage or nemesis? Oxford: Blackwell; 1979; 91.
90. Ibid, 147.
91. Kennedy I. The unmasking of medicine. London: Allen & Unwin; 1981; ix.
92. Ibid, 20.

93. Ibid, 25.

94. Ibid, 27.

95. Ibid, 125.

96. Miller H G. Medicine and Society. London: Oxford University Press; 1973.

97. The Edinburgh Declaration 1988. Lancet 1988; 2: 464.

98. Report of a working party on the teaching of medical ethics, Institute of Medical Ethics, 1988, Chairman Sir Desmond Pond.

99. Ibid, 3.

100. Ibid, 35–40.

101. GMC. Tomorrow's doctors: recommendations on undergraduate medical education. London: General Medical Council; 1993.

102. Consensus statement by teachers of medical ethics and law in UK medical schools. Teaching medical ethics and law within medical education: a model for the UK core curriculum. J Med Ethics 1998; 24: 188–92.

103. Mattick K, Bligh J. Teaching and assessing medical ethics: where are we now? J Med Ethics 2006; 40: 329–32.

104. Das A K, Mulley G P. The value of an ethics history? J R Soc Med 2005: 98: 262–266.

105. Evans M, Louhiala P, Puustinen R. Philosophy for medicine: applications in a clinical context. Oxford: Radcliffe Medical Press Limited; 2004.

106. Calman K C, Downie R S, Duthie M, Sweeney B. Literature and medicine: a short course for medical students, Med Educ 1988: 22: 265–9.

107. Osler W. Aequanimitas: with other addresses to medical students, nurses and practitioners of medicine. New York: McGraw Hill; 1906; 211.

108. Chekhov A. Letter to Suvorin, 1888.

109. O'Donnell M. Doctors as performance artists. J R Soc Med 2005: 98: 323–4.

110. Calman K C. A study of storytelling, humour and learning in medicine. London: The Stationery Office; 2000.

111. Mann, T. Magic Mountain.

112. Holmes O W. The Professor at the Breakfast Table. London: Routledge & Sons; 1905; 29,

113. Nuffield Provincial Hospitals Trust Conference on Postgraduate Medical Education. BMJ 1962: 1: 466–7.

114. Lister J. Regional postgraduate medical centres. BMJ 1968; 3: 736–38.

115. Lister J. Postgraduate medical education. Rock Carling Fellowship. Nuffield Provincial Hospitals Trust; 1993.

116. Lister J. History, aims and acknowledgements of the postgraduate centre movement. Update. Dec 1986; 20–25.

117. Dorman T. Osler, Flexner, apprenticeship and the 'new medical education'. J Roy Soc Med 2005: 98: 91–95.

118. Pickles W. Epidemiology in country practice. Bristol: John Wright and Sons; 1939; 9.

119. Bowles M D, Dawson V P. With one voice: The Association of American Medical Colleges 1876–2002. Washington: AAMC; 2003.

120. Mission statement of Academic Medicine. AAMC. Weekly Report. May 26, 1988.

121. Whitcomb M E. A new goal for the journal. Academic Medicine 2005; 80: 515–6.

122. Ibid.

123. Journal of Medical Education 1966. Vol 1.

124. Aims of 'The Clinical Teacher'. The Clinical Teacher. London: Blackwells.

125. Ellis J. ASME. Brit J Med Educ 1966: 1: 2–6.

9

Even more change: the last 15 years, 1990–2006

We have had to accept, for our purposes, the virtual absence of systematic factual information about the practical processes of medical teaching in Britain and their effectiveness; we have recommended that provision be made for proper study of the aims and methods of medical teachers, as part of a substantial research effort in medical education in the coming years.[1]

The Royal Commission on Medical Education (The Todd Report) 1968

Medical education research is dominated by assessment of trainee performance followed by trainee satisfaction. Leading journals in medical education contain little information concerning the cost and products of medical education, that is, provider and patient outcomes. The study of these medical education outcomes represents an important challenge to medical education researchers.[2]

Prystowsky and Bordage, 2001

INTRODUCTION

The last 15 years have seen an explosion of interest in medical education, and take us from the 1990s to 2006. As a subject it has come of age. Research units have been set up, conferences grown in size, journals developed and new innovations pioneered. The policy developments have been considerable, but it is perhaps too early to evaluate their overall significance. This short section will set out the context of the changes and then give brief descriptions of the major developments in both basic (undergraduate) and specialist education.

Before proceeding it is perhaps worth commenting on the two quotations at the beginning of this chapter. Both make the point that medical education needs a much stronger evidence base, and that even the ones available miss important components and consequences of learning: the impact on patient care.

THE CONTEXT

So much has changed it is difficult to know where to begin. Consider first the NHS: it has been subject to major on-going changes in its structure, management and functions. These changes have had a significant impact on educational processes. For example, the move to more outpatient work has meant fewer patients in hospital (very good for patients), providing less opportunity for students and trainees to observe and take part in the processes of care. The European Working Time Directive has restricted the hours for training and thus resulted in further diminished opportunities for learning. Shift work and the loss of some of the identity in clinical units have made it more difficult to provide feedback on performance, as the players continue to change. These issues and many more can be overcome with more emphasis on community practice and better integration in follow-up processes, and can result in innovative ways of delivering learning. The following summarises some of the changes and challenges of the last 15 years:

+ Enormous increase in the knowledge base.

+ Research seen to be more important than teaching as

estimates of research quality determine the funding for universities.

- Greater emphasis on skills and, in particular, communication skills.

- Changes to the curriculum, with new subjects appearing and greater emphasis on well-developed subjects (e.g. changes to anatomy teaching, ethics, arts and humanities, medical anthropology).

- Greater emphasis on inter-professional education and the recognition of the importance of teamwork.

- Rise in interest in educational research, and the respectability of research in education.

- Innovation in teaching methods: problem-based teaching, skills labs, new methods of assessment (OSCEs), computer-based learning, access to information through the Internet.

- Emphasis on competence, mastery learning, new theoretical frameworks for learning. Developments in educational psychology and the principles of learning, especially adult learning.

- Teaching the teachers. This is a fairly recent development and is discussed in a subsequent chapter.

- Renewed interest in methods of selection for medical school and for specialist training.

- Renewed interest in rural medicine, with new medical schools emerging as the prime focus of learning. This has been an important initiative for developing and developed communities.

- Much greater interest from the public and politicians in the performance of doctors. Greater use of targets, objective setting, league tables, work plans, audit and the publication of outcomes.

- A very large number of agencies and public bodies have been set up, providing guidance to the professions on all aspects of health, medicine and healthcare. These include the National Institute of Clinical Excellence (NICE), the Human Genetics Commission and the Human Fertilisation and Embryology Authority. National service frameworks have been developed for many disease groups, and professional bodies have produced their own guidance. The doctor is overwhelmed with evidence.

+ Public expectations have grown and there is a much greater wish to be involved. Patient choice is an increasingly important thread which goes through all health service work.

+ Radical changes to the NHS, its operation and governance.

+ The increasing importance of patient choice.

+ Increasing number of women entering medicine.

+ A general interest in the arts and health, and a resurgence of philosophy and ethical issues in medicine. The role of literature, philosophy, the social sciences and the humanities are all now being re-examined. Courses and conferences exploring the role of books, film, poetry, art and architecture in the care of patents and the education of the doctor are now expanding.

+ The above also relates to the need for wisdom and judgement as part of clinical skills. The generalist, someone who can span a number of disciplines, is becoming more important as specialisation develops.

+ Specialties which have not had as much attention—such as mental health and the care of the elderly—are being looked at afresh.

THE MAJOR POLICY CHANGES

Changes in policy have been considerable in the last 15 years, and this section summarises the major ones. These change are, of course, ongoing and difficult to evaluate from the perspective of the early 21st century. Indeed, there is a fascinating history to be written in 25 years about what occurred in this period. Many of those involved are still active and still trying to improve medical education. It is to be hoped that this will continue.

Tomorrow's Doctors: GMC recommendations on undergraduate medical education[3]

Tomorrow's Doctors appeared in 1993 and proved a landmark in medical education. Publication of the recommendations saw significant changes in medical education: a radical re-think of most undergraduate courses in the UK to a much more student-centred learning process. This coincided with the beginnings of a radical restructuring of the NHS. Funding to carry forward the recommendations was tight but some was found (personal communication K.C.Calman). Ten years on, these changes are still ongoing. Tomorrow's Doctors was updated in 2003 and is a remarkably clear document. Re-reading the report is interesting, particularly the Introduction:

> Given the pace at which the horizons of medical science and technology expand, we can be certain that the doctors of tomorrow will be applying knowledge and deploying skills which are at present unforeseen. We cannot teach science that is at yet undiscovered, nor can we forecast its future implications. But some of the present day art and science of medicine is fundamental to its practice and will certainly endure…For the rest, we can at best strive to educate doctors capable of adaptation to change, with minds that can encompass new ideas and developments and with attitudes to learning that inspire the continuation of the educational process throughout professional life…Whereas the focus of medical education during the present century has been mainly on the understanding of disease processes as they affect individuals, on their diagnosis and management, there

is an evident re-awakening of the wider interest of our forebears in the health of populations...Public Health, temporarily lost from the vocabulary, has been firmly reinstated as a priority in the planning of medical services in this country and abroad, and the undergraduate curriculum must reflect this important change in emphasis.

The report notes once again the burden placed on medical students due to the over-crowding of the curriculum and recommends special study modules, and a reduction of the factual content as a way forward.

Hospital Doctors: Training for the Future. The Calman Report, 1993[4]

This report, initiated because of changes in European legislation, took the opportunity to revise postgraduate education and to build a framework for subsequent developments in re-accreditation. The document emphasised the continuum of medical education, and most of its recommendations were not new:

+ Competitive entry to the specialist grade.

+ Continuity of the period of specialist training with appropriate planning of the experience.

+ Regular supervision of the trainee and feedback on performance.

The only new aspect (and one which has been particularly valuable in the development of the process of revalidation) was that the outcome of the process would be based on competence to practise. This assessment would be made by the specialist bodies, which would also set out the experience required to be an independent practitioner. Each trainee would be given a training number to ensure some human resource planning in each specialty, and at the end of the process trainees would be awarded a Certificate of Completion of Specialist Training (CCST). There was some concern at the time at the use of the word 'completion', as the feeling was strong that the process was not completed but continuing. However, this was the term used in the European legislation.

The length of training for each speciality was determined by the appropriate body (college or society), as was the curriculum. The profession, therefore, had the opportunity to consider how such programmes would be put together, how they would be evaluated, and what competencies and minimum length of training would be required to achieve them. This process was overseen by a body (the Specialist Training Authority (STA) of the Medical Royal Colleges), and the individual who had achieved the CCST was placed on the Specialist Register by the GMC, who had been designated as the competent authority. Over 12,000 trainees in 53 specialties went through this process between 1996 and 1997, and the process is ongoing. Recently, a Postgraduate Medical Education and Training Board has been set up to replace the STA (2004).

Good Medical Practice[5]

This important document was first issued by the General Medical Council in 1998. It sets out the duties and responsibilities of the doctor including:

+ providing a good standard of practice and care
+ decisions about access to medical care
+ keeping up to date
+ maintaining your performance
+ teaching and training
+ relationships with patients—consent, confidentiality, trust, good communication
+ dealing with problems in medical practice—conduct of colleagues and complaints

+ working with colleagues—treating colleagues fairly, working in teams, leading teams, sharing information with colleagues, delegation and referral

+ providing information about services, writing reports, research, conflicts of interest, and financial interests

+ the health of the doctor and putting patients at risk.

This is an important basic document with sets out the framework within which doctors operate. Some of the background to this is set out in *The Doctor's Tale* by Donald Irvine (2003).[6]

Other publications by the GMC

Over the last 15 years the GMC has produced a range of other documents on topics such as:

+ continuing professional development

+ seeking patients' consent: the ethical issues

+ serious communicable diseases

+ HIV and AIDS: the ethical considerations

+ confidentiality

+ advertising

+ the duties of a doctor.

The establishment of several new medical schools

In 1998 the government announced that it was to set up a series of new medical schools to meet the demand for more doctors. These were established in Exeter and Plymouth (the Peninsula School), the University of East Anglia, Leicester–Warwick, Keele, York–Hull, Brighton–Sussex and Newcastle–Durham.

This provided an opportunity to re-think the curriculum again, with many considering community based programmes and problem-based learning. The arts and humanities and the social sciences have also been given prominence. The first graduates from these schools emerged in 2006.[7] There is a great opportunity to innovate at these schools and try new and interesting methods of approach.

Revalidation, accreditation and mandatory re-licensing[8]

This builds on the GMC document, *Good Medical Practice and Maintaining Good Medical Practice*. It is a major initiative begun in the last few years and initiated in April 2005. All doctors must now hold a licence to practice, and to retain that licence must undergo a process of 'revalidation'. Doctors must demonstrate at regular intervals that they remain up-to-date and fit to practise. Revalidation is an important part of demonstrating accountability to patients and the wider public. It will shift the emphasis away from qualifications alone towards a regular assessment of whether the doctor remains competent to practise. It will require all doctors to reflect meaningfully on their practice, using information gathered through audit and other means, and to seek the views of others on their performance, throughout their medical careers.

Modernising Medical Careers: The Curriculum for the Foundation Years in Postgraduate Medical Education and Training, 2005

This is an important new development spearheaded by Sir Liam Donaldson, chief medical officer. It deals with the early years of postgraduate education, often seen as the 'lost tribe'. It proposes a broad curriculum with core competencies, and has a particular emphasis in the second year of the programme on acute care. It will provide a firm basis for the specialist training period.

Creation of a new body to oversee all professional education in health

The Council for the Regulation of Healthcare Professions (CRHP) came into being following the Bristol Inquiry into cardiac surgery in children (chaired by Sir Ian Kennedy). It was implemented through the NHS Reform and Healthcare Professions Act and came into being in 2003. It brings together nine regulatory bodies, including the GMC, the General Dental Council, the Nursing and Midwifery Council and the Royal Pharmaceutical Society of Great Britain. Its function is to promote the interests of the public and patients in the field of regulation of health professionals, and it reports annually to Parliament.

Future changes to the GMC

As this book is being written, the GMC is once more under scrutiny. This has resulted from the 'Shipman' case, in which a doctor murdered an unknown number of patients, perhaps in the hundreds. Several reviews have been undertaken to see why these crimes went unidentified and where the failures lay. Dame Janet Smith produced a major report on this in several parts, and this is now being actively debated.

New innovations in teaching and the preparation of teachers

As will be discussed in the section on teaching and training in a later chapter, the major innovation from the Dearing Report[9] was that preparation for teaching would be part of the professional development of all staff in universities.

CONCLUSIONS

The last 15 years have seen huge changes. Those responsible for medical education have responded by adapting and modifying the curriculum at undergraduate and postgraduate levels. Major issues remain, notably achieving a satisfactory solution to the issue of revalidation. The external environment is continually changing, and this too will require those involved to adapt. There is a much greater sense that the public want to know what is going on, and want to be involved. This, as has been discussed before, is a positive aspect of the changes, and the profession should rise to the challenge and help patients and the public to become more involved. When the history of this period is written some time in the future, it is to be hoped that those who write it will be sympathetic to the efforts made to improve both the process of learning and patient care.

REFERENCES

1. Royal Commission on Medical Education. Royal Commission on Medical Education, 1965-1985. Report, etc. [Chairman, The Rt. Hon. the Lord Todd]. London; 1968; 20.
2. Prystowsky J B, Bordage G. An outcomes research perspective on medical education: the predominance of trainee assessment and satisfaction. Med Educ 2001; 35(4): 331–6.
3. General Medical Council. Tomorrow's doctor's: recommendations on undergraduate medical education issued by the Education Committee of the General Medical Council in pursuance of Section 5 of the Medical Act 1983. London: General Medical Council; 1993.
4. Department of Health. Hospital doctors: training for the future. The Calman Report. London: Department of Health; 1993.

5. General Medical Council. Good medical practice. London: GMC; 1998.

6. Irvine D. The doctors' tale. Oxford: Radcliffe Medical Press; 2003.

7. Howe A, Campion P, Searle J, Smith H. New perspectives—approaches to medical education at four new medical schools. BMJ 2004; 329: 327–31.

8. General Medical Council. Licence to practice and revalidation. London: GMC; 2003.

9. Higher education in the learning society. Report of the National Committee of Inquiry into Higher Education. The Dearing Report. 1997.

PART 2
The Present

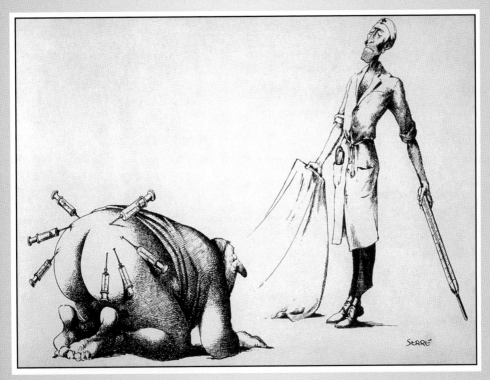

The dominance of the doctor and the submissiveness of patients. From 'Humour noir et hommes en blanc' by Claude Serre©Glenat. Reproduced with permission.

10

The themes

But how the subject theme may gang
Let time and chance determine
Perhaps it might turn out a sang
Perhaps turn out a sermon

Robert Burns in an *Epistle to a young friend*, 1786

INTRODUCTION

*T*his chapter identifies what are considered to be the major themes of this book (first raised in Chapter 1) and discusses them in the next few chapters. They are not new themes; indeed, most of them can be identified from earliest times. They could have been put together in different ways, and this classification represents a particular vision of the current issues in medical education. The names used for them have changed over the years, as has the scope of each theme, but the fundamental issues remain the same. This introductory chapter sets them out and deals with the relationships between them. They cannot be considered in isolation; they are all mutually dependent on each other (as will be discussed). For some of the major themes, ways forward will be suggested; for others, answers await.

All of these themes should be benchmarked against the public's views and interests in medicine. They should 'belong' to the public, as the public are integral in coming to a solution to some of the most difficult issues in medicine. The themes and the solutions are 'public property', and as will be stated several times, the profession has nothing to fear from the active involvement of patients, the public and other professions in determining the role and boundaries of medicine. The profession should lead this debate and not be forced into positions by others. If, as will be discussed shortly, the role of medicine is to help patients and the public and to serve the common good, then this external involvement is essential. Inevitably much of this section will focus on the UK, though the topics are likely to be relevant to elsewhere.

THE THEMES

This section briefly summarises the next few chapters and sets them in a general context.

1. The roles and boundaries of medicine (Ch. 11)

This chapter will include a discussion on defining the good doctor and the concept both of a profession and professional. This seems the logical place to start. What is medicine for? Does it have a purpose? Is it a science or an art? Inevitably, this leads to a discussion on the purpose of medical education, and this will be picked up later. There is considerable discussion on the concept of a profession. Numerous groups in the last 10 years have been attempting to set out what it means to be a doctor, and the values behind medicine. These are important debates and should be encouraged. Leadership emerges as an important issue.

Defining a 'good doctor' inevitably leads to a consideration of the role of the public and patients in decisions around medicine and medical practice. Just as important, however, is the relationship between medicine and the other professions: the 'hard' sciences, social sciences and the arts. This is a rapidly developing area and one in which medical practice can only benefit from and extend its role. There is an increasing amount of interdisciplinary work—in clinical care, in teaching and learning and in research. In the search for the unity of knowledge, the boundaries and overlaps become increasingly irrelevant as knowledge increases.

Another key issue is that of research and the importance of the curiosity of the doctor to explain and change health and illness. Indeed, medicine could be said to have two purposes. The first is to take existing knowledge, skills and attitudes to improve practice and public health, and through learning put them into practice for the benefit of patients and the public. This is the healing component of medical practice. The second purpose is to discover new knowledge and transmit this knowledge (handing it on to others) for the benefit of the whole population.

The role of the doctor in society might be seen as a subset of the role of medicine, and is a subject less often discussed than it might be. Apart from healer, the doctor can also be seen as educator, advocate and agent of change. These are ancient roles and deserve more prominence. They are associated with how the public understands clinical and research issues, such as resource allocation, ethical problems and public health dilemmas. The doctor has an important role in setting out the issues but also acting as an advocate and agent of change.

2. The quest for competence: the search for the 'good' doctor (Ch. 12)

This chapter will consider how best to assess competence and what makes a good doctor. Discussion here will relate back to the roles and boundaries of medicine, and will link this to the concept of a profession, and that of a professional. Competence is a key issue. With the development of new specialties and sophisticated techniques and treatments, assessment is no longer a simple matter, yet it is at the heart of patient confidence and trust in doctors. Part of this debate will consider how best to grow and cultivate a good doctor.

3. Who should become a doctor? Selection for medicine (Ch. 13)

One must first adequately define the role of medicine and the competencies required before being able to determine the best criteria for selection. It is an age-old problem and recent commentators have often found it too difficult to discuss. A particular issue for medical education is can these competencies—once defined—be learned by all; or can only some people be a good doctor? Can knowledge, skills and attitudes all be learned? If they can, selection is irrelevant; anyone can be a doctor. If not, then some form of selection will be required.

4. Handing on learning: the learning environment (Ch. 14)

The public require assurance that competence is being maintained. Once it is clear what medicine is for, what competencies are required and how best to select students, the issue then is how to provide a learning environment within which the student can grow and flourish. This horticultural allusion relates back to the discussion on the cultivation of the doctor in the section on competence. New methods of learning will be explored and compared to those which have been present for generations. The use of IT, simulators and clinical skills laboratories are all part of this. This chapter will also cover the role of the book in the 21st century.

The curriculum is an amalgam of content, method and assessment techniques. These are all discussed in some detail, though it will be argued that the content is perhaps best discussed at local level and is likely to vary considerably from time to time and place to place. In each instance it is essential that we return to the purpose of medicine to help define the content. The content will probably vary between different countries and with a different range of health problems. A key philosophical issue is how 'success' of a course at undergraduate or postgraduate level is assessed.

Part of this discussion will relate to the role of the teacher, and the historical debates on this topic will be reviewed, as will the definition and characteristics of a good teacher. There is an important relationship between the learner and the teacher at all levels of clinical practice, and this will be discussed in some detail. In a similar way there will be a discussion about the relevance of inter-professional education.

A further question which will be examined is how those who teach should be prepared for the process. As before this topic will be discussed in an historical context, recognising that in the great scheme of things it is a relatively recent development. The discussion will be in a UK context. This also relates to a current debate about the relationship between teaching and research: how relevant is it and does it matter?

5. Beyond learning: dealing with new medical knowledge (Ch. 15)

One of the most obvious facts about learning is that you only learn what other people know, or in some instances what they do not know. Learning, as has been described, can be delivered in many ways. One important aspect of learning is the development of the ability to ask questions, to be curious and to challenge assumptions. This means going beyond learning into the discovery of new knowledge, methods, service delivery and even new methods of learning. Historically, this has been a fundamental part of the role of the doctor in trying continually to improve the care and treatment of patients and the public. It is about both research (discovering new things) and development (implementing new developments and modifying them). It includes the better understanding of disease and the nature of health and illness. It is about continually pushing back the frontiers. It is about innovation and doing things differently.

Like other aspects of these themes, dealing with new knowledge has a strong patient and public focus, and requires not only the understanding by patients of the research to be carried out but their commitment and courage in taking part in such research. However, without the curiosity to understand and explain, and the wish to make things better for patients, medicine would just be like any other technical career. With such interests, medicine is taken beyond facts and figures and becomes a profession, and indeed defines the role of the profession.

Medical magnets

One of the striking features that emerges from a review of the history of medical education is how individuals have journeyed—often long distances—to receive the 'best' education. Over the centuries these 'centres of excellence' have moved around the world and continue to do so. Today, at the start of the 21st century, this is perhaps less relevant to undergraduate study, as most medical schools provide a very adequate grounding. It is at the specialty level that this is still noticeable. Where is the best teaching/research centre for cardiology in this country, or in Europe, or in the world? If I really did want to be a neurologist or an oncologist, where are the 'centres of excellence' that would attract me and encourage me to be part of that team? Much of this is about leadership and providing a learning environment at the sharp end of a new and developing subject area. Personal influence is critical, and those who plan education programmes need to reflect on the importance of having a faculty with 'drawing power'. Over the years the names of medical magnets have been remembered in the creation of travelling clubs and specialist societies to continue the fellowship and camaraderie which grew up around such individuals. Of particular relevance to medical education is the same question: where would I go to expand my learning in this subject? There is little doubt that these examples show the importance of medical leadership in the development of new areas of health and healthcare.

11

The aim of medicine: the roles and boundaries of the profession

Life is short, and the Art long; the occasion fleeting,
experience fallacious and judgement difficult. The physician
must not only be prepared to do what is right himself, but
also to make the patient, the attendants, and the externals
cooperate.[1]

Hippocrates

INTRODUCTION

D efining the aim of medicine and its role is a fundamental task which needs to be explored before considering what kind of education is required to produce
a medical practitioner or specialist; it is essential that there is a
clear view of the role of medicine and of the doctor. Without such
a vision of the aim of medicine it becomes impossible to plan
an educational programme and to assess whether or not it has
been effective.

F.N.L. Poynter makes the interesting point that this aim has
never really been clear:

Medical education reflects the organisation of the profession
and its institutions and just as vestigial features are very
prominent in the profession in England, so they may be clearly
seen in the system in education. This has never been

designed and planned as a whole for its purpose. Indeed, nobody is agreed on its purpose, that is, what type of doctor the system is intended to produce. To take an industrial analogy, it is rather as if a great variety of machine tools were assembled from a number of different car factories and linked together in the belief that the ultimate product would be a motor car of some kind, though nobody was at all sure what it would look like or how it would perform. The product does indeed work and does indeed pass the different kinds of inspectors, each of whom is supplied with a different blue print for his tests.[2]

The historical review in this present volume suggests that it might be possible to define the aims and roles of medicine and of the doctor in a form which most doctors are likely to agree. Crucially, this also requires the agreement of patients and the public. In achieving the role and purpose of medicine, the doctor is seen as the primary mechanism through which these are realised. Such definitions raise issues around the concept of a 'professional' and what that means.

The roles and the aims also begin to define the boundaries of medicine. Where does it begin and where does it end? How is the knowledge base of medicine related to other disciplines and branches of knowledge: for example, the development of advanced practice roles of other health care professionals? What role do the arts and social sciences play in the education of the doctor? How does the doctor interact with other professional groups? These are important questions and, like the definition of the aim of medicine, lay the ground-work for subsequent themes in this section of the book: the quest for competence, selection for medicine and the learning environment. Without such a debate, the comment make above by Poynter will continue to remain true.

Setting out the aim of medicine

With the historical review described in Part 1 of this book as a background, it is possible to summarise these discussions and set out aims for medicine and the roles of the doctor.

It is suggested that the **aim of medicine** is to assist in the process of healing in its broadest sense—both of individuals and of communities. This is the primary function of the doctor. Doctors do this by improving quality of life, providing care, relieving suffering, promoting health, and preventing illness and disease. This aim is grounded in the understanding of health and the mechanisms of illness and disease, which then forms the basis of effective and appropriate treatment. Doctors must do this in full cooperation with the patient, public and other providers of health care.

Put another way, the **purpose of medicine** is to serve the community by continually improving health, healthcare and quality of life for the individual and the population. This is accomplished by understanding disease, promoting health, preventing illness, providing treatment and care, and making effective use of resources, all within the context of a team approach.

There is a philosophical issue around such aims. Are they timeless, or do they change as the environment, culture and knowledge base change? Stated as above these aims could be considered enduring yet with a need for interpretation and modification to fit the more detailed objectives of doctors working at any particular time or context.

Defining the roles of the doctor

Three roles thus follow from the aims set out above:

1. To be a healer and to understand the processes of care and to intervene when appropriate. To wish to help others and to see medicine as a vocation.

2. To understand people and use this to provide better care, with cooperation and involvement of patient and the public, should they wish. To communicate as effectively as possible. To be an advocate for health.

3. To understand the reasons for illness and disease and to use

this knowledge to improve health, healthcare and quality of life and well being.

The kind of doctor required is one whose qualities fit these roles: that of the healer, people-centred and curious about health and illness. By defining the qualities required, not the type of doctor, it becomes easier to see a way forward. There is no single 'type' of doctor. There may be several 'types', but they should all have the qualities listed above.

Not all doctors will spend an equal amount of time in each of these roles, nor will they have specific expertise for all, but every doctor will have some part in them and will ensure that their work is directed towards the aims as set out above. For example, the pathologist may spend much time examining the process of disease but will still have an interest in how this is applied to the process of care. The research scientist will operate in the same way. The psychiatrist may put greater emphasis on understanding people, as may the doctor interested in changing the public health. The general practitioner will have a more even spread, while some specialist clinical colleagues will spend more time on care processes such as treatment. The 'ideal' doctor may be an illusion. What we may need is a range of doctors with a series of qualities which are expressed in different degrees in different individuals.

The aim of medicine set out above will now be discussed in some detail, followed by a review of the roles of the doctor. This will link to, and be the foundation for, subsequent sections on selection and development of the curriculum. It will also create the backdrop against which the issue of 'competence' can then be explored.

THE AIM OF MEDICINE
The concept of 'healing'

The definition as set out above has several concepts enmeshed within it. The first of these is that of 'healer', a rather old-fashioned term but one which illustrates a tangible objective, that of helping people to become whole again. In the 1752 edition of Samuel Johnson's dictionary, 'Physick' was defined as the science of healing. This healing may be of the body, the mind or even the spirit. Medicine has this goal because of the unified nature of the individual and, indeed, of the population. Whole communities may need healing, hence the relevance of this to the role of the public health doctor. But is 'healing' now a long dated concept, alien and foreign and steeped in mystery? The argument here is that it is at the root of medicine. Healing is where medicine began: an attempt to alleviate suffering. Advances in biomedical science have made it possible to heal more effectively and in some instances effect cures, but at its heart, medicine is still about healing and will remain so until all of the uncertainty is removed and all illness understood. Many illnesses remain difficult to understand and control. The art of medicine is partly about knowing what can and cannot be treated effectively. The art remains part of the healer's repertoire.

In the words of a French saying of disputed origin:

Guèrir quelquefois

Soulager souvant

Consoler toujours

Which translated is: 'To cure sometimes, to relieve often, to care always'.

Related to healing is the concept of care, something so fundamental to medical practice that it hardly needs to be stated. Yet it must be. What all doctors can do—irrespective of the patient, the population, the illness or the disease—is to care, and to show that they care. To demonstrate that the person in front of them is important, important enough to listen to and to try to understand his or her problems. It is about improving the quality of life of the individual. The very act of taking time, of being interested, of showing that you have a real concern for someone else, is important. To show compassion and a wish to help sends vital signals to patients and communities. To act as advocate for them when they are in difficulty is an essential part of medicine. Caring is not a passive process but a very active one, and one which can drain the doctor and take all his or her resources; hence the need for all medical practitioners to be able to refresh themselves and retain their own quality of life.

Relieving suffering is a more active part of this process. It may help to listen and understand, but care is likely to go beyond this. Active intervention may be required, and in this instance it becomes important to be clear about the objective of that intervention. Is it to completely remove the problem, effect a cure, to tackle the disease by directing therapy against it; or is it to relieve the symptoms of the disease without affecting the underlying pathology? Such objectives are not mutually exclusive, and during the course of the illness, different aims may be pursued at different times in an attempt to continually improve the quality of life of the individual— a topic which will now be discussed.

Quality of life

Quality of life is difficult to measure or even to define. Clearly, it can only be described and measured in individual terms, and depends on present lifestyle, past experience, hopes for the future, dreams and ambitions. It must include all areas of life and experience and take into account the impact of illness and treatment. A good quality of life may be said to be present when the hopes of an individual are matched and fulfilled by experience. The opposite can be said to be true—a poor quality of life occurs when hopes do not meet with experience.[3]

Quality of life changes with time and under normal circumstances can vary considerably. The priorities and goals of an individual must be realistic and would therefore be expected to change with time and be modified by age and experience. To improve quality of life therefore it is necessary to try to narrow the gap between the hopes and aspirations, and what actually happens. The aim is to help people reach the goals they have set for themselves, or to reduce their expectations. A good quality of life is usually expressed in terms of contentment, satisfaction, happiness, fulfilment, and the ability to cope.

Certain implications follow from this definition of quality of life:

+ It can only be assessed and described by the individual—what I mean by quality of life may be different from your concept.

+ It must take into account many aspects of life.

+ It must be related to individual goals and aspirations.

+ The goals must be realistic.

+ Improvement is related to the ability to identify and achieve these goals.

+ Illness and treatment may well modify these goals.

+ Action may be required to narrow the potential gap. This action may be taken by the patient alone or with the help of others.

+ The gap between expectation and reality may be the driving force for some individuals.

+ As each goal is achieved, new ones are identified, opening up the gap once again. It is a constantly changing picture.

Quality of life is, therefore, a measure of the difference at a particular moment between the hopes and expectations of the individual and the individual's present experiences. Quality of life has many dimensions, covering all life areas including home and garden, work, hobbies, family, financial issues, body image, diet, mobility, ambitions, spiritual issues and concepts of the future. Part of the role of the doctor in caring for patients is thus to assist in improving quality of life.

A related concept in the role of the doctor is that of service. To serve patients and the public is a key aspect of the doctor's work. This will often come into conflict with other aspects of medical care, such as resource allocation, but this does not remove the obligation of a professional to serve the individual. Indeed, it is this principle which is at the heart of medicine.

Determinants of health

Before describing some of the other facets of the 'aim of medicine' we should return to the determinants of health, a topic first raised in Chapter 1. In broad terms, there are five factors which determine health, and these can help to define the range of learning required of the doctor before practising medicine.

1. **Genetics and the biological makeup of the individual.** While it may not be possible to modify our genetic makeup at present, new tools will become available in the next few decades. Even now, stem cell therapy is beginning to show how such things can change.

2. **Social and economic aspects of life.** It is well recorded that such factors can exert a profound influence on health.

3. **Environmental factors.** Such factors, including infectious diseases, have a major influence on health.

4. **Lifestyle.** What we eat, drink, how we behave and what excesses and habits we indulge in can have a very significant impact on health.

5. **Health services.** This includes the way in which healthcare is delivered and what diagnostic and treatment services are available.

The first of these factors is essentially about the understanding of disease and illness. It is a research-based area which tries to determine which factors in the pathogenesis of disease are most crucial and how they can be influenced. The relevant sciences include genetics, pathology, microbiology, molecular biology and many others. This is an area which should be of interest to all doctors, and indeed defines the role of the doctor as much as that of a healer. Greater understanding leads to the development of more rational treatments, improved therapies and novel ways of diagnosis and intervention. This leads to more effective and appropriate treatments.

Promoting health is the next component of the aim of medicine. This is an active process and one which can be overlooked by doctors. It concerns providing the individual or population with the knowledge and skills to make choices: what they eat, how they behave, what exercise they take, what habits they pick up and how they might deal with such issues. Importantly, there is a need for a much greater evidence base to determine not only which factors are important, but what interventions are effective in changing health. This is a key research question which needs an answer.

Health promotion is a positive way of improving well-being. The opposite side of the coin is the prevention of illness and disease, including early diagnosis. There are a range of possible interventions: screening, immunisation and changes in health behaviour in relation to lifestyle. While this may be seen as an area of special expertise, all doctors should consider what factors can prevent disease. It is not just about primary prevention but includes secondary and tertiary prevention.

All of this highlights, as did Hippocrates in his first aphorism, and serves to emphasise that the practice of medicine requires the 'full co-operation of the patient'. This is such an important part of the role of the doctor that it needs to be stated over and over again. Involvement implies communication, a two-way process in which listening by the doctor is a key element. Part of this process relates to the social function of the doctor, as advocate, teacher and agent of change and this is a topic which will be discussed in a subsequent section.

Hippocrates first aphorism also emphasises the involvement of 'attendants'. In more modern terminology this is about team work: about working with, learning from and listening to other health professionals who bring skill and expertise to the care of

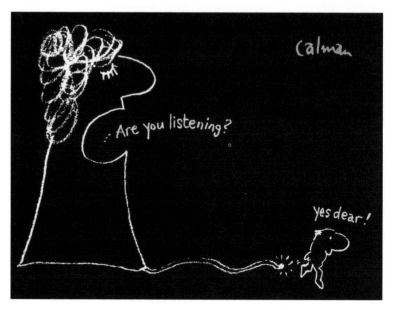

The importance of listening. Patients sometimes shout at us but we don't hear. S & C Calman ©. Reproduced with permission.

patients. Team working is now a part of all specialties, in all settings. Learning together or 'inter-professional learning' will be discussed in a subsequent section of this book but raises a broader issue—that of the boundaries of medicine. This is a concept which can be considered in several ways as described in the introduction to this section.

The aims of the medical Royal Colleges

The original medical Royal Colleges were established between the 16th and 18th centuries. It is instructive to look at their charters in relation to the aims described in this chapter and to consider how they stand up to modern scrutiny.

Royal College of Surgeons of Edinburgh, 1505

"He must be worthy and expert in all the subjects belonging to the said crafts, diligently and knowledgeably examined and admitted by the masters of the said craft...that he know anatomy, the nature and complexion of every member of the human body...for every man ought to know the nature and substance of everything with which he deals, or else he is negligent; and that we may have once a year a condemned man after death to perform anatomy on, whereby we may have experience, each one to instruct others...No masters of the said craft shall take on an apprentice or hired man in time to come to use the craft unless he can both write and read...Beseeching on this account Your Lordships and Wisdoms...that you will take into consideration these our simple desires...and with the Grace of God we shall do such service and favour to the King's Grace and good town that you shall be satisfied of it."[4]

Note the references to understanding disease, standards and in particular to serving the town of Edinburgh.

Royal College of Physicians of London, 1512

"For as much as the science and cunning of Physik and Surgery (for the perfect knowledge whereof be requisite both great learning and ripe experience) is daily within this realm exercised by a great multitude of ignorant persons...Therefore that no person within the City of London nor within seven miles of it should take upon him to "exercise and occupy" as a physician or surgeon except he were first examined, appointed and admitted by the Bishop of London or by the Dean of St Paul's "calling to him or them four doctors of physik and for surgery other expert persons in that faculty".[5]

This was revised on several occasions, and the one in the reign of James II (1686–7) notes 'the public good and common benefit of all our loving subjects' and gives the College 'full and sole power, privilege and liberty and authority and is authorised to write and print books and pamphlets on medicine and surgery".

These early documents note the poor quality of practice 'by the multitude of ignorant persons' and gives the College rights to regulate practice in London and beyond. It should be noted that the formal examination is approved by a lay person, the Bishop, although assisted by doctors. The phrase 'public good and common benefit' is an important one, as is the ability to print books.

Royal College of Physicians and Surgeons of Glasgow, 1599

"James, by the Grace of God, King of Scots...with the advice of Our Council, understanding the great abuses which has been committed in time bygone, and yet daily continues by ignorant, unskilled, and unlearned persons, who under the colour of Chirurgeons, abuse the people to their pleasure, ...it shall not be lawful to any manner of person within the said bounds to exercise medicine, without testimonial of a famous university where medicine is taught...That the said Visitors, their brethren and successors shall convene every first Monday of ilk month at some convenient place, to visit and give counsel to poor diseased folks gratis."[6]

This charter has interesting references to the poor quality of practice, the territorial limits of the new charter, the need for a university degree, and that the poor would be visited and treated gratis. To the present day this last statement ends all meetings of the College Council.

Royal College of Physicians of Edinburgh, 1681

"Charles by the Grace of God of Great Britain France and Ireland...Know ye in as much as we out of our natural goodness and paternal indulgence towards our people...and are most desirous and providently careful not only of the rights properties and passions, and other enjoyments whatever of our subjects be secured and provided for...but also (what is of greatest value to them and most nearly concerns them) their life and health of all external benefits the foundation and subject, should be preserved by God's blessing accompanying the ordinary means, the diligence of honest faithful and approved physicians, and their faithful endeavours to cure and prevent the numerous dangerous diseases incident to human frailty."[7]

Note the comment on prevention and the importance of health.

Royal College of Surgeons of England, 1800

"George the Third, by the Grace of God...and whereas it is of great consequence to the Common Weal of this Kingdom that

> the Art and Science of Surgery should be duly promoted. And whereas it appears to us that the establishment of a College of Surgeons will be expeditious for the due promotion and encouragement of the study and practice of the said art and science...The Oath...that you will diligently maintain the Honour and Welfare of the said College...and act equally and impartially according to the best of your skill and knowledge, So help you God."[8]
>
> Note the reference to the art and science of surgery and the values determined in the oath.
>
> The importance of belonging to a College, Guild or Craft has been noted earlier in this book. The rituals associated with initiation have changed over the years but the power of being part of a professional organisation which conducts and controls standards remains.

THE PROFESSION OF MEDICINE

Over the last few decades much has been written about professions, professionalism and the competence of doctors. This literature takes the aim and roles of medicine and puts them in a broader context of those who practice medicine (the profession), and considers how individual practitioners (doctors) fit into this concept as professionals. The concept of competence will be explored further in the next chapter and will be related to clinical practice.

This section therefore considers three issues. The first is that of quality: how it is defined and possibly measured. The second is the concept of a profession, and that of a professional. Third is a brief discussion on competence and how it relates to the first two topics. Competence, it will be argued, is one of the mechanisms by which quality and professionalism come together in clinical practice; its assessment integrates a complex, real-life, problem-based environment and the ways in which doctors respond to such issues. Finally, there is a summary and discussion on how such issues determine the learning process.

Defining quality

Much of this discussion will relate to the concept of 'quality', a term which is particularly difficult to define.

> *I know there is such a thing as quality, but as soon as you try to define it, it goes haywire and you can't do it.*[9]
>
> Robert Pirsig in *Zen and the Art of Motorcycle Maintenance*

The following definition sets out one way of considering quality:

> *Quality is a concept which describes in both quantitative and qualitative terms the level of care or service provided. Quality therefore has two components. The first is quantitative and measurable, and the second qualitative, though assessable and associated with value judgements. Quality is a relative not an absolute concept.*[10]
>
> Calman, 1992

Quality is therefore not just an analysis of activity in isolation. It must always be described in comparison with something else, either a similar activity or the same activity measured at another time. It also implies measurable consistency, reliability and validity over time. Thus, quality (as a relative concept) can always be improved, and this potential is at the heart of all quality initiatives: the process of continual improvement. It also involves judgements based on experience of similar issues in similar places. Those who regularly visit hospitals, schools and local authorities not only obtain evidence for quality in the form of reports and papers, they can 'feel' quality when present. This subjective approach can often be seen as an internally focused view by doctors based on the erroneous experience elsewhere, but most, including the public, could agree that it is important. In due time there may be better ways of defining this aspect of quality but for the moment these qualitative views remain important.

Quality can be related to the achievement of specific aims, objectives and standards. These standards should not be seen as fixed, as they will inevitably change as medical advances arise and improve the outcome of care. Quality is about doing things right first time and working for continual improvement. There is no 'gold standard', only doing better than you are at present.

The definition of a profession and a professional

Much has been written on this subject over the years, and it is well to remember the article by Burnham in this context.[11] He makes the point that writings on medicine and the profession have been altered by writers to illustrate the ideal and to place the great figures of medicine in the best 'professional' light. In spite of these warnings, the concept of being part of a profession is a powerful one and, in contemporary terms, is exercising much thought. Nineteenth century writers such as Osler would have had no difficulty in discussing and writing about the concept (and did). In more recent years, the subject has generated a spate of papers, conferences and books. This has been helpful in defining the profession and professionalism, and setting the concept in a wider framework. Much of this effort is a search for a new Hippocratic Oath, a statement of beliefs and values which the profession can hold on to.[12,13] Other important recent thinking is listed in the Bibliography.

Some of the work over the last 50 years will be reviewed in the section below, followed by an attempt to bring together the main strands of thinking. This review considers mainly the literature on doctors, but it is recognised that there is a much wider literature on other professional groups, and from different perspectives.

'Towards a definition of a profession'[14]

This paper by M I Cogan in the *Harvard Educational Review* is one of the earliest reviews of the concept of a 'profession'. He takes at first an historical approach and considers a range of definitions of profession, and concludes (as others have) that it is very complex. *Webster's New International Dictionary*, for example, excludes some specific work groups and notes that the word 'profession' is traditionally applied to the 'three learned professions of divinity, law and medicine'.[15] Cogan himself notes that 'it may be observed that the traditional professions mediate man's relationship with God, and man's relationship to man and state, and man's relationship to his biological environment'. Others have broadened the range of activities covered by the term 'profession'. For example, Beatrice Webb (quoted in Cogan) states that there are five classes of professional associations:

1. The learned professions: law, medicine, teaching.
2. Technicians of industry: engineers, architects, chemists, etc.
3. Technicians of the office: accountants, clerks etc.
4. Manipulators of men: managers, foremen etc.
5. Professional artists: painters, musicians, actors, writers etc.

There is a clear hierarchy in the list and this is beautifully illustrated in a quotation in Cogan's paper. It is from the play *Sylvester Dangerwood* by George Colman the Younger:

> *My father was an eminent button maker...but I had a soul far above buttons...I panted for a liberal profession.*

Cogan interestingly cites Flexner, who said that the most important and indispensable criterion of a profession is devotion to the interest of others and a denial of the mercenary spirit. Finally, having reviewed all of this material he gives his own definition:

> *A profession is a vocation whose practice is founded upon an understanding of the theoretical structure of some department*

of learning or science, and upon the abilities accompanying such understanding. This understanding and these abilities are applied to the vital practical affairs of man. The practices of the profession are modified by knowledge of a generalised nature and by the accumulated wisdom and experience of mankind, which serves to correct the errors of specialism. The profession, serving the vital needs of man, considers its first ethical imperative to be altruistic service to the client.

This definition is reflected in many subsequent ones and seems to capture the essence of the concept.

The Boys in White: Student culture in medical schools

This book by Becker and others is one of the earlier sociological studies of a medical school. It follows a group of students through observation and interviews, and records the findings. Carried out in the late 1950s and early 1960s, the study describes the way in which the culture develops and the opportunities, constraints and rites of passage in which 'men turn boys into fellow men fit to be their own companions and successors'.[16] Even 50 years ago there was concern about the quality of entry into medicine: are students of poorer quality or less devoted to their work than previous generations, or are they better?

Several points made are very striking even half a century on. For example, in the following quotations we see how rapidly students become socialised.

1. In spite of all our efforts, we cannot learn everything in the time available.

2. We work just as hard as ever, but now we study in only the most effective ways, and learn only the things that are important.

3. Some students said: We will decide whether something is important according to whether it is important in medical practice. Other students said: We will decide whether some-

thing is important according to whether it is what the faculty wants us to know.[17]

They retain important values:

We have already seen that medical students enter medical school with broad and idealistic concerns. They are not interested in medicine as a way of getting rich; this may be because they feel so sure of doing well financially in medicine…they come in with a complement of ideas about healing the sick and rendering service to mankind. They resent any hints that they may have crasser motives. They are determined to learn all the facts that the medical school can give them, in order that they may do the best possible job of caring for the patients they will later have. They work long hours and are willing to work even longer hours.[18]

In another section the students were asked about their ideal physician:

We supposed that the answer to this question would be likely to provoke materialistic answers: references to large incomes, large houses, and large cars. We erred in making this assumption, for 87% of our 62 interviewees gave answers that could only be categorised as idealistic. They typically spoke of the successful doctor as one who really helped his patients, as a man who worked hard and acquired all the skill and knowledge necessary to give such help.[19]

One of the key conclusions relates to student culture. They worked hard, together, and wanted to do well. They retained, though changed the focus, of their idealistic aspirations. They were able to manage the culture in the medical school and change and adapt to it over the course. They are strongly committed and cannot think of any other career for themselves— the wish to do medicine. They would regard failure as a great disgrace. They regard their teachers as men who really know what is best for them. For this reason the medical student is more likely than any other kind of student to do what his faculty wants him to do and be whatever his faculty wants him to be.

This is a remarkable example of the power of the hidden agenda and of the socialisation of the medical student. This book makes a fascinating read, presenting as it does a snapshot of the life of medical students with some powerful messages.

The Profession of Medicine

This book was written in 1970 by Eliot Freidson. It reviews medicine from a sociological perspective and begins to define the difference between a profession and an occupation, high-lighting autonomy and the right to control one's own work as most relevant. He makes the point (and perhaps an uncomfortable one) that:

> *A profession attains and maintains its position by virtue of the protection and patronage of some elite segment of society which has been persuaded that there is some special value in its work. Its position is thus secured by the political and economic influence of the elite which supports it.*[20]

This is an interesting and relevant comment, as we can see in political regimes across the world, which in a stroke can completely change the professional status of doctors. Freidson also makes the point that:

> *Unlike science and scholarship, which create and elaborate the formal knowledge of civilisation, practicing professions have the task of applying that knowledge to everyday life. Practicing professions are the links between a civilisation and its daily life and as such must, unlike science and scholarship, be in some sense joined to every day life and the average man.*[21]

Freidson then discusses the formal characteristics of a profession, based on the work of Cogan and others, and explores other issues, such as determining its own standards, licensing and admission boards manned by its own members, and being free from lay evaluation.

Physicians for the twenty-first century[22]

This supplement to the *Journal of Medical Education* was published in 1984 by the Association of American Medical Colleges, and is subtitled: *Report of the Project Panel on General Professional Education of the Physician an College Preparation for Medicine.* The project panel offered five major conclusions and a number of specific recommendations for discussion. Those which are particularly relevant to the profession of medicine are summarised here and the report should be consulted for full details.

✦ **Purposes of a general education.**

'In the general education of the physician, medical faculties should emphasise the acquisition and development of skills, values and attitudes by students at least to the same extent as they do acquisition of knowledge'.

'Medical faculties should adapt the general professional education of students to changing demographics and the modifications occurring in the health care system. Future practice will be shaped more by these changes and modifications than by traditional medical care systems of the past three decades.' 'Medical students' general professional education should include emphasis on the physician's responsibility to work with individual patients and communities to promote health and prevent disease.'[23]

✦ **Baccalaureate education.** The key feature here was the need for students to come into medicine with a broad background in the natural and social sciences, and in the humanities. There is also an interesting discussion on the process of selection.[24]

✦ **Acquiring learning skills.** Here the emphasis is on independent learning skills, and allowing sufficient time for reflection. Problem solving should be part of this process, and the evaluation of performance should reflect this. Thus 'the evaluation of students' academic performance should be based on large measure on faculty members' subjective judgements of students' analytical skills rather than their ability to recall memorised information'.[25]

+ **Clinical education.** Much of this section is concerned with evaluation, planning and selecting appropriate settings. There is an emphasis on the integration of educational programmes.

+ **Enhancing faculty involvement.** This is essentially about the organisational setting and the need for mentoring and leadership in staff, at faculty and institutional level.

This thorough review sets the direction of medical education: integrated, concerned with health and illness and with a strong emphasis on leadership.

The Goals of Medicine: Setting new priorities[26]

This important document by the Hastings Center was published in 1996. It was the product of a major international project involving 14 countries. The premise was that the 'ends' and not just the 'means' of medicine are at stake. What is medicine for? Advances in medicine which change the natural history of disease present a double-edged sword: longer lives may come at a price in terms of illness and the costs of treatment and care. The balance is crucial. The project thus tried to set out the goals of medicine: the aims and implications and where to go from here.

The goals are defined as:

+ The prevention of disease and injury, and promotion and maintenance of health.

+ The relief of pain and suffering caused by maladies.

+ The care and cure of those with a malady and the care of those who cannot be cured.

+ The avoidance of premature death and the pursuit of a peaceful death.

These four goals allow a more focused discussion on biomedical research, the design of healthcare systems and how physicians should be trained. It encourages a more epidemiological and public health view of research to provide a broader understanding of diseases in society. Efforts to provide healthcare systems should begin with a 'solid core of primary and emergency care, and consider the needs of society's most frail humans'. Medical students should be taught that death is inevitable and 'that they will not always be able to cure. They must learn to address the problems of chronic illness'. There is a need for a broad education, including such subjects as economics and the humanities.

There is a particularly important conclusion about public health. The report makes the comment that most of the uses of medical knowledge are good, but may be misused. For example 'the use of public health information to justify undemocratically coercing large groups of people into changing their "unhealthy behaviours"' may not be appropriate. The point is also made that at the other extreme, medicine cannot have as a goal 'ultimate well-being', beyond the aim of good health for every individual. Medicine they comment 'is also incapable of determining the overall good for society'.[27]

In looking forward they suggest that medicine as a profession should aspire:

+ To be honourable and to direct its own professional life.
+ To be temperate and prudent.
+ To be affordable and sustainable.
+ To be just and equitable.
+ To respect human choice and dignity.

This report is a most valuable summary of thinking internationally at the end of the 20th century. It contains very useful pointers to the future.

Professing medicine: strengthening the ethics and professionalism of tomorrow's physicians[28]

This volume, published by the American Medical Association (AMA) in 2002, is a series of essays on topics related to professionalism, some written by staff and some by students. It is a commemorative issue of *Virtual Mentor*, the AMA's online ethics journal. It is a fascinating collection, full of personal experiences and old and new wisdom. Much of the volume relates to the issues around the teaching of medical ethics, and the changes over the years. It finishes with a 'Declaration of Professional Responsibility: Medicine's Social Contract with Humanity'.

We, the members of the world community of physicians, solemnly commit ourselves to:

1. *respect human life and the dignity of every individual*

2. *refrain from supporting or committing crimes against humanity and condemn any such acts*

3. *treat the sick and injured with competence and compassion and without prejudice*

4. *apply our knowledge and skills when needed, though doing so may put us at risk*

5. *protect the privacy and confidentiality of those for whom we care and breach that confidence only when keeping it would seriously threaten the health and safety of others*

6. *work freely with colleagues to discover, develop, and promote advances in medicine and public health that ameliorate suffering and contribute to human well-being*

7. *educate the public and polity about present and future threats to the health of humanity*

8. *advocate for social, economic, educational, and political changes that ameliorate suffering and contribute to human well being*

9. *teach and mentor those who follow us for they are the future of our caring profession.*[29]

Medical professionalism in the new millennium: a physicians charter[30]

This document (2002) is the product of the Medical Professionalism Project, brought together by European Federation of Internal Medicine, the American College of Physicians, the American Society of Internal Medicine and the American Board of Internal Medicine. These organisations recognised the need for a renewed sense of professionalism, one that is 'activist in reforming health care systems'. They therefore set up a group to develop a charter to 'encompass a set of principles to which all medical professionals can and should aspire'. The charter is intended to apply to different cultures and systems, and is summarised in the box below.

Medical professionalism in the new millennium: a physicians charter

The fundamental principles

+ The primacy of patients' welfare
+ The principle of patients' autonomy
+ The principle of social justice

A set of professional responsibilities

+ Commitment to professional competence, which includes life-long learning
+ Commitment to honesty with patients
+ Commitment to patient confidentiality
+ Commitment to maintaining appropriate relationships with patients
+ Commitment to improving quality of care
+ Commitment to improving access to care
+ Commitment to a just distribution of finite resources

+ Commitment to scientific knowledge
+ Commitment to maintaining trust by managing conflicts of interest
+ Commitment to professional responsibilities

The charter ends with a challenge to all doctors: 'This Charter on Medical Professionalism is intended to encourage such dedication and promote an action agenda for the profession of medicine that is universal in scope and purpose'.

The Doctors' Tale

Sir Donald Irvine has written widely on the medical profession and professionalism (see the Bibliography). In this book he summarises a long and distinguished career in medicine. At times he is critical of the profession and its inability to change, and he ends his book with a call for a 'new professionalism'.

So how does the new professionalism differ from the old? It starts by recognising the importance of the autonomy of the patient. A sound ethical foundation, scientific and technical competence, the interests of the patient and the notion of service are still fundamental core values. However, it embraces now evidence-based medicine rather than clinical pragmatism, the recognition of the importance of attitudes and behaviour, partnerships with patients, and accountability rather than professional autonomy. At the same time professionalism is about teamwork, rather than individualism, collective as well as personal responsibility, transparency rather than secrecy, empathetic communication and above all respect for others. An unreserved commitment to quality improvement through clinical governance is fundamental.[31]

He finishes this paragraph by returning to Freidson (referred to earlier in this section), who said that medicine must be 'enthused with a spirit of openness, driven by the conviction that one's decisions must be routinely open to inspection and evaluation, like the openness that pervades science and scholarship'.[32] Over this 30-year period we have returned to consider some very basic values.

Attributes of medical graduates

This important paper was published in 2003 by the Australian Medical Council. It covers in list form:

+ knowledge and understanding

+ skills

+ attitudes as they affect professional behaviour.

Most of the list is covered in the publications above, although it is useful to note that it does cover 'systems of provision of health care including their advantages and limitations, the principles of efficient and equitable allocation and use of finite resources'.[33] It emphasises the ability to interpret medical evidence in a critical and scientific manner, and to use libraries and other information resources to pursue independent inquiry relating to medical problems. It refers to a skill, not required by Hippocrates, as 'the ability to appropriately use information technology as an essential resource for modern medical practice'. It recognises the importance of teamwork and the need to prevent one's own personal or religious beliefs from interfering with patient care.

Doctors in Society: Medical professionalism in a changing world[34]

This document published in 2005 is a further major contribution to the debate. The document aims to stimulate debate, and in the summary (p. 56) notes '...our collective and abiding aim is to put medical professionalism back on the political map of health in the UK'.

There is a subsequent paper on this topic as it relates to trainees.[35] The authors emphasise the importance of professionalism.

The profession of medicine, presented in the light of the documents listed above, is seen as positive and a good for society. However, we should not forget that at times professions, and individual professionals, can be arrogant, secretive and exclusive.

Defining a profession: a summary

One way of defining the qualities of a 'profession' is to set out the characteristics which seem to be most appropriate. Using the work cited above, and the paper by Calman (1994)[36], these might include:

+ Medicine is a vocation or calling, and implies service to others. This remains an important part of being a doctor. The wish to be a doctor and to help others may seem old-fashioned in a time of increasing commercialisation in medicine, but it remains central. When we consider how best to select medical students and young doctors for particular specialties this will be an important factor to note.

+ Trust and respect are two key aspects of a profession. The patient and the public must trust the doctor, and there should be mutual respect. These two factors (trust and respect) can be difficult to establish and require considerable care and hard work. They can be easily lost, and in the words of the proverb: 'Trust comes on foot and goes on horseback'.

+ Medicine is an art as well as a science and requires judgement and wisdom to make decisions with patients in the face of uncertainty.

+ Respecting the value of human life. This is an important value. Doctors are in a privileged position which can allow them to take advantage of those who are vulnerable.

+ Maintaining privacy and confidentiality. Those who consult a doctor expect to have their privacy protected and their health information confidential.

- Acting as an advocate for the patient and the public in health-related matters. This is a matter which will be discussed in more detail in a subsequent section. It recognises that the doctor has a role as advocate, supporter, agent for change and educator.

- Medicine has a distinctive knowledge base which is kept up to date. This knowledge base comes from the sciences, arts and social sciences. It is broad and constantly changing. This requires that the doctor must continue to learn and keep up to date.

- Medicine has a special relationship with those it serves, patients or clients, in which trust is important. This is not just a client or customer relationship. It is deeper and grounded in values and based on trust.

- Medicine has particular ethical principles—the ethical base. This is of fundamental importance, and has been central to clinical practice for generations. These are set out in various ways through codes, oaths and sets of principles.

- Setting standards and examinations. This has been a part of professional practice for centuries, set and assessed by the profession. Slowly this will change as the public have a hand in the standards set.

- Medicine is self regulating and accountable to patients, clients and the profession itself. This is perhaps the issue most debated at the present time. How far can the profession continue to be accountable to itself, and how much can it relinquish this to those not part of the profession? The view of this author is that involvement of patients and the public in a tangible way will only strengthen the profession. There is nothing to hide or be afraid of.

- Medicine is open and available for evaluation. This is the corollary to the discussion on self regulation: the need to be open and transparent in relation to outcomes of care and public health practice.

+ Medicine works closely with other professional groups. The importance of teamwork and of recognising the skills and expertise of others is very much part of being a profession and will be discussed in more detail later.

+ Ability to lead and determine direction of the clinical team. This must be earned by the demonstration of many of the qualities listed above.

These then are some of the characteristics of a profession, although there are some who would argue that in the 21st century, medicine is no more than a trade, a series of skills which can be easily mastered and bought at a price. This is not what a profession should be. It has at its core a commitment to people and a strong vocational aspect, without which it would just be another job. It follows from this that respect for the value of human life is a given, as is privacy and confidentiality. Acting as an advocate may seem again to be out of place, but as will be discussed in another section it is increasingly important. Perhaps the most contentious is that the profession should sets its own standards and be self regulating. In the 21st century the public should be part of this, and self regulation could be seen to perpetuate an inward looking club, with no responsibility to the public. But these views are not incompatible with public involvement in such bodies as the General Medical Council and, increasingly, in the Royal Colleges provides a means for such input. Medicine should not be afraid of such ventures as it can only strengthen the profession when those outside see the effort involved. As Freidson noted, medicine should not be 'free of lay evaluation'.

One issue that has exercised the medical profession over the last few years is the use of resources and the role of the doctor as a manager. Today there are even greater managerial pressures on doctors to consider broader issues in healthcare; not just doing their best for an individual patient. How can these factors be resolved in the light of the statements above? Having to deal with finite resources is not a new issue. Doctors have always had to decide how best to use their time and skills. Health care is now so complex that some kind of consideration needs to be given in terms of how overall resources can and should be used. This inevitably leads to a discussion on how the public should be involved in such issues, and the topic then becomes a political one.

The list above attempts to define some characteristics and qualities of the profession, but what about professionals? Clearly they should subscribe to the list of characteristics above; so these then need to be translated into personal values. Such values might include the ability or willingness to demonstrate:

- the clear wish to be a doctor and to see it as a vocation; to be committed
- respect for human life and an interest in people
- care, compassion and concern for patients and the public: empathy
- ethical consideration of all issues
- an interest in health as well as illness
- communication skills and those of advocacy
- the desire to be an educator and advocate of change
- the courage to take difficult decisions
- equanimity in the face of difficult issues and stressful circumstances
- a wish to learn and undertake continuing professional development, to be reflective in practice and learn from experience
- confidentiality and privacy
- an understanding of teams and the value of colleagues in other disciplines
- the ability to analyse and solve complex problems—clinical reasoning
- intellectual resourcefulness and initiative in the handling of unusual or unexpected situations

+ teaching ability—for other professionals, patients and the public

+ a recognition that accountability to patients, the public and the profession are important

+ curiosity and an interest in research and development

+ humility, to recognise when things could have been done better

+ the desire to act as an advocate for health

+ leadership in promoting health.

Such a list can of course be debated, discussed and refined. Its potential value lies in the selection of those who wish to study medicine or who wish to proceed up the career ladder. Such a set of characteristics might be useful in this process and will be discussed later in the section on selection.

THE BOUNDARIES OF MEDICINE

If the aim of medicine is primarily to heal and the role of the doctor is to be an instrument of that healing, how does this relate to other branches of knowledge and other professional groups? What is it that is distinctive about being a doctor? How does medicine fit into the wide range of interests in the arena of health?

Medicine and related disciplines

Perhaps the first (and to some extent the easiest) aspect is the relationship between the science base in medicine and other areas of knowledge. Medicine is not a discrete science and, indeed, it could be said that there is no such thing as 'medical research', only research into medical and health problems. To enhance our understanding of disease and its control requires a very wide range of scientific interests, and there should be no boundaries in this regard. The purely medical role in this relates to direct patient contact and research at the bedside, clinic or operating theatre. But even here, other professional groups may have an equally important role in some aspects of this work. Perhaps of more relevance is the role of the doctor in posing the question and in setting out what needs to be done and how it might influence care. This is not an insignificant role and provides those in close contact with patients and the public with opportunities for identifying new approaches. Similarly, the implementation of new treatments is most likely to be carried out by doctors, though not in all instances.

In a similar way, the social sciences have a huge amount to contribute to our understanding of illness, how people respond and react to bad news and how we can improve the ways in which we can assist the healing process. The arts also have a part to play. There is an increasing interest in the ways in which the quality of life can be modified and improved through music, literature and the visual arts. The humanities allow us to think with a philosophical perspective on ethical issues, the value of life and the nature of human existence (see Bibliography). In one sense this is the justification for basic medical education being carried out in a university setting. It brings medical students into contact with students and staff from other disciplines and broadens their horizons.

Each of these broad areas affects our understanding of people, disease and how we can respond to the needs of patients and the community. In seeking to improve health and well being there are no boundaries and no barriers to searching for solutions, wherever they may be. The unity of knowledge is the important issue, and we should not set up artificial boundaries where none need exist. It follows from this that the doctor is only one part of a broad team seeking new ways to improve health. Medical practitioners have a particular role at the science–patient interface.

Boundaries within medicines

A second and more complex area is the relationship between doctors and other health professionals. The first and most obvious point is that working as a team must be taken as a given. Modern care requires the skills and expertise of many professionals. This is likely to become even more relevant as the complexity of care increases. But what are the distinctive and specific roles of the doctor in the multidisciplinary team? And if there are distinctive features, how does the learning experience assist in developing them? While this latter aspect will be discussed in more detail in a later chapter, some conclusions can be drawn at this stage.

1. **Training.** Doctors generally have longer periods of learning at both undergraduate and graduate levels. The specialty training programmes are comprehensive, organised and associated with regular assessment. Continuing professional development is an integral part of this, and revalidation is an accepted part of professional practice. These factors alone do not make doctors distinctive, but there is generally a difference in the length and breadth of the formal training programme. The educational implications of this conclusion are that at each stage of the process the learning should be relevant and supported. Life-long learning should be recognised from the very beginning as part of professional practice and should not be an 'add-on'. The acquisition of (and the wish to have) the skill to learn is a fundamental part of being a doctor.

2. **The wish to be a doctor and not another type of health professional.** This may seem obvious, but it is highly relevant. People choose to be a particular type of health professional.

3. **Growing role of other health professionals.** Certainly doctors do not have a monopoly on caring and compassion. Nor do they have all the skills of other professional groups:

speech therapists, physiotherapists, pharmacists, nurses, midwives, psychologists and all of the other wide range of expertise available. While they have a special role in treatment, particularly in interventional management such as surgery, other groups have an increasing role. Even in surgery non-medical health care staff are taking a greater role.

4. **The diagnostic process.** However, doctors do have a particular role in diagnosis, and especially in the implications for, and consequences of, whatever label is placed on the problem presented. These labels may change with time, and from the historical review it could be said that 'the history of medicine is the re-classification of disease'. The key issue is the range of uncertainty surrounding a diagnosis. Once the diagnosis is made, then intervention protocols can be set in motion and it is possible that other members of the team will deal with these aspects of care. However, people rarely present with a clear and obvious diagnosis, and tests are not always conclusive and need to be interpreted in the light of the patient's story. There is often doubt and debate about the outcome. To deal with this requires judgement and wisdom, two subjects not easily learned or assessed. In such instances, breadth of experience, a wide vision and the ability to come to a conclusion become crucial. Single diagnostic techniques—blood tests, endoscopies or imaging—do not constitute a diagnosis. They are only part of a wider investigation which must be grounded in listening to the patient. Similar issues surround the investigation of a public health problem. In both, decisions may have to be made on uncertain and inadequate evidence. It is doctors who generally take this broader view and who bring such experience to the making of a diagnosis. The consequences of coming to a diagnosis in such circumstances may also be difficult. What is the patient to be told and when? How do you describe uncertainty and present this in a way which assists the patient or the population to make choices? In

situations which are not black or white, and where there is uncertainty, how are choices presented? With such uncertainty, what is the 'truth'? These are not new issues, and from the point of view of the learning process how is the doctor to be exposed to the ways in which decisions are reached? How is the experience gained? There are several ways in which this can occur, at all levels of clinical practice:

+ Personal experience, and noting and recording the outcome as experience is developed.

+ Observing and reviewing the work of others— apprenticeship.

+ Keeping up to date at seminars, workshops and by reading and reviewing the literature.

+ Continually challenging assumptions and looking for new ways of care.

+ Mentoring is another way in which regular feedback on performance and quality of care can be provided.

5. **Understanding disease and rational treatment.** This is another component of the role of the doctor. It is not sufficient to treat illness without having some form of rationale or paradigm on which to base such interventions. This review has shown that over the centuries the understanding of health and illness has continually changed and is likely to do so again. Treatments which we currently consider sophisticated and avant-garde will in a few years seem crude and old fashioned. The key is that medicine is always changing and it is imperative that doctors are involved in leading such changes. The lessons of **not** changing are very clear to see and will be discussed more fully in the section on 'Beyond learning and innovation'.

6. **Medicine: science or art?** Debate over whether medicine is a science or an art is generations old. In truth it is both. The scientific method allows the maximum to be gained by investigation and examination. The art comes in synthesising

this information in the context of individual patients, their wants and needs, and coming to a shared judgement (with the patient) as to the best way forward. Patients with identical 'diagnoses' may have different 'interventions' based on the judgement at the time.

7. **Other distinctive aspects of being a doctor.** If diagnosis is one distinctive part of the role of the doctor, are there any others? The doctor as a healer has already been discussed. Other professionals are also part of this process: using existing knowledge to improve the care of the patient. A second and related role is keeping abreast of new knowledge and, in particular, to discover new knowledge and use it for the benefit of patients and the community. This is the importance of curiosity, of seeing things differently, of continually questioning conventional wisdom, of understanding disease. This is part of the distinctive role of the doctor, although other professions are heavily involved in research in their own areas of expertise. So how is this aspect of practice to be learned? It must begin at the beginning, in medical school where an atmosphere of inquiry and questioning is the norm. It requires a range of learning experiences to be provided which stimulate original thought and push learning to the limits. As a postgraduate, the learning should be in an environment of checking the evidence, of ensuring that all avenues have been pursued. It means being involved in original work and in writing it up. This is not just about 'publishing or perishing', it is about exercising the imagination and building up expertise and wisdom.

THE DOCTOR IN SOCIETY

This is a subset of the general aim of medicine and the role of the doctor. The doctor is a citizen as well as a physician and, therefore, has an important role in society. Indeed, the doctor may have several different roles.

The advocate

In this role the doctor has a responsibility to put forward the case for the patient or the public, to stand up for them and support their needs. This has been a long-standing role. Over the generations, doctors in various ways have supported the case for better public health, treatment facilities, the needs of patients in particular groups or with particular diseases. Such advocacy may be within a professional setting, in a public forum or in the political arena. It is an important function of the doctor. The actions may be directed at resources required for care or public health measures or greater recognition of special needs and concerns. Other actions might include supporting the rights of prisoners, speaking out against torture or poverty, supporting vulnerable groups, commenting on environmental issues, vaccination, health promotion (cigarette smoking), risks, etc. It is uncomfortable to be in such positions and requires courage to continue the advocacy in the face of significant opposition. All of this may require the doctor to lobby government (local or central), local health or environmental agencies, and to deal with the media. Those who have read Ibsen's *Enemy of the People* will know what this means (see p. 190).

The ability to present the case, to convince the authorities to change, requires special skills of rhetoric and persuasion, and courage. The doctor must believe in the cause and use a variety of methods to bring the issue to the attention of the public.

Of particular concern to the doctor, especially those in public health medicine, is how far the doctor can go with a particular policy if the professional consensus suggests that it may be damaging health, or is providing suboptimal treatment or care. What does the doctor do in such circumstances, other than provide advice and present the evidence to policy makers and the public? One course of action is to resign, not something to consider lightly. However, it may be the only way in which the doctor can reconcile his or her own conscience and ethical views.

The educator

In addition to having a role as an educator (teacher) of students and doctors, there is also a responsibility for the education of patients, the public and politicians. This is a most important role, as without knowledge and the skills to act on this knowledge, patients and the public will have increasing difficulty in making choices. Sources of information on illness and disease have never been easier to get—books, the media including television and the Internet. There is a need for dispassionate advice built on experience, as without this patients and their families will not have what they need to make choices. Doctors have a public role in disseminating information about their special interests. They need skills in public speaking, in explaining and in helping others to understand the possibilities and limitations of procedures and outcome. This is not easy, as the following splendid poem illustrates:

> She asked me if she took one pill for her heart and one pill for her hips and one pill for her chest and one pill for her blood how come they would all know which part of her body they should go to.
>
> I explained to her that active metabolites in each pharmaceutical would adopt a spatial configuration leading to an exact interface with receptor molecules on the cellular surfaces of the target structures involved.
>
> She told me not to bullshit her.
>
> I told her that each pill had a different shape and that each part of her body had a different shape and that her pills could only work when both these shapes could fit together.
>
> She said I had no right to talk about the shape of her body.
>
> I said that each pill was a key and that her body was ten thousand locks.
>
> She said she was not going to swallow that.
>
> I told her that they worked by magic.

She asked me why I didn't say that in the first place.[37]
Glenn Colquhoun, in *Playing God Steele Roberts*,
Aotearoa, New Zealand, 2002

The agent of change

Related to the above discussion is the role of the doctor as an agent of change. This requires the doctor to produce evidence and present it effectively to those who matter. It can be a lonely and a long-term task to change the health of the public. However, it is part of professional practice: whether it is changing the service, improving the quality of care, developing new treatments or improving the health of the public. It requires trust to be established, and an ability to present risk issues in ways which are understandable and help people make informed choices. It also requires the ability to say 'don't know' when there are uncertainties.

The private citizen

Is it possible to separate the doctor as citizen from the doctor as professional? Do the standards of behaviour of a doctor in a professional role differ from those in a 'private' role as citizen? Do we expect higher standards of behaviour in doctors than we would expect from the public generally? Should doctors not smoke or eat too much or be violent to others just because they are doctors? There is little doubt that public expectations are high and that, as with other professional groups, doctors are expected to 'set an example', however unrealistic this may be.

The leader

In many instances doctors are expected to assume positions of leadership, and some preparation for this is essential. This might come from working with other effective leaders, or by learning through experience or relevant courses. The key issue is that leadership needs to be earned and cannot be assumed. To retain the position as leader of a particular team will require more than the title 'doctor'.

SUMMARY AND CONCLUSIONS

The objective of this chapter was to develop a definition of the aim of medicine and to consider its consequences. A secondary aim was to consider the boundaries of medicine and the roles of the doctor, and to define their distinctiveness. It was to investigate why we need doctors.

It was concluded that:

1. The aim of medicine is to assist in the process of healing. Doctors are one of a group of practitioners who have a role in this.

2. Medicine is a vocation and associated with the concept of service.

3. The distinctive features of the medical practitioner are:

   + the wish to be a doctor
   + the length and breadth of the learning process, including an understanding of the determinants of health and the process of disease
   + the ability to deal with the complexity of diagnosis, prognosis and their consequences; as part of this a recognition of the importance of people and the community
   + the experience and skill necessary to deliver a range of interventions, some of which were only performed by doctors
   + a recognition of the need to consider health as well as illness
   + an active approach to continuing learning and revalidation

- ✦ a sense of curiosity and the wish to do things better
- ✦ the development of judgement and wisdom, through experience, and to deal sympathetically with patients and their families at times of uncertainty and anxiety
- ✦ the ability to work in a team and share expertise and skills with others
- ✦ the skill and courage to act as an advocate for health and of change, and to have a role as an educator of patients, the public and the profession.

Such a list is no more than a starter. The work going on in many places represents the beginning of a renaissance in thinking about what medicine is and how it can maintain its high standing in the community. It will only do this by retaining humility and a respect for the views of others. Now is a time for change.

Medical practitioners sometimes suffer from the disease, mural dyslexia—the inability to see the writing on the wall. They cannot see that this is no time for complacency, but for vigorous and positive action. The profession must return to its roots and embrace public involvement as a signal of the determination to act as healers and assist people in need.

REFERENCES

1. The Aphorisms of Hippocrates, Aphorism 1, Translated by Francis Adams. Baltimore: Williams and Williams; 1939.
2. Poynter F N L. Medical education since 1600. In : O'Malley C D. ed. The history of medical education. Los Angeles: University of California Press; 1970; 235–6.
3. Calman K C. Quality of life in cancer patients—an hypothesis. J Med Ethics 1984: 10: 124–127.
4. Charter of the Royal College of Surgeons of Edinburgh, 1505.
5. Charter of the Royal College of Physicians of London, 1512.
6. Charter of the Royal College of Physicians and Surgeons of Glasgow, 1599.
7. Charter of Royal College of Physicians of Edinburgh, 1681.

8. Charter of the Royal College of Surgeons of England, 1800.

9. Pirsig R M. Zen & the art of motorcycle maintenance: an inquiry into values. London: Bodley Head; 1974.

10. Calman K C. Quality: a view from the centre. Quality in Health Care 1992: 1: 28–32.

11. Burnham J C. How the idea of profession changed the writing of medical history. Med Hist Suppl 1999; 43(2): 155–72.

12. Calman K C. A study of storytelling, humour and learning in medicine. London: The Stationery Office; 2000.

13. Tallis R. Hippocratic oaths: medicine and its discontents. London: Atlantic Books; 2004.

14. Cogan M I. Towards a definition of a profession. Harvard Educational Review 1953: XXIII: 33–50.

15. Webster's New International Dictionary.

16. Becker H S, et al. The Boys in White: Student culture in medical schools. Chicago & London: University of Chicago Press; 1961; 4.

17. Ibid, 111.

18. Ibid, 422.

19. Ibid, 429.

20. Freidson E. The Profession of Medicine. New York: Dodd, Mead and Company; 1975; 72.

21. Ibid, 74.

22. Association of American Medical Colleges. Physicians for the twenty-first century. Report of the Project Panel on the General Professional Education of the Physician and College Preparation for Medicine. Washington DC: AAMC; 1984 (Published as supplement to the Journal of Medical Education Vol. 59); .

23. Ibid, 6–5.

24. Ibid, 7–10.

25. Ibid, 11–13.

26. The Hastings Centre. The goals of medicine: setting new priorities. The Hastings Center Report; 1996.

27. Ibid, Executive summary.

28. AMA. Professing medicine: strengthening the ethics of professionalism of tomorrow's physicians. American Medical Association; 2002.

29. Ibid, 131.

30. Medical Professionalism Project. Medical professionalism in the new millennium: a physicians' charter. Lancet 2002; 359: 520-22.

31. Irvine D. The doctors' tale: professionalism and public trust. Oxford: Radcliffe Medical Press; 2003.

32. Ibid, 206.
33. Attributes of medical graduates. Australian Medical Council; 2003.
34. Royal College of Physicians. Doctors in society: medical professionalism in a changing world. Clin Med 2005; 5: Suppl 1.
35. Chard D, Elsharkawy A, Newbery N. Medical professionalism: the trainees view. Clin Med 2006; 6:68–71.
36. Calman K C. The profession of medicine. BMJ 1994; 309: 1140-3.
37. Colquhoun G. Playing God Steele Roberts, Aotearoa, New Zealand; 2002.

12

The quest for competence: defining the professional

First the proper person to judge whether a piece of medical work has been properly done is the same sort of person as is actually engaged on such work, of curing the patient of his present sickness—in other words the medical practitioner himself. And this is equally true of the other skills and empirical crafts. As then it is amongst doctors that a doctor should give account of himself, so also should professional men among their peers.[1]

Aristotle, *Politics*, Book III

Medicine is difficult not only after acquiring all the knowledge, for much skilfulness and long training in the treatment of the sick. That is the physician, after encompassing all of the knowledge mentioned above and establishing it firmly in his memory so that he can recall it easily whenever he wants to, possess the capability to apply all the general laws he knows to individual cases and adjust them to the patient and the treatment.[2]

Ibn Jumay

DEFINING COMPETENCE

*I*n the context of quality and professionalism, why is defining competence so important? What is it for and how does it fit in? Competence can be considered to be relevant to three groups:

+ For the public—to give assurance of the quality of care and public health to be provided.

+ For patients—to ensure individual high quality of care.

+ For the medical profession—as an impetus to maintain high professional standards.

Competence can be recognised as the endpoint of the process of defining quality and of the assessment of the individual doctor as a professional.

What then is competence?

It is the ability of the individual doctor, within the context of a team, to demonstrate the integration, in practice, of a series of characteristics and qualities, and of knowledge, skills and attitudes in improving health and health care. This includes the ability to apply such characteristics to real problems in real time, and assess and present the outcomes. Competence is a measure of quality and of professionalism. It must integrate all of the characteristics and qualities listed in Chapter 11. It is inextricably related to learning and understanding, and to continuing education.

Competence is not something tested like an MOT (from the car road test by the Ministry of Transport). This test assesses the functions of the car under some circumstances but makes no allowances for the complexity of tasks, the uncertainties and problems faced by the doctor.

There is also an assumption that terms such as 'competent' or 'capable' or 'good' are synonymous with infallibility. This is

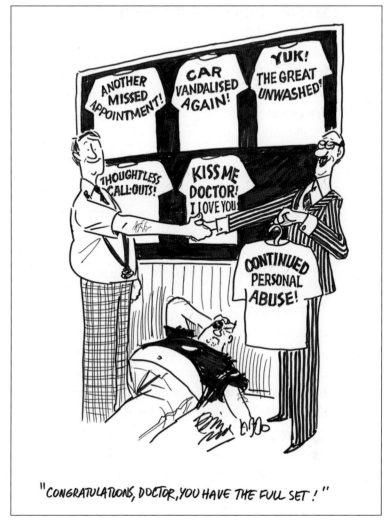

The competences required of doctors at the start of the 21st century as depicted by Bill Tidy. Note there are no clinical skills required, only social ones. By permission of Bill Tidy.

not the case. In issues of uncertainty where judgement is required, it is always possible for errors to be made. There needs to be a system for dealing with such issues and ensuring that they are minimised. There may also be conflicts of opinion between doctors, reflecting different views on complex issues. Such conflicts are no different in other professional groups, such as lawyers, teachers and ministers of religion, and the public need to recognise this. Competence should, therefore, not be equated with infallibility; dealing with complexity and uncertainty will inevitably involve differences of opinion and mistakes. However, systems should be available to reduce these to a minimum. Bad doctors are those who make recurrent errors and should be picked up by such systems. However, this should not be the principal function of formal assessment, which is the regular upgrading of knowledge, skills and attitudes in the majority of doctors.

Competence also varies with time and expertise. The newly qualified doctor will be less 'competent' than an experienced one—hence the need to ensure that assessment takes these factors into account. This relates back to the definition of quality, which addresses the issue of comparisons between different groups.

The assessment of competence is thus based on two assumptions. First, that the vast majority of doctors do an excellent job and wish to continue to improve their performance by learning in a practice-based way, related to particular patient problems, experience of a wide range of conditions and changes in knowledge. The second assumption is that learning leads to changes in knowledge, skills and attitudes, and this results in changes in the management of a particular patient or patient group. This is an important assumption, but one based on a significant amount of evidence: a notable achievement of education.

Words related to competence

In the assessment of competence, a wide range of related terms have been used, each with particular meanings, although these meanings may not always have been well articulated. They include: safe, capable, competent, expert, good, quality, attributes, mastery, effective, performance, outcome-based, problem solving and professionalism. They all mean slightly different things. For example, the 'good' doctor seems to represent more that the 'competent', and may reflect human skills, such as 'bedside manner' and the personal attributes of the doctor.

Some analogies may be useful in this analysis of levels of competence. For example, I might be competent to play 'club' golf, but not 'competition' golf. Similarly, I might be able to play the piano for the family and my own interest in a competent way, but not on the concert platform. Using the word competent, therefore, needs to be qualified by the level of skill and expertise involved. Indeed, even a very competent golfer playing at the highest of levels may have a poor round of golf or miss a shot.

The assessment of competence

What the doctor needs is a range of abilities, some of which are listed below and relate back to the previous discussion on the role of the doctor. It is this range which needs to be assessed. A doctor should be able to:

+ Solve complex problems—there may be no simple solutions and considerable uncertainty.

+ Listen to and interpret what someone else (the patient or population) feels, wants and needs.

+ Integrate knowledge, skills and attitudes in real situations and in real time.

+ Make judgements and take appropriate action in the face of uncertainty and inadequate information, and on the basis of a knowledge base and expertise which changes with time.

+ Demonstrate intellectual resourcefulness and initiative in the handling of unusual and unexpected situations; to be able to work under pressure.

+ Publish outcomes which are seen to be relevant to patients, public and peers, and to one's own self esteem.

+ Continue to learn and change with time and increasing responsibility.

✦ Reflect on practice, outcomes and experience and learn from this.

✦ Consider the ethical implications of making clinical decisions.

Competence always implies feedback on performance (reflection) and completing the loop on a regular basis.

The CanMeds2000 project

The Royal College of Physicians and Surgeons of Canada's 'Skills for the New Millennium' project is an excellent example of defining competence. The project has been taken up and modified by a number of countries, including Australia and New Zealand. The authors of the project report define the essential roles and key competencies as follows:

1. **Medical expert.** Able to demonstrate diagnostic and therapeutic skills for ethical and effective patient care. Access and apply relevant information to clinical practice. Demonstrate effective consultation services with respect to patient care, education and legal opinions.

2. **Communicator.** Establish therapeutic relationship with patients/families. Obtain and synthesise relevant history from patients/families/communities. Listen effectively. Discuss appropriate information with patients/families and the healthcare team.

3. **Collaborator.** Consult effectively with other physicians and healthcare professionals. Contribute effectively to other interdisciplinary team activities.

4. **Manager.** Utilise resources effectively to balance patient care, learning needs, outside activities. Allocate finite healthcare resources wisely. Work effectively and efficiently in a healthcare organisation. Utilise information technology to optimise patient care, life-long learning, other activities.

5. **Health advocate.** Identify the important determinants of health affecting patients. Contribute effectively to improved health of patients and communities. Recognise and respond to those issues where advocacy is appropriate.

6. **Scholar.** Develop, implement and monitor a personal continuing education strategy. Critically appraise sources of medical information. Facilitate learning of patients, house-staff/students and other health professionals. Contribute to the development of new knowledge.

7. **Professional.** Deliver highest quality of care with integrity, honesty and compassion. Exhibit appropriate personal and interpersonal professional behaviours. Practice medicine ethically consistent with the obligations of a physician.[3]

This is an important piece of work and provides a most useful basis for competency assessment. It has been used in the UK to assess surgical trainees.[4] The main themes are reflected in the sections which follow.

Who should assess competence?

This is an important issue: if only doctors assess doctors, those outside the profession might reluctantly conclude that medicine is a closed shop with no room for a wider input. In practice, although much of the assessment is likely to be carried out by doctors, there is growing involvement of other groups, such as other professions (well recognised in specialties such as obstetrics where nursing staff have an important role), patients (through direct involvement and satisfaction surveys; there is much more that could be done here) and the wider public, who are now beginning to make use of published data on outcomes. The profession has nothing to fear from such activities; it can only gain. However, there can be a simplistic view about such assessments which, if not carefully handled, could lead to the drawing of inappropriate conclusions. For example, if the case mix or the age and complicating factors are not taken into account the wrong conclusions may be arrived at. Surgeons in the UK have taken an important lead in this by producing results based on case mix as reported by individual surgeons.[5,6,7,8,9] While the publication of mortality rates from hospitals has been routine in America, it is only in very recent times that this has occurred in Britain, with St George's Hospital in London leading the way. It is important that the profession, in association with managers and other health professionals, take the lead in this area. In 2006, mortality rates for surgeons and hospitals in Scotland were made publicly available.

Revalidation is a subset of this and is the process by which there is a regular review of competence, validated by peers, to give assurance to the public and the profession that individual doctors are up to date, and still learning and modifying practice based on new evidence of effectiveness. This process also needs public scrutiny to make it effective and build up trust.

Assessing competence is not a new issue. For example, Aristotle in Book III of *Politics* writes:

> *First the proper person to judge whether a piece of medical work has been properly done is the same sort of person as is actually engaged on such work, of curing the patient of his present sickness—in other words the medical practitioner himself. And this is equally true of the other skills and empirical crafts. As then it is amongst doctors that a doctor should give account of himself, so also should professional men among their peers.*[10]

In an article on 'The function of praise in the contract of a medieval public physician', which looks at the history of contracts between the civil authorities and doctors, drawing on Greek and Roman experience, Sistrunk writes:

> *Roman policy makers faced the same basic problems that the Greeks had encountered before them. How could they develop a meaningful mechanism to evaluate the proficiency of a member of a profession that possessed a specialised*

knowledge beyond the ken of the uninitiated? Or, to put it more simply, how could lawyers recognise expertise outside their own province?

The Romans found, as the Greeks had, that the most practical way to discover whether or not an applicant was qualified for a civic position was by the hazy criterion of public renown. In the absence of any professional licensing body, the Romans had to rely on the good reputation of the physician and to determine this they utilised the testimony of teachers, friends and grateful cities as well as public contests…and to choose men to whom they must entrust themselves and their children when ill.[11]

An interesting and contemporary view in some ways. We now have a licensing system, and our patients still trust us and are our greatest allies. If we involve them more then trust will build. The quotation from the 20th century novel *Mona Maclean*, noted in Chapter 6, fits well here. She comments that one of the reasons for becoming a doctor is to know to whom to refer one's friends.

Patients and the assessment of competence

In the early 1800s, Robert Owen was piloting a new way of changing the quality of life in a population by providing work, education, food and board, and a moral approach in the model community of New Lanark, some 30 miles south of Glasgow in Scotland. The work consisted mainly of weaving, and as a way of monitoring the moral charter of the weavers, Owen located a small coloured cube at each loom. The colours from white to black signified the moral charter of each weaver. Each Monday he changed the colour for each worker, depending on his assessment of the worker's character, and this was on public display. He notes that over the years the colours changed from dark to light with the impact of work, education and religion.

The author of this book has often wondered if this might be a useful way of patients recording their satisfaction when leaving a consultation. They could change the colour on a cube outside the office and let other patients see their estimate of value.

The assessment of competence is essentially one of the management of complexity. It is relevant to all professional groups, not just medicine. If you try to examine competence in a formulaic way over several different grades of doctor (student, trainee, specialist, general practitioner, etc.), with 40-plus specialties and a wide range of knowledge, skills and attitudes required, it becomes almost impossible. There are too many categories, too many subsets and the process is probably too restrictive. Even if each category and specialty had its own defined competencies, it remains very complicated for patients and the public to follow. A new paradigm is required to deal with this complexity.

THE NEW PARADIGM

This paradigm is based on an analysis of the doctor's work pattern and the decisions that need to be made in dealing with problems in clinical or public health practice. It would be the same process with any other professional group. The key is making records of outcome of care available to peers and the public, together with a clear process for dealing with the most common conditions met by the doctor. An explanation of how such data are derived is essential. This will allow comparisons to be made with other groups and individuals of equivalent status. It must be acknowledged in this model that variations will exist and, as has been said already, that doctors are not infallible. However, a commitment to the public presentation of results should ensure that such variations will be minimised. Patient preferences, choices and case mix must also be taken into account, as these may vary and may not fit into patterns, and may be the cause of such variations.

The paradigm is a essentially a problem-based approach in which the doctor has to make a diagnosis, consider the prognosis and possible active management, while at the same time deal with the individual concerns of the patient.

In dealing with an individual patient who seeks help, the following questions might be asked:

1. What is the problem? Can I come to a provisional diagnosis? Do I need further investigations to be carried out?

2. Can I deal with it? Am I familiar with this problem, or do I have the capability to deal with it if it is a new one? If not, should it be referred elsewhere?

3. What will happen to the patient? What is the natural history or prognosis of this problem? What will happen if I do nothing in the way of active treatment?

4. Is this likely to be a one-off episode or will continuing care be required over a long period?

5. What will I discuss with the patient? Have I kept the team informed? Are there ethical issues involved?

6. Do I need the assistance of the wider team? Do I need further help in diagnosis, investigation and management? Should it now be referred elsewhere?

7. How should the problem best be managed? If active management is to be considered, what is the evidence base?

8. What happened to the patient? Do I have a good record of care? Can I assess the outcome of care?

9. What can I learn from this problem? Could I have done it better? The CPD component.

10. Can my peers and the public have access to my record of care?

Such a list can be matched by that of the patient who will want to know:

1. What is wrong with me? The diagnosis.

2. What does this mean for me? The prognosis.

3. What can you do for me? The treatment.

4. What if the treatment is not successful or not available? Will you still care for me?

5. What can I do to help? The need for personal involvement.

A similar list can be drawn up to cover public health issues. See the box below for some examples to illustrate these principles, and the public presentation of data.

Examples

Patient 1: a young man of age 14, presents to the general practitioner with right-sided abdominal pain and fever. The story in this instance is probably concluded at stage 2 listed above, and the patient is referred to hospital. The outcome will be noted some days later when the GP can confirm, or otherwise, that the patient had an acute appendicitis, the probable diagnosis. If it turns out to be something different (e.g. early Crohn's disease), this is not a mistake but an appropriate referral from which learning can occur. The key is closing the loop on the issue, and in this instance there may be a significant learning experience.

Patient 2: a 45-year-old woman presents to the breast clinic with a 2 cm lump in the left breast. There is a clear protocol to be followed, and this is explained to the patient and her partner. She agrees, and further discussion takes place between the patient and the nurse counsellor. The patient is admitted the following day for a biopsy; the result is positive and the patient informed. Following further discussion, the patient does not agree to go ahead with the standard treatment but requests a further opinion. This is arranged and the patient transferred elsewhere. The opportunity to discuss this is taken at the next meeting of the team, and arrangements are made to obtain information on follow-up to learn from the process. This could be marked as a failure to complete a patient protocol, and the doctor could be seen to be at fault. This is not the case if it is seen as the proper exercise of patient choice.

> **Patient 3**: a 65-year-old man presents to his general practitioner with a recurrent cough. He is a heavy cigarette smoker. A provisional diagnosis of chronic bronchitis is made and he is started on antibiotics. The doctor considers the question of lung cancer, but as it is the third patient with a similar problem seen that day she decides not to request a chest X-ray at this stage. The patient returns 10 days later with no change in his condition, and on this occasion he is sent for an X-ray which returns one week later showing a suspicious lesion. The patient is told and referred to a specialist unit. One week later the patient is admitted and the diagnosis confirmed. The following day the patient's son arrives at the surgery to complain about the delay in treatment. A perfectly reasonable decision was made by the doctor, but it could have been different.

How then do we measure competence? Competence is measured by the ability to put into practice the knowledge, skills and attitudes which have been learned and understood. It is this integration in practice which is the crucial part, not simply the acquisition of knowledge and skills. The integration occurs in two contexts:

1. Process—how the care is delivered, attitudes to patients, etc.
2. Outcomes—audit of the clinical and public health outcomes.

In essence, however, it is learning which is at the heart of this. Learning implies not only the acquisition of knowledge and skills, but their understanding and the ability to put them into practice.

Thus, competence can be measured in several ways:

+ Appraisal interview and review of practice—the professional input.
+ Satisfaction of patients—the patient input.
+ Publication of outcomes—the public presentation.

In setting this out in practice, some or all of the following may be helpful. This is not intended as a complete list but one for debate and discussion, and it is likely to vary from specialty to specialty.

1. A clinical record system to document patient records and outcomes.

2. Identification of major procedures, diseases, etc. seen by the clinician or unit: for example, to list the 5–10 commonest issues dealt with.

3. Available guidelines, frameworks or standards for each of the above. These may vary according to patient choice and should include procedures for follow-up if appropriate.

4. Audit procedures in place to monitor quality. These should be available for peer review.

5. Documentation of all new procedures introduced, with evidence of evaluation available. Research and development and the continuing improvement in practice are key components of high-quality medical care.

6. Demonstration of patient involvement in the work of the unit. This might range from the provision of information and participation groups to regular patient surveys.

7. Staff appraisal to give feedback on performance.

8. Documentation of educational programmes available and evidence of participation.

9. Teamwork. Evidence of involvement of other professional groups in the work of the unit.

10. Management of resources. Clinical work inevitably involves the use of resources. Evidence should be presented on how such resources have been managed.

With these factors as a basis for discussion, what are the kinds of questions which might be taken forward at an appraisal interview?

1. In the context of the process of delivering care:

   ✦ What are the major changes in practice, if any, over the past (year)? What have been the major developments in the subject? How have they influenced practice? These questions assess awareness of recent developments and their impact on personal practice.

   ✦ What CPD activities have been undertaken, and what if anything has changed in practice as a result?

   ✦ What changes have there been in the management of the delivery of the service? For example, changes in out-patients activities have been changed, changes to follow-up of patients, etc.

2. In the context of measuring the outcome of care and the integration of the factors above:

   ✦ How are outcomes measured in the major clinical issues noted above?

   ✦ How is patient input assessed?

Competence is thus the endpoint of a process by which the quality of the individual doctor is assessed in practice. This naturally relates to the concept of a profession and a professional. A profession is thus defined by the characteristics and qualities listed in the previous chapter. A professional is a person who meets these criteria AND who can demonstrate this through the assessment of competence.

Such a definition does not mean that mistakes will not be made (they will) or that behaviour and attitudes will be perfect on all occasions (they will not). What it does mean is that the doctor will recognise such problems, rectify them where possible, and learn from them. With experience and continual learning, the frequency of such problems will reduce, but can never be zero. When the range of problems is larger than expected as compared to peers, or where there is a particular problem which is not being dealt with by the individual, then more effective action will be required by the individual or appropriate professional body.

CULTIVATING A GOOD DOCTOR

The major theme which runs through this book is that education is at the heart of the process of developing the doctor. In searching for a way of describing this process, the horticultural analogy was identified, and the word cultivation substituted for education in order to assist in illuminating the way in which doctors learn. The whole phrase, 'cultivating a good doctor', is of significance; each word is important and will be examined separately (though not in order).

First then consider the word 'doctor'. What do doctors do? This has been a theme throughout the book and might best be defined as follows. Medicine is a profession practised by doctors. It draws its knowledge, skills and attitudes from the sciences, social sciences and the arts. It is thus both an art and a science. It deals with all aspects of healing, health and illness in populations and individuals, and is part of a long tradition of healing. Within this wide domain, doctors may specialise in one or other branches of professional practice. As it is a profession, medicine has a special relationship with patients and the public. It has a strong value base, and the practice is infused with ethical principles. There is an important international dimension to the concept of a medical profession. The other characteristics of a profession are listed in Chapter 11.

Note that the second word is 'a' not 'the' doctor. This implies that each doctor is a unique individual and requires individual cultivation. Not all doctors will be the same, nor would it be desirable to have a series of clones of the 'ideal' doctor. Each 'seed' representing the individual doctor will grow differently depending on the environment and the learning experiences encountered. Such experiences can be shaped and modified to expose the doctor to different influences, and cultivation can influence the basic genetic material. Mentoring is one way in which the cultivation is improved.

The third word to consider is 'cultivating': this signifies growth, tending, care and development by labour and skill. This is the process of education. It begins with the young plant—tending and nurturing it, providing nourishment and different conditions within which to grow and flourish. These influences are not just in the medical school or in practice, but in the home and school, among friends and outside interests. These are all relevant in shaping and cultivating the individual doctor. Sometimes pruning will be required as medical knowledge and skills are replaced by new developments and interests. Growth is an inevitable consequence of proper cultivation and one which lasts throughout the whole lifetime of professional practice. Even the most experienced doctor needs cultivation. The contribution by the medical system to cultivate the doctor is nicely summed up by Shakespeare in *Macbeth*: 'Welcome hither. I have begun to plant thee and will labour to make thee full of growing'.

There is another interpretation of the word 'cultivation', rather more old-fashioned and not used often. It refers to the person who is educated and who continually improves the mind by study and learning. It is a word which Osler would have recognised. This interpretation remains relevant to the doctor and is the internal and personal equivalent of the external cultivation by others, and is equally important.

In more conventional terms, medical education is the process by which those intending to practise, or who are already in clinical or public health work, learn the skills, knowledge and attitudes required to practise medicine. It is a continuing process, and this is one of the important characteristics of the medical profession.

Much more difficult to define is the word 'good'. It is a value-laden word and depends on whom one asks and which characteristic of the doctor is being examined. Several other words or phrases have been used in similar ways. These might include 'competent' or more interestingly, 'the kind of doctor I would go to'. How are such doctors recognised? And if they can be recognised, how can all doctors be 'cultivated' to achieve the same accolade? Does the characterisation 'good' depend on who makes the judgement? Is it the doctor, the patient or the public?

The process by which such value judgements are made is complex and not easily analysed. This chapter has tried to define competence in a way which assists this discussion, but it is likely that newer and better ways will be found. We must continue to cultivate our thinking on this matter.

SOME CONCLUSIONS

Defining competence is not easy. It boils down to an assessment of the ability of the doctor to practise to high standards on a day-to-day basis. By defining qualities, characteristics and processes rather than detailed targets, the method can be adapted to different circumstances and different specialties. It is predicated on the publication of both processes and outcomes for the consideration of other professionals and the public. The public must trust doctors and (based on the aim of medicine described in the previous chapter) the assessment of competence is the endpoint of the process which is publicly driven. It also allows doctors to know whether or not they are doing a good job.

REFERENCES

1. Aristotle, Politics. Book III. Translated by Barker E. Oxford: Oxford University Press; 1940; 125.
2. Jumay I. Treatise to Salah ad-din on the revival of the art of medicine. Translated by Hartmut Fahndrich. Wiesbaden: Kommissionsverlag Franz Steiner GMBH; 1983; 13.
3. The Royal College of Physicians and Surgeons of Canada. Skills for the New Millennium. Royal College of Physicians and Surgeons of Canada; 2000.
4. Rowley D I. The surgeon's job: how should we assess the trainee? J Roy Soc Med 2004: 97: 363–65.
5. Baxter N N. Monitoring surgical mortality. BMJ 2005; 330; 1098–99

6. Thompson A M, Stonebridge P A. Building a framework for trust: critical event analysis of deaths in surgical care. BMJ 2005; 330: 1139–43.

7. Bridgewater B. Mortality data in adult cardiac surgery for named surgeons: retrospective examination of prospectively collected data on coronary artery surgery and aortic valve replacement. BMJ 2005; 330: 506–510.

8. Keogh B E, Dussek J, Watson D, Magee P, Wheatley D. Public confidence and cardiac surgical outcome. BMJ 1998; 316: 1759–60

9. Treasure T. Mortality in adult cardiac surgery. BMJ 2005; 330: 489–90.

10. Aristotle. See Reference 1.

11. Sistrunk T G. The function of praise in the contract of a medieval public physician. J Hist Med Allied Sci 1993: 48: 320–34.

13

The selection of medical students

He never showed signs of a lively imagination, nor of a quick intelligence you find in some; but these were qualities which lead me to foresee that his judgement would be strong, a quality essential to the exercise of our art...eventually after much hard slog, he succeeded in graduating with glory; and I can say without vanity that, in his two years on the benches, no candidate has made more noise than he in the disputes of our school. He has made himself formidable, and no thesis can be advanced without his arguing the opposite case to its ultimate extreme.[1]

Molière, *Le Malade Imaginaire*. M. Diafoirus speaks of his son
the doctor

For a man to be truly suited to the practice of medicine he must be possessed of a natural disposition for it, the necessary instruction, favourable circumstances, education, industry and time. The first prerequisite is a natural disposition, for a reluctant student renders every effort vain.[2]

Hippocrates

INTRODUCTION

One of the most contentious issues in medicine at the present is how to choose medical students. But it is not a new issue; the Egyptians and the Greeks were concerned about it. In the early days, a commitment to medicine and a wish to learn were the key issues. There were few constraints in terms of numbers, and until the 18th century the classes were small and selection limited perhaps to a bachelor's degree in the arts or, in many instances outside the university centres, little in the way of book learning. By the 18th century the classes had become large, often attracted by a particular lecturer or professor (the 'medical magnet'). As this was mainly a system of teaching with limited bedside or laboratory experience, the need to limit numbers was less important. However, with the rise of scientific knowledge, an expanding knowledge base and a need for clinical teaching and laboratory work, some form of selection became necessary. As fees were essential, only those who could afford it were likely to be considered and entrance was subject to an increasing list of requirements. These included a range of subjects to be passed at school level, which might include the sciences and the classics.

Until the beginning of the 20th century, many medical schools required a bachelor's degree in the arts, which in Scottish universities would include logic, rhetoric and moral philosophy.[3] The loss of an arts degree as a preliminary to medicine was regretted by many. For example, in an emotional plea to medical students at an Introductory Address made in 1870 at the University of Glasgow, Professor Young said:

> *Time was when MD presupposed the possession of the degree of BA; the abolition of this halting point is by many, as by myself, regretted; its restoration, let us hope will not be long delayed...If the Medical Council replaced Latin and Greek with French and German, the acquaintance of the profession generally with contemporary Continental discoveries and modes of thought would be increased.*[4]

However, as the range of those wishing to study medicine increased, as grants became available and the number of medical schools increased, a real surplus of those wishing to study medicine developed: in many cases 10 applications or more to one place. It is in this light that the following discussion is placed.[5–10] In the context of the early 21st century, with a surfeit of candidates to study medicine, how can appropriate selection be achieved? The specific issue of women in medicine is important. In UK medical schools it is not unusual for over 50% of entrants to be women. The careers of such women are increasingly well documented[11] as are remaining difficulties.

THE CHARACTERISTICS OF A PROFESSIONAL

In an earlier chapter the aims of medicine were set out, and subsequently the characteristics of a professional were defined. These are listed again below:

+ The wish to be a doctor and to see it as a vocation, to be committed.

+ A wish to learn and to undertake continuing professional development.

+ Respect for human life and an interest in people.

+ Care, compassion and concern for patients and the public—empathy.

+ Ethical consideration of all issues.

+ To be interested in health as well as illness.

+ Communication skills and those of advocacy.

+ Courage to take difficult decisions.

+ Equanimity in the face of difficult issues and stressful circumstances.

+ Confidentiality and privacy in work.

+ An understanding of teams and the value of colleagues in other disciplines.

+ Ability to analyse and solve complex problems—clinical reasoning.

+ Intellectual resourcefulness and initiative in the handling of unusual or unexpected situations and work under pressure.

+ Teaching ability.

+ Accountability to patients, the public and the profession.

+ Curiosity and an interest in research and development.

+ Humility and the ability to recognise when things could have been done better.

+ An advocate for health.

+ To be a leader in promoting health.

As in previous discussion in other chapters, we need a range of types of doctor and thus a range of qualities. This should be borne in mind in relation to selection.

There are two fundamental questions which arise from such a list:

1. Is it possible to assess such characteristics or qualities in candidates age 18–19?

2. Can such characteristics be learned or are they fixed by the genes or by personality, and thus cannot be acquired?

A further problem of selection arises because of public concerns about the quality of doctors. In addition, because of the large numbers applying for medical school or into particular specialities, there is a need to make choices. It is instructive to take each of the issues listed above and test them against the two questions.

The wish to become a doctor. This is one of the most longstanding criteria, from Hippocrates onwards. It is well illustrated in the *Boys in White* study referred to in an earlier section.[12] Above all, if the person does not wish to be a doctor or a specialist, or follow some other branch of medicine, that individual is likely to become frustrated and not perform at his or her best. But how does one test the strength of commitment? Asking at interview or in written form allows the truth to be easily manipulated. Some evidence of an understanding of medicine might assist: placements in hospital or in the community, visits to surgeries and clinics, and evidence in the student's response. Certainly, there should be some evidence of thought as to what being a doctor means. However, like many of the issues to be discussed, this may disadvantage those who have difficulty in gaining such experience due to family background, lack of funding or opportunity. This will need to be taken into account. The fact remains that if the individual does not wish to be a doctor and enters the profession because of parental pressure or other reasons, disappointment is likely. But it is also possible that someone who has not thought about medicine can and will grow to love it. However, with the pressure on places, it is perhaps best to select those who have made an active choice.

The wish to learn. Learning medicine is a life-long process. It requires acceptance of the responsibility to continue to learn and, as we discussed at the beginning of this book, to develop a love of learning. The student and doctor need to be able to see the value in such learning and its impact on the care of patients. But the question again arises: how can this be assessed? The proxy is the ability to pass examinations and get good results. This demonstrates ability but not necessarily the wish to learn. It can also disadvantage those who have not had appropriate learning experiences in school or college. Much experience has shown that academic ability is important but not necessarily the only criterion. In his essay on the Masterword in Medicine, Osler sets out the importance of 'work' in the career of the doctor.[13] This is another component of the wish to learn. Many of the articles cited in previous chapters have argued for a 'balanced education' prior to entering medicine. By this is meant that the entry qualifications should not all be in science.

Respect for human life and an interest in people. This is more difficult to assess from a written statement or at interview. The ability to converse, meet people and interact is important but again will disadvantage those whose experience is limited. Evidence of work in the community in youth organisations or in school activities would suggest that they can meet others and be part of a team. Can such skills be learned? The answer is probably yes.

Care, compassion, concern and empathy. This is such an important part of being a doctor that there needs to be some assessment of the student's ability. But how, and can it be learned? At the age of 18 or 19 this is an extraordinarily difficult aspect of life to assess and will depend of life experiences to date, family background and values. These may not have been articulated at home or in school (why should they have been?). How can they be evaluated on paper or brief interview? Perhaps this can be done in a qualitative way by interview as a subset of ability to communicate. The contention is also that it can be learned by working with a master and a team during which the hidden agenda of medicine becomes clear.

Ethical issues. The same can be said for ethics. Students may not have been exposed to such issues, though they are likely to have come across some of the dilemmas in medicine through the media. They will learn much more during the medical course and begin to develop an awareness of their own values and beliefs. They will learn to argue the case for a particular view and understand when others disagree. However, it is difficult to assess at the start of a career though it might be possible to structure questions which would allow discussion of such issues.

Be interested in health as well as illness. This is very difficult to assess other than in a superficial way. It is part of the learning experience, which will demonstrate this and show its value.

Communication skills and advocacy. Of all of the criteria which relate to medicine, this is the one which patients and the public comment on most. Why can't doctors communicate properly? Why can't I understand what they mean? Why do they treat me in such an off-hand way? These comments and many others put communication skills at the top of the agenda. The question is whether or not it is an innate ability or can be learned? There is good evidence that it can be made better and is something which can be learned.[14] So how can it be assessed at interview and at admission? The answer is probably with difficulty, and assessments are likely to favour those whose family background encourages discussion, debate and conversation. The use of non-medical members of admission panels can add a different dimension to the process and is likely to exclude people, rather than include them. This may be one way of reducing numbers. As an aside, the textbook of clinical skills used by the author of this book contains the following advice on communication—not necessarily to be followed:

> *The interrogation of the patient. The object of interrogation is to elicit information regarding the patient's present illness, the state of his previous health and that of his family. The interrogation must be patiently carried out, the patient being allowed, as far as possible, to tell his story in his own words. One patient is a good witness and another poor. One gives an excellent history. Another has to have the history of his illness dragged out of him by methods of slow extortion, and even then a great deal of what he says may prove irrelevant. Some patients may seem quite unable to give any precise account of what they feel to be wrong. This may be due to stupidity or to the effects of disease on their mental faculties.*[15]

The courage to make difficult decisions. This is one of the key functions of the doctor. The ability to prioritise, identify the issues and act in the most appropriate way. In a clinical setting this can range from triage in an accident and emergency department to the care of those seriously ill and dying. This is not something that can be readily assessed at entry to medical school, but is relevant at specialty training level.

Equanimity. In his great essay on this subject, Osler describes equanimity as the ability to remain calm and in control when everything else is in chaos, or when there are moments of great tension or stress.[16] Equanimity is one of the hallmarks of the medical leader: no panic, just clear and effective action. The assessment of this in medical students is almost impossible unless they are faced with a significant challenge, or perhaps placed on an adventure course with others and evaluated in this light.

Confidentiality and privacy. This could be raised at interview but it is something which is learned and part of professional practice.

Working in teams. As medical practice has developed, so working in teams becomes the norm. Doctors will be part of a team and may lead the team. Assessment of this in the student might focus on teamwork in school or leisure activities. Doctors need to be able to recognise the skills of others. Much of this can be learned, and the experience could be assessed at the time of admission.

Ability to analyse and solve complex problems. This is at the heart of what doctors do and is sometimes referred to as clinical reasoning. It can be assessed in various ways, such as puzzle solving or the use of games. It is a function of the intelligence of the individual (not the knowledge base) and could therefore be used to identify those whose educational experience may not have been optimal but who still demonstrate potential.

Ability to work under pressure and handle unusual and unexpected situations. This could be assessed by reference to past experience, or the use of a test of rapid thinking by giving the student, for example, a short time to make a response to a problem or to a written question.

Teaching ability. The doctor as the teacher and educator is a concept which has been raised in a previous section. It is part of the ability to communicate and is something which can be learned and improved on.

Accountability to patients, the public and the profession. This is part of professional practice and cannot be assessed at the beginning of a career. There is also a managerial component related to the use of resources and a strategic view of the clinical service.

Curiosity and an interest in research and development. This is another aspect of medicine which is of fundamental importance. Its assessment at the level of the medical student will not be about medical research (though that might be touched on at interview) but about what interests them, what makes them excited, their hobbies, wider interests and involvement. How curious are they about the world? Do they question things and ask for explanations? This can be assessed at interview and can lighten up an individual who might then talk about their real interests.

Humility. This was raised as a characteristic and quality of a professional in that it showed the ability to recognise the possibility of being wrong, and the potential to do better. It is the ability to reflect on practice and oneself, and explore improvement. It is not easy to assess but can be probed by asking what individuals are most, and least, proud of.

Advocate for health. This characteristic relates to the ability to represent patients and the public in the wider public arena, to support the need to improve health and to speak up for those who are vulnerable. It would be difficult to assess at the very early stages of a career in medicine, other than via communication skills.

Leader in promoting health. Leadership is an important part of being a doctor. However, at this stage in the career, it is difficult to evaluate. There will be some proxy measures that can be assessed, such as leadership in school or community activities, awards for such activities and public recognition of achievements.

SELECTION: SOME ALTERNATIVES

The relevance and importance of selection have been emphasised, and the ability to assess those entering medicine has been related to the characteristics and qualities defined in previous sections. The process is not an easy one: so what are the alternatives?

There could be a case raised for 'not bothering': accept everyone who wants to do medicine in the first year of the course and weed them out at a later date. This happens in some countries. However, it is expensive and may raise false hopes of selection. As a method it would only be suitable for a first year which is classroom-based and does not involve community or clinical involvement as most courses now do.

A second mechanism is to place all those who wish to be a doctor into a general course for all health professionals, with some form of selection being undertaken early on in the course. This is certainly possible, but one of the main motivating factors for doctors is to be a doctor, and this may discourage entry to such a course, though it is a valuable route to explore.

A third possible mechanism is graduate entry to all programmes. This would show that the individual was capable of learning and was motivated to do additional training to be a doctor. It would provide greater opportunities to test other skills and experiences, including curiosity, communication skills and a wider interest in medicine. Another advantage is that a wide range of graduates from backgrounds in the arts, social sciences and science can be admitted to medicine. If this became restricted to only science graduates it would remove some of the interesting benefits. Graduate entry programmes therefore have considerable advantages. However, there are some downsides. The course will generally be longer in total and the cost higher. Another major drawback is that there is still likely to be an issue of selection if there are more applicants than places; some form of assessment of ability and qualities for entry to medicine will still be necessary. Graduate entry programmes reduce the requirements for selection but do not eliminate them. An interesting paper by Eva et al reports on a pilot programme of mini-interviews consisting of 10 short objective structured clinical examination (OSCE) type stations with scenarios that require applicants to discuss a health-related issue. Both examiners and applicants thought this was useful and the concept could be developed further (see later).[17]

The Council of Deans of Medical Schools in the UK (2004) has produced a statement of principles for selection to guide the process.[18] These include, in summary:

+ Selection for medical schools implies selection for the medical profession. Fitness to practice must be considered.

+ Identification of core academic and non-academic qualities of a doctor.

+ A high level of academic attainment will be expected.

+ The practice of medicine requires the highest standards of professional and personal conduct.

+ The practice of medicine requires the highest standards of professional competence.

+ Candidates should demonstrate some understanding of what a career in medicine involves and their suitability for a caring profession.

+ The selection process should be transparent and involve procedures that respect obligations under relevant diversity and equality legislation.

+ The primary duty of care is to patients. For example, there will be a need to comply with health and safety regulations and consider health conditions of the students.

+ Failure to declare information that has a material influence on a student's fitness to practise may lead to termination of their medical course.

Searching for the evidence that selection processes do indeed result in an appropriate outcome is more difficult. Turnbull et al considered evidence from the University of Adelaide which included an oral assessment process and improving equity of access. They found positive outcomes with the methods used.[19]

There is also an important question as to who should select medical students, and doctors as their careers progress. As far as medical students are concerned, experience of lay members of the public being involved in the process can be found in a

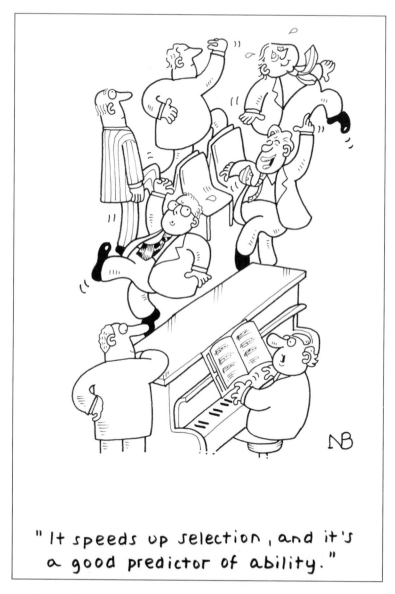

"It speeds up selection, and it's a good predictor of ability."

Another method of selection, faster than selection panels and assessment boards. By permission of Neil Bennett, published in *The Times*.

number of places such as Newcastle, Australia and Durham, England.[20] This has proved to be a useful way of providing a different view, and it ties the local community into the medical school. As careers progress, there is a greater degree of outside scrutiny of appointments, with external assessors and lay representatives. This should generally be a good thing.

SELECTION: A SUMMARY FOR MEDICAL STUDENTS

Having reviewed the information how can we best proceed? First, the graduate entry programmes can assist but do not eliminate the assessment process. Of the characteristics set out above, some can be assessed on paper, some at interview and some with additional techniques. Much will depend on the resources available, the student population and the experience of admission staff. Below are the characteristics of the doctor, divided into groups in order to assist the process:

A written statement. It should be possible to assess:

+ educational attainments

+ experience of the health sector

+ evidence of outside activities, team working and leadership.

The interview. It should be possible to assess:

+ the wish to be a doctor, motivation

+ the wish to learn

+ outside interests, curiosity, communication skills

+ interest in people, work in teams, leadership

+ ability to deal with crises (equanimity), to learn lessons from experience (reflective practice) and humility.

These issues could be developed further using the OSCE-type approach discussed above. This would allow a structured approach to the assessment and provide opportunities to raise some of the issues listed above. There is a cost to this, but an improved outcome would be worth the additional outlay.

Other mechanisms. If facilities are available, there could be team-working exercises, assessment of problem solving and analytical skills, and ability to communicate.

What cannot be assessed. There is a range of other qualities and characteristics which cannot be assessed in this way and which must be learned during the educational process or become part of professional practice.

What really matters? At the end of this process some things really matter:

+ a real wish to do medicine, to see it as a vocation and have values and ideals

+ the wish and ability to learn and be curious about health and illness, and a wish to continually improve the care given

+ to be a communicator and be part of a wider healthcare team

+ the ability to handle crises with equanimity and reflect on performance and experience

+ the experience and skills to handle complex and difficult problems.

Helping those from disadvantaged groups. Time and again there is concern raised that those who come from disadvantaged groups will not have the experience for interviews or skills assessment. They may not be able to communicate as well, or have the people skills of those who are more privileged and who have been tutored in the 'correct' responses. They need to be handled with sensitivity. Many of the role models in medicine came from such backgrounds and have contributed enormously with their own experience. In an interesting report, McLachlan makes the point that outreach might be better than selection for increasing diversity.[21]

Postgraduate and specialty selection. By the time the doctor is moving into specialty education and training, it should be possible to asses all of the characteristics listed above: accountability, ethical issues, respect, communication skills, research and development, manual skills, teaching ability, ability to solve problems, analytical skills, equanimity, dealing with crises, reflective practice and many others. With postgraduates, the written submission and interview may not be sufficient to differentiate and other methods of assessment may be more useful: for example, references and reports from members of staff, portfolios of work and evidence of proficiency.

SOME CONCLUSIONS

Following the discussion on the roles and aim of medicine and the definition of competence, the selection of those who are taken into medicine was the next logical step. The characteristics of the doctor were listed and an attempt made to define which of these could be assessed at undergraduate and at graduate and specialty level. Some key elements were identified, notably the wish to become a doctor and the willingness to learn. Many of the other characteristics and qualities could be learned as part of the process of becoming a doctor and being a specialist. There is a need to refine these and to develop newer and better instruments to do this. The model discussed above might be one way of doing this.

REFERENCES

1. Molière. *Le Malade Imaginaire*.
2. Hippocratic writings. Translated by Chadwick J, Mann W N. London: Penguin Books, 1978.
3. Davie G E. The Democratic Intellect: Scotland and her universities in the nineteenth century. Edinburgh: Edinburgh University Press; 1961.
4. Introductory Address delivered at the opening session of the University of Glasgow 1870-71. Edinburgh and London: William Blackwood and Sons; 1870; 66–7.

5. Turnbull D, Buckley P, Robinson J S, Mather G, Leahy C, Marley J. Increasing the evidence base for the selection for undergraduate medicine; four case studies investigating process and interim outcomes. Med Educ 2003; 37: 1115–1120.

6. Morrison, J, How to choose tomorrow's doctors. Med Educ 2005; 39: 240–42.

7. Lumsden M A, Bore M, Millar K, Jack R, Powis D. Assessment of personal qualities in relation to admission to medical school. Med Educ 2005; 39: 258–65.

8. Paterson F, Ferguson E, Norfolk T, Lane P. A new selection system to recruit general practice registrars: preliminary findings from a validation study. BMJ 2004; 330: 711–4.

9. Peile E, Carter Y. Selecting and supporting contented doctors. BMJ 2005; 330: 269–30.

10. McManus I C, et al. Intellectual aptitude tests and A levels for selecting UK school leaver entrants for medical schools. BMJ 2005; 331: 555–60.

11. Allan I. Women doctors and their careers; what now? BMJ 2005; 331: 569–71.

12. Becker H S, et al. Boys in White: student culture in medical school. Chicago: University of Chicago Press; 1961.

13. Osler W. Aequanimitas: with other addresses to medical students, nurses and practitioners of medicine. London: H K Lewis, 1904; 347–71.

14. Fallowfield L, Jenkins V. Communicating sad, bad, and difficult news in medicine. Lancet 2004; 363: 312–19.

15. Huthchison R B, et al. Hutchison's Clinical Methods. 13th edn. London: Cassell; 1956; 2.

16. Osler, 3–11.

17. Eva K W, et al. An admissions OSCE: the multiple mini-interview. Med Educ 2004; 38: 314–26.

18. Council of Deans of Medical Schools in the UK; 2004.

19. Turnbull D, et al. Increasing the evidence base for selection for undergraduate medicine: four case studies investigating process and interim outcomes. Med Educ 2003; 37: 1115–20.

20. Powis D, Bristow T. Selection of medical students at Newcastle. In: Henry R, Byrne K, Engel C, eds. Imperatives in medical education: the Newcastle approach. Newcastle, UK: Faculty of Medicine and Health, University of Newcastle; 1997.

21. McLachlan J C. Outreach is better than selection for increasing diversity. Med Educ 2005; 39: 872–75.

14

Learning and teaching in medicine

*I was sickening; but once you attended me Symmachus, with
a train of a hundred apprentices. A hundred hands frosted by
the north wind have pawed me; I had no fever before
Symmachus; now I have.*[1]

Martial, *The Epigrams*

*There are three types of teaching in all, each with its place
in order. First is that which derives from the notion of an
end, an analysis. Second is that from the putting together
the findings of analysis. Third is that from dialysis (the
separating out) of a definition; and this is now what we will
embark on. This type of dialysis may also be referred to as
unfolding, simplification or explication.*[2]

Galen

*Again, in the habits and regulations of schools, universities
and the like assemblies, destined for the abode of learned
men and the improvement of learning, everything is opposed
to the progress of the sciences; for the lectures and exercises
are so ordered, that everything out of the common track can
scarcely enter the thoughts and contemplation of the mind.*[3]

Francis Bacon

In short, the teacher in a university is the pivot of the method. He must be learned in his subject, skilled in craft, competent in administration, experienced in research, and catholic in mind. He should reach his post not by favour, by merit of age or seniority, by social convention, but chiefly because he is a teacher and leader of men.[4]

Sir George Newman, *Notes on Medical Education*

INTRODUCTION

The title of this book includes the phrase, 'Handing on learning'. As discussed in Chapter 1, this comes from the Hippocratic Oath and is symbolic of the process of learning whereby the teacher facilitates the handing on of their own knowledge, interpreting that of others, and also handing on the love of knowledge. It is generally a very efficient process but can be dominated by the assessment method rather than in-depth (deep) learning. If the methods are inappropriate they can turn off the learner, particularly those who see thinking and reflection as being more important that rote learning. A good example of this is Sir James MacKenzie, a man who revolutionised general practice and cardiology. He received his medical education in Edinburgh and didn't like it. He notes:

There are two very distinct qualities of the human mind: memory and the power of reasoning…the outcome of teaching today is to hail the student with superior powers of memorising…the other individuals…possess more of a power of reasoning…this type of mind is slow in acquiring knowledge…but can appreciate the bearing of one fact on another.[5]

Learning must therefore enthuse and inspire the student or graduate. Learning is normally formalised around a curriculum, a topic which will be discussed below in some detail.

Entering medical school can be daunting. The student, perhaps used to different methods of learning in school, can be confused and disoriented. The classification used by Perry is useful. This divides the learning experience into different stages. In summary it notes that:

1. *The student sees the world in polar terms of we-right-good vs. other-wrong-bad. Right answers for every thing exist in the absolute, known to authority whose role is to teach them. Knowledge and goodness are perceived as qualitative accretions of discrete rightness to be collected by hard work and obedience.*

2. *The student perceives diversity of opinion and uncertainty, and accounts for them as unwarranted confusion in poorly qualified Authorities or as mere exercises set by Authority "so we can learn to find the Answers for ourselves".*

3. *The student accepts diversity and uncertainty as legitimate but still temporary in areas where Authority "hasn't found the Answer yet." He supposes Authority grades him in these areas on "good expression" but remains puzzled as to standards.*

4. *The student perceives legitimate uncertainty (and therefore diversity of opinion) to be extensive and raises it to the status of an unstructured epistemological realm of its own in which anyone has a right to his own opinion, a realm which he sets over against Authorities realm where right-wrong still prevails or the student discovers qualitative contextual reasoning as a special case of "what They want" within Authority's realm.*

5. *The student perceives all knowledge and values (including Authority's) as contextual and relativistic and subordinates dualistic right-wrong functions to the status of a special case, in context.*

6. *The student apprehends the necessity of orienting him-self in a relativistic world through some form of personal*

commitment (as distinct from unquestioned or unconsidered commitment to simple belief in certainty).

7. *The student makes an initial commitment to some area.*

8. *The student experiences the implications of commitment, and explores the subjective and stylistic issues of responsibility.*

9. *The student experiences the affirmation of identity among multiple responsibilities and realises commitment as an ongoing unfolding activity through which he expresses his life style.*[6]

Students go through some or all of the above phases as they progress through medical school and into independent professional practice. Those involved in planning need to be aware that such phases exist.

THE CONCEPT OF A CURRICULUM

The curriculum is determined by defining both the role of the doctor and the competencies required, subjects discussed in previous chapters. The curriculum is related to the selection of students and their background knowledge and experience. The curriculum is often seen at the heart of the process of medical education, but it is in fact the delivery system for the roles and competencies which have been defined. It is the endpoint, the effecter arm, rather than the driver.

The curriculum for each medical school varies considerably, as do the missions and objectives. The range is fascinating, allowing for different styles of learning and emphasis across the content. There is no such thing as a standard curriculum; they all seem to be different and based on concepts agreed by each individual school. Some reflect a scientific bent, others are very community linked, and still others allocate significant time to research or self-study modules. The choice is important for

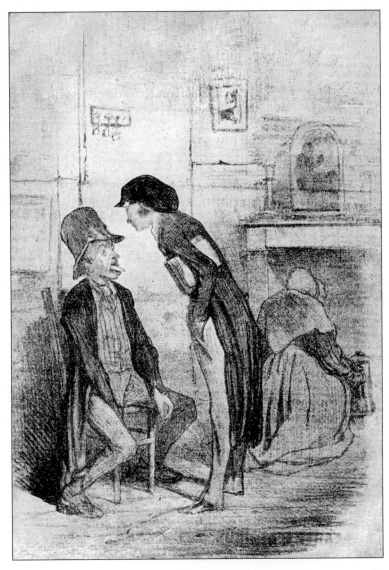

The gauche medical student asks the patient to stick out his tongue, and while it is out, he asks the patient to tell him how he is feeling. French, 19th century.

students and in a comparative sense to use these differences to learn from the experience.

The curriculum can be considered to have three major components:

1. The content—what is to be learned?

2. The methodology of learning and the resources available—how is it to be learned?

3. The methods of assessment—how will I know I have achieved the learning goals?

A fourth, related, component is the preparation of teachers of medicine to carry out their role effectively; this will also be discussed in this section, with particular reference to work in Britain.

Each of these topics will be examined though there will be less weight given to the content, as this is likely to change with time as new knowledge and skills become available, and with both place and culture. The need to keep the curriculum up-to-date and, at the same time, to not overburden the student will be emphasised. The curriculum is essentially a package to assist learning. It provides a structure into which the learner can find the beginning of the journey through the range of subjects and their interactions with other areas of knowledge. The curriculum provides a route map, learning resources and methods of assessment by which the learner can identify where they are and where they need to go. The concept applies equally to undergraduate and postgraduate education. In the context of CPD, it is the practitioner's own responsibility to plan and implement such learning as will be required.

Shaping the outcome

There is an assumption that setting out the curriculum in the manner described above will result in effective learning and equip the student, postgraduate and practitioner with all that they need. However, it is well to note that there are others factors operating which may be equally powerful. These include:

+ **Role models—the hidden agenda in the curriculum.** This is one of the most powerful forces. Having been through a learning experience which changes the way you think, or which increases the knowledge base of the doctor, such new ideas can be readily quashed in the 'real' world. There may be a different culture in the clinical setting, or the values may not be the same. This provides a problem for the doctor, and the conventional way forward is to fit in and not rock the boat. It is possible that the sophistication of students to make choices as to their role models will overcome such 'hidden agendas', but it is difficult and they badly need to have the curricular messages reinforced.[7]

+ **Personal experience and personality.** While much can be learned in medicine, the personality of the doctor and their life experiences are also very relevant. These can cloud the acquisition of new knowledge, skills and, of particular concern, attitudes. The interaction of one's own values with those of others is an important part of learning.

+ **Methods of assessment.** As will be discussed later, the assessment process drives the learning. No matter how one might regret this, if at the end of the day the measure of success is to pass examinations, this will be the motivation for learning and will determine the type of learning. This argues, of course, for better methods of assessment.

+ **The learning experience.** The ways in which the content of the curriculum is presented to the student are also critical. If the content is presented in a didactic way (e.g. 'this is the only answer to the problem' or 'I, the professor know best'), this process will be perpetuated when the student someday takes on responsibilities as a teacher.

+ **The link between teaching and research.** This is discussed elsewhere. Exposing students to an environment in which research takes place can enhance learning, and the 'teaching' component is less relevant to a highly motivated group of students.

+ **Relationships and development of other professional groups.** This is an important driver for change. Other groups, such as nurses, pharmacists, physiotherapists and speech therapists, all have an important part in the clinical team. As the knowledge and skills of such professional groups grow and their roles expand, there will be increasing overlap with the role of the doctor. This has already been discussed, and will be picked up later in terms of learning methods.

+ **The role of the teacher.** This will be discussed in more detail later, but at this stage it is important to record its importance. Teachers act as role models and provide the student or young doctor not only with a learning resource (that's what they are) and a facilitator for their learning, but a person to whom they can relate and perhaps emulate. They are a subset of the overall role models met by students, but are particularly important ones.

+ **The healthcare system.** The organisation of the health-care system, and the pressures to meet targets and objectives, can also affect the methods of learning and, indeed, the experience offered to students. Shorter stays in hospital, more outpatient and community work are all effective ways of improving the care of patients. However, unless this is factored into the curriculum, experience may be lost to the student and the postgraduate.

+ **The process should be seen as an educational one, and not simply training.** The distinction between the two has been made on many occasions over the years.[8,9] One phrase neatly sums this up: 'To be trained is to have arrived. To be educated is to continue to travel'.

+ **Ethical issues in medical education.** There are clearly issues of introducing patients to young students or young doctors. Such ethical matters are generally handled by explaining the issue to patients and ensuring full consent to history taking or clinical examination. There are particularly sensitive issues around the examination of the genitals, and procedures undertaken during anaesthesia.[10]

These factors (and there may be many others) will impact on the learning experiences and the opportunities available.

The outcome is also relevant in terms of what is to be 'produced', and at each stage in the planning process there should be a return to a basic consideration of the knowledge, skills, qualities and attitudes required. There is a danger that the process becomes one of technical training rather than education.[11] Leinster's article is a response to funding issues and who might dictate the curriculum. He argues that students must be exposed to research, and that academics should continue to be involved in teaching, service delivery and research. This debate is taken further by Rees[12], who discusses who controls medical education and argues for a cooperative approach with all of the bodies concerned, including the learners and patients. Two further articles on this subject emphasise the effect of sources of income on the course and the need for greater research on the outcomes.[13,14] The Newble paper provides a model for curriculum development and a mechanism for taking on board the requirements of other bodies, such as the GMC.[15] There is also a danger that we produce 'oven-ready' graduates who lack the ability to think and deal with new and complex problems.

THE CONTENT OF THE CURRICULUM

As has been noted, the content will vary from time to time and is likely to change regularly. New subjects will develop, as will new concepts and skills, and they all need to be considered and debated. It is instructive to look back at one's own curriculum and consider the content and indeed the methods of learning and assessment. Much has changed already. It is for this reason that regular reviews are essential to gauge the balance of subjects, the level of learning required and the relationship between branches of learning. The latter is of importance if the concepts, depth of knowledge and skills are to be effectively related to wider scientific and social issues. Major changes in science, the arts and social sciences can have a profound effect on the medical knowledge base. This is one of the main arguments for carrying out medical education within the context of a university where such interdisciplinary learning can occur.

One major issue raised over the generations is the amount of knowledge required to practise as a doctor. Medical education is often criticised as being too detailed; students become filled with facts but are given insufficient time to reflect and think about what they do. This also relates to the methods of learning and assessment. In a book on the history of medical education it would be unwise to set out any kind of curricular content. That is a decision for each school in each country, with each specialty and each postgraduate organisation. What must be clear is that the content reflects practice (another frequent criticism), allows time for reflection and some in-depth study, and is not overloaded.

A second major issue is the balance between the sciences, the social sciences and the humanities. All are important, of course, and the conflict has often been expressed in the debate between the views of Osler (the humanists, espousing the art of medicine) and Flexner (the importance of science).[16,17] In some ways this is a false antithesis. Both are important, though if people ask for advice on a disease or illness it is useful to know what it is and how it might be alleviated before considering what and how to communicate this to the patient. The knowledge base is vital. There is, in addition, the need to understand electronic methods of communication and the use of information technology in medical education.[18]

The content must also reflect the knowledge of the student when the learning begins. This is one of the golden rules of medical education: always begin at the level of the learner and do not make assumptions about prior knowledge.

METHODS OF LEARNING

The emphasis in medical education should be on learning rather than teaching. At all levels, from undergraduate to continuing professional development, we are dealing with a highly intelligent and motivated group. Given the resources and the guidance, they should be able to learn much on their own or with their peers. If one of the roles of medicine is to continue to produce doctors who are reflective, problem solvers and action-orientated, such characteristics need to be seen as part of the outcome of the learning process.

Over the centuries, as this book has demonstrated, the methods of learning have gradually evolved, though most change has occurred in the 20th century. If Galen had returned at the beginning of the 20th century he would have been astonished at the new knowledge (he may not have agreed with it), but he would have recognised much of the methodology. Laboratory work and dissection would have been new, but small group teaching, lectures and the use of books would all have been familiar.

Some things have gone: the role of aphorisms and poetry in learning, and the use of question-and-answer methods seem to have lost favour, but still surface occasionally. Mnemonics still remain useful in some areas of learning, but are probably frowned upon.

Case histories and problem-solving methods are increasingly being used. These allow more self-directed learning and evaluation, exercising the student's powers of reasoning, synthesising and presenting issues. Students in this model work together, learn together and share knowledge: skills they will need in clinical practice. Developing the teaching resources for such learning can be time consuming but provides the basis for one of the key skills defined earlier, that of problem solving and being able to put such knowledge into practice. It should be noted here that the ability to solve problems is not the same as problem-based learning. They may be related, but are distinct and this leads to a discussion of the broader issue of the value of problem-based learning (PBL).

PROBLEM-BASED LEARNING: FROM WHERE TO WHERE?

This is the title of an article by Hamilton[19], and it is an important contribution to a current debate: does problem-based learning (PBL) work? Hamilton traces the background from Flexner to the present day. As we have noted before, problem-based learning is not the same as the ability to solve problems (though it is related). It is a method (long used under other names) to stimulate learning by presenting the student with a problem to work with and learn from.[20] The debate about its value has been ongoing for some time. For example, Hinduja et al[21] found that students in a traditional course show higher levels of anatomical knowledge than those on an integrated PBL course. Prince et al[22] from Maastrict in the Netherlands noted that students reported that they felt deficient in some science areas, notably anatomy. Other studies from the same school are not so clear.[23, 24]

In a commentary, Fergusson tries to put things in perspective. She notes that 'after repeated attempts to establish problem-based learning (PBL) as superior to traditional teaching methods, even PBL's staunchest supporters acknowledge that PBL has fallen short of initial expectations'.[25] A study by Dolmans et al argues that the failure might be due to poor implementation, and that research on PBL might give better insight into effective learning, especially around self-directed learning skills, communication skills and group work.[26] In addition, Iputo and Kwizera showed that those from a disadvantaged background had lower attrition rates and progressed faster when on a PBL programme.[27] The student view is also important.[28]

So what does all of this mean? Perhaps, as Norman has suggested, it means that there are potential benefits from both small-group learning as well as the more traditional curriculum.[29] People learn in different ways. Perhaps they need a range of mechanisms to ensure that learning is both organised and integrated, and that structure as well as method is important. Both traditional and PBL emphasise different skills and experiences, both of which are important.

THE ROLE OF CLINICAL TEACHING

Clinical teaching remains important. Listening to a real patient or public group with a problem to bring forward is a clear learning activity, as well as a privilege. Notes made at the time allow reflection and a connection between this individual and the rest of the medical knowledge base. Small group clinical teaching allows the demonstration and practice of clinical skills, and (with the patient's consent) on-the-spot feedback on performance, reinforcing the learning brought by the immediacy and relevance of the clinical problem.

The apprenticeship model fits into this method of learning and takes small group clinical teaching a stage further. It allows real contact between the master and the apprentice in which learning is demonstrated and shared. In spite of the many pressures on time and energy, this is of great value in building role models, and exciting and enthusing the student for a particular specialty and professional direction.

More recent developments have included the use of patient volunteers, simulators and computer-based models, and clinical skills units. Each of these has a very important role in learning. Patient volunteers, for example, can be used to hone and reflect on interviewing skills. Video feedback allows the patient to discuss with the student how they performed and how they might improve. Simulators come in all shapes and sizes and provide practice in activities ranging from basic clinical skills, taking blood pressures, examining the eye or removing blood, to vaginal and rectal examinations. Such simulation systems prepare the patient for the real thing and provide confidence and safety. If students are encouraged do these procedures in groups on the simulator, they can learn from each others' mistakes.[30,31] Clinic-based reviews of clinical issues carried out at the patient's beside or outpatient area with computer access to databases and information can provide another mechanism of real-time learning, integrating the knowledge base with patient needs.[32]

The more complex systems (and it is likely that such innovations will develop considerably) can already simulate operating theatre practice in which an entire surgical team is involved, having to work together to deal with a patient problem. Such interdisciplinary learning is particularly valuable. Surgical skills in suturing and endoscopy can be developed using similar models, and it is likely that their role will grow and expand.

CURRICULUM DEVELOPMENT IN DIFFERENT SETTINGS

Significant differences in the curriculum may be required to meet different needs, although the principle will remain the same. In the developing world, for example, the range of diseases, the community setting and the health service needs may all be very different from those encountered in a medical school within a developed country. This provides an exciting opportunity for the use of innovative courses and methods, and, in particular, medical education in a community setting.[33–36]

More recently (particularly in Australia and Canada) there has been increasing interest in rural medicine and curricula designed specifically to enhance the role of rural medicine and provide an appropriate experience in settings which provide the background for learning. These courses are patient-centred and case-based, using 'smart' classrooms, video conferences and online learning. Like other aspects of learning, the relationship between the teacher, the student and, in this case, the community is crucial. It is described as being 'dispersed community engaged team teaching'. Rural medicine programmes are now operating in Japan, Australia, Norway, the Philippines and Canada. Such programmes are relevant to many other countries with remote and rural populations, and provide a way of encouraging medical students and doctors to work in such settings and develop the specific knowledge and skills required. They become true generalists, able to deal with many conditions (or know when not to), and this will be an issue picked up in the conclusions of this book.[37]

MEDICAL ILLUSTRATIONS

The earliest illustrations used to assist learning were in the form of paintings, line drawings or woodcuts. Some of these, such as in Vesalius' *De Fabrica* and William Hunter's *Anatomy of the Gravid Uterus*, were works of art. In the preface to Hunter's text, in addition to thanking his younger brother John, 'whose accuracy in anatomical researches is so well known', he notes the following:

> *The art of engraving supplies us, upon many occasions, with what has been the great desideratum of the lovers of science, a universal language. Nay it conveys clearer ideas of most natural objects, than words can express; it makes stronger impressions on the mind; and to every person conversant with the subject, gives an immediate comprehension of what it represents.[38]*

What a splendid description of the role of illustration and the visual media in medical education. Until the 19th century, little changed in medical illustration, but with the advent of the microscope and the camera the range was expanded. Eventually, moving images were used, and film and video became part of the repertoire of the lecturer. The role of medical illustration is well described in the biography of Max Brödel who worked at Johns Hopkins.[39] Lantern slides were replaced by 35 mm slides, and then computer-generated presentations created in programs such as PowerPoint. Moving images and computer-generated graphics were only a short step on the way. Real time simulators of clinical issues are now a possibility: a long way from the woodcut and the diagram, from talk and chalk to computer-generated images. The question remains as to whether or not such developments have improved the learning process. More research will be needed.

PATIENT INVOLVEMENT IN CURRICULUM DEVELOPMENT

At various points in this book the case has been made for more patient and public involvement in medicine. In the case of undergraduate medical training, reference has already been made to the role of the public in the selection of medical students. In a similar way, patients and the public need to be seen as partners in curriculum development. The contribution can be in several different ways, including patient/public involvement in learning (as actual or simulated patients), providing feedback to students on performance, or being part of the curriculum team.[40,41]

INTERPROFESSIONAL EDUCATION

For many generations the medical profession was the only group of health professionals with organised educational programmes for its learners. While there have been other groups, notably priests in the early days and religious foundations which encouraged the care of the sick, there were no others until relatively recently. The apothecaries were certainly part of the broad group of medical practitioners but they transmogrified into the general practitioner, as well as (more recently) the pharmacist. There were nurses and midwives, bonesetters and herbalists, but none of these occupational groups had any real form of educational provision for their practitioners. Medical education grew up, therefore, as a single form of learning. In the last century, with the growth of other professions and the expansion in their roles and expertise, and the growing emphasis on teamwork in patient care, the concept of interprofessional education is now being examined in many places. Buchan and Calman have described how such 'advanced practice roles' have developed and will continue to do so.[42] They examined the cost effectiveness of the new roles and came up with mixed results. They note that many of the results relate to the nurse substituting for the doctor when the diagnosis has been established, and questions remain unanswered when the diagnosis is unknown.[43] As roles become widened and boundaries blurred, it becomes increasingly necessary at the beginning of the process to agree the particular role of the doctor in the healthcare setting. This is undoubtedly likely to change over the next few decades as new professional groups develop, and skills and expertise are shared and brought together for the good of the patient. This, after all, is the key factor: what is best for the patient.

We have already tried to define what it is that doctors do that others don't. It was concluded that they have a special interest in diagnosis, in determining prognosis, in setting out the management plan and in developing new and improved methods of diagnosis and treatment—the curiosity factor. They also have broader roles in communication, advocacy, treatment etc., but these may well be shared by others. With this as a background, how can we achieve the necessary understanding of the role and expertise of each member of the healthcare team? It should be said at the outset that such teams already operate well in clinical practice. In areas such as diabetes, caring for the elderly, palliative care and many specialty practice settings, each member of the team is seen to contribute fully to the process of care. The development of clinical skills units and the use of simulation techniques have enhanced this. Leadership of the team varies and depends on the problem and the skills required. How then can we ensure that this becomes the norm and not the exception? Much of the debate is around the relationship between medical and nursing education, but it is much wider than this. For example, the anatomical knowledge of the head and neck required of the speech therapist is much greater than that required of the medical student, and in a similar way the knowledge base of the pharmacist is different and more extensive than the undergraduate medical student.

A wide range of models is already available and many more are being assessed at present; it is a very active part of research in clinical education (e.g. see Carlisle et al[44]). The following is a brief outline of the kind of models which are available. Time will tell which is the most effective.[45]

Basic education. Options include:

+ The integration of all health professional groups with joint teaching on many subjects.

+ The integration of specific aspects of the course: ethical issues, communications skills, clinical skills, organisation of health service etc., but not all aspects.

+ Integrated teaching of topics by staff from a variety of professional groups, based around specific diseases or procedures.

+ Integration of learning by different student groups around particular problems through which each group learns about the expertise of the other.

Postgraduate education. This is often very effectively related to case-based, team-based learning and is associated with actual problem solving. In many places this would be a daily occurrence.

Continuing professional development. Team-based learning, joint seminars and research work are likely to be the ways forward.

There is much work going on in the field of inter-professional education, and many different models are being evaluated. The best way forward remains to be seen. What is not in doubt is that working in teams enhances patient care and brings to the patient the skills and experience of many different health professionals.

BOOKS AND LIBRARIES

Much of the history of medical education has been concerned with the transmission of the written word. This has brought, in Osler's words, the author 'mind to mind' with the reader. In the great age of Chinese medicine, in Egyptian medicine and in Greece, while some of the transmission was oral and the learning related to that, it was always considered appropriate that the doctor could read and write. Libraries grew and provided focus for the transmission of ideas. Education grouped around such places, and even in the 17th and 18th centuries some of the impetus for the formation of medical societies and colleges was the creation of a mutual library as a learning resource. The details of the books in such libraries, private or communal, make fascinating reading. The advent of mass paper production and subsequently the invention of printing completely revolutionised the way in which knowledge could be readily and portably transmitted.

With the increase in knowledge, specialist publications in the form of journals became available in all specialty areas, allowing clinicians and scientists to keep up to date. Specialities come of age when a journal is created to cater for special interests and developments. It is interesting to note that medical education itself is now served by a series of journals. *Medical Education*, the British born journal, celebrated its 40th anniversary in 2006 (see Ch. 8).

With the introduction of the computer, the Internet, the World Wide Web and the digitalisation of print media, books could become redundant, as libraries (original copies of any book in the world) become available at home on a laptop. So what then is the future of the book? Is there a life beyond the book? Will libraries still be necessary? What will happen to those who like the feel and the smell of books and the pleasure of browsing, not knowing what might be found? Will there be a post-book era?

First, the assumption is that libraries will still be essential even in the post-book era. There will still be need for a place where printed material—the written word—is collected, catalogued and able to be searched. In the future, much of this will be Web-based, with access to original work, or copies of that work, being easily available. As computers become smaller and more portable, they will become as accessible and easily usable as books. We will simply download a few books for the train or plane journey, or for research purposes. Journals are already moving that way and the process is likely to increase.

This may be appropriate for 'new' books, but for older ones and manuscripts, the marginal notes, comments and ownership may be even more valuable, and we must not lose that aspect of scholarship.

What then of the book itself? Will there still be a need for books? If books are conceived as the presentation of a subject using the written word by one or more authors, then there is no a priori need for these to be printed on paper and bound as books; they could equally be produced in digital form. The concept of the book, however, remains as a method of presenting a subject in an accessible and organised way, which guides the reader through a topic and relates it to others. Books might become shorter and refer to papers and other media on the web. They might become guidebooks which take the learner in a graduated way through a subject and how it relates to other scientific and knowledge-based work. This has always been the characteristic of the great textbook: the way in which the knowledge is organised so that the learner gets most out of it. In this they follow good educational principles, and take the learner to a different level of knowledge and understanding. So books, as a systematic collection of knowledge organised in a way which facilities learning and which is connected to many other resources, is likely to be the way forward. In this process the smell and feel will be lost. Some will think that this is progress; this author might not agree.

THE ASSESSMENT OF LEARNING

Over the centuries many different ways of assessing learning have been used. Sometimes they have been modest, and a Class Ticket from the University of Glasgow in the 19th century recorded the learning outcomes as: 'Attended with regularity, behaved with propriety and duly performed the work of the Class'.[46] Not quite enough for today's quality assurance systems.

Examinations sometimes do not discriminate sufficiently. There is an apocryphal story told of Sir William Macewen who had described a triangle behind the ear from which to treat mastoid disease. At a surgical fellowship interview he was asked to describe the triangle and the examiner disagreed. He retorted that he was Macewen and therefore should know. He was failed for disclosing his name.

Assessment methods have included:

+ Oral examinations in private or in public—defending the thesis.

+ Written examinations. These have included essays, mini-essays (short answer questions), reflective writing and portfolios of work including case-based analysis.

+ Multiple choice questions (true/false and single best option) and patient management problems.

+ Dissertations and reviews on set topics or in special study areas. This might include areas of original work and research.

+ Laboratory based work including practical and experimental work in areas such as anatomy, physiology and pathology.

+ Computer-based assessments.

+ Clinical examinations including 'short' and 'long' cases, objective structured clinical examinations (OSCEs).

Such techniques are well described in standard texts and journals. It might be thought that with this range of methods, some of which have been used for thousands of years, we would be clear about their respective roles and value. However, it is clear that this is not the case and more work is required, and the need is clear.[47] In general, it would be safe to say that a range of methods is likely to be more effective that one single technique.

There is little doubt that the methods of assessment drive the learning process. If a subject is not examined then it cannot be important.

In more recent years, reflective learning has been more readily used.[48] This consists of students developing reflective portfolios on subjects within the curriculum. It is clear that some students have found these confusing, and it has taken a little while to establish the method. In a recent paper, Rees and Sheard reviewed a group of second year students and their portfolios on communication skills. Those who found it a positive experience were more likely to get good marks and were more confident about other reflective portfolio assessments.[49]

A further area of interest is the development of clinical reasoning skills. As we have noted, this skill is an important part of the competency required of the doctor. Norman has reviewed the traditions associated with such skills. He concludes that:

It becomes evident that expertise lies in the availability of multiple representations of knowledge. Perhaps the most critical aspect of learning is not the acquisition of a particular strategy or skill, nor is it the availability of a particular kind of knowledge. Rather, the critical element may be deliberate practice with multiple examples which, on the one hand, facilitates the availability of concepts and conceptual knowledge (i.e. transfer) and, on the other hand, adds to a storehouse of already solved problems.[50]

In short this is about experience and exposure to a wide range of problems, with feedback on the outcomes.

EVALUATING THE OUTCOME OF MEDICAL EDUCATION

This is one of the most important areas of medical education, yet the least developed. In the late 1960s, Kilpatrick presented a model of evaluation based on four steps which were not specifically intended for medicine.[51] They have been modified and evolved, and in summary are:

Step 1. Reaction. This covers issues such as student satisfaction with the teaching, programme etc.

Step 2. Learning. This includes knowledge, skills and attitudes.

Step 3. Behaviour. Has the student's behaviour changed and are they doing things differently?

Step 4. Results. Have these changes in knowledge and behaviour altered patient care? Have the outcomes of care improved?

It will be clear that much of the educational research is built on Steps 1 and 2. They are the easiest to measure: student satisfaction and learning outcomes. Some have dealt with behaviour change but very few with the key issue—that of changes to the outcome of care. This is well documented in a paper by Prystowsky and Bordage. They analysed 599 articles and most (49.4%) were on student performance, 34.1% covered student satisfaction, 2.3% focussed on cost and only 0.7% measured patient outcomes.[52] This is of course a challenging area but the critical one. The learning of doctors is for a purpose—to improve patent care—and while it could be assumed that adequate learning as measured by testing at levels 1–2 might be a proxy for this, it is by no means obvious. As the authors of this paper make clear:

> *Medical education research is dominated by assessment of trainee performance followed by trainee satisfaction. Leading journals in medical education contain little information concerning the cost and products of medical education, that is, provider performance and patient outcomes. The study of these represents an important challenge to medical education researchers.*

An interesting comparative study of the differences and similarities in curriculum and outcome between two countries (Canada and France) shows that some of the variations are related to history and national values.[53]

So there is a real challenge to do better and to complete the loop between learning and better patient outcomes.

RESEARCH IN MEDICAL EDUCATION

One of the great indictments of medical education is that while practising evidenced-based learning the evidence base itself is limited.[54] This was forcibly brought out in the Todd Report of 1968 (see Ch. 8), where one of the first comments made was a lack of evidence of effectiveness in medical education. The research base is weak both in terms of capacity and capability. It is not a well-funded area and those involved are often working in an isolated way, with short-term grants and changing personnel.[55,56]

The International Handbook of Research in Medical Education provides an important basis for further work.[57] Not all is bad, and in a positive light Norman has written about the ways in which the process has developed and improved.[58] Medical educators have much to learn from other fields, such as anthropology, education and the social sciences, and closer involvement with such disciplines might be helpful. Part of the research needs to be devoted to better ways of facilitating learning by teachers, and their preparation for the task. The *British Medical Journal* has produced guidelines for evaluating papers on educational interventions.[59]

There is no shortage of questions waiting to be answered. They range from the methods of selection of students to the assessment of CPD programmes, and everything in between. We need more people engaged in such research and funded on a long-term basis. In carrying out this research there is a need to reflect on the ethical issues involved.[60]

Perhaps the biggest contribution which could be made to the care of patients and the public would be a strong research and evidence base in education upon which to build best practice. Investment in this area might see substantial gains in the effectiveness of learning and the more rapid diffusion of new knowledge.

POSTGRADUATE AND CONTINUING EDUCATION

The discussion above is not specific for undergraduate prog-rammes but reaches across the whole continuum of learning. This includes CPD and life-long learning. How do we keep up to date while practising in a busy clinical subject? Where do I find the time, and what do I need to know that is new and different? There is an equal impetus to improve the educational evidence base in postgraduate learning. It is salutary to review again the numerous reports on medical education discussed in Chapter 8 and ask the question as to how many of the recommendations were based on evidence and how many on the views of the committee believing that the changes proposed seemed like a good idea at the time. Once again, numerous questions still remain to be answered.

PREPARING TO BECOME A TEACHER

Introduction

One of the most fascinating aspects of the process of learning is the amount of preparation teachers require in order to be effective. For centuries the qualities of a good teacher have been extolled and set out, yet there is scant evidence of any form of educational programme for the preparation of teachers. In early Chinese literature there is a good account of how teachers would be punished if their students were not successful, but little else appears. A recent publication on the learning histories of experienced medical teachers is illuminating.[61] The role of the critical friend in medical teaching has recently been described.[62]

In Billroth's book on the medical sciences in 19th century Germany there are a few paragraphs on 'teaching the teachers'. However, closer inspection shows that this is really about teaching those who lecture to be better research workers: not quite the same.

In Britain the education of school teachers began in the early 19th century, often from a Sunday school perspective linked to the churches. This developed and became formalised by the turn of the 20th century. But for university teachers there was nothing.

In Osler's essay, 'Teacher and Student', delivered to the University of Minnesota in 1892, he emphasises the importance of the teacher, including (and here he quotes Cardinal Newman) their personal influence on the learner.[63] He passes judgement on the poor quality of medical education in the past. He comments on the growth of new ideas in medical education, and in methods of teaching, including improved equipment, clinical and laboratory, and 'the kindlier spirit of generous rivalry which has replaced the former debased method of counting heads as a test of merit...'.

He interestingly paraphrases the words of Matthew Arnold when he says that the:

...function of the teacher is to teach and to propagate the best that is known and taught in the world. To teach the current knowledge of the subject he professes—sifting, analysing, assorting, laying down principles. To propagate, i.e. to multiply the facts on which to base principles— experimenting, searching testing. The best that is known and taught in the world—nothing less can satisfy a teacher worthy of the name, and upon us of the medical faculties lies a bounden duty in this respect, since our Art, coordinate with human suffering, is cosmopolitan.

While Osler does not mention 'teacher training', that comment comes as close to a mission statement for teachers as might be required.

In addition to describing their roles, he notes that teachers have not been sufficiently recognised as compared to the clinician and research worker, and this is a common theme in many of the reports which have been written about teachers and teaching.

Osler's contemporary, William Welch, also comments on teaching. In his address on 'Humane aspects of medical science' delivered on the 10th anniversary of Johns Hopkins University, Baltimore, April 26th 1886, he notes:

Experiment and observation of nature have taken place, in the medical as well as other sciences, of deductive reasoning and appeal to authority. In former times medical teaching consisted chiefly in didactic lectures which were for the most part commentaries on the great medical writers of antiquity. Useful as didactic lectures may have been in mediaeval medical instruction their value for the present time has been greatly lessened by the multiplication of good textbooks in every department of medicine. With the decadence of the purely didactic lecture as the main feature of the system of medical education, the importance of laboratory instruction, of clinical teaching, and in general of demonstrative and objective methods of imparting knowledge has become better recognised.[64]

A very powerful statement indeed. He also, in a subsequent address, comments on the importance of the student being brought into contact with those who are 'not merely teachers but investigators'.[65]

Finally in an address on the 'Advancement of Medical Education' to the Harvard Medical School in 1892, Welch comments:

One of the most hopeful signs of the advancement of medical education in this country is the elevation of the standard, not only of those who study, but also those who teach medicine. A few books and some oratorical gift no longer suffice to make a medical teacher, and the aspirants to professorial honors are no longer expected to begin their apprenticeship with teaching materia medica and to climb up gradually the various chairs until perhaps they reach that of medicine or surgery. It is true that profound learning does not carry with it of necessity the special gifts of a teacher, but I believe that this point of view has been too much emphasised. The well-trained students and the fruitful investigators in their special departments, even if they do not possess the greatest facility of expression, are generally the soundest and most satisfactory teachers.[66]

These comments from Osler and Welch, two great teachers at the turning point between the 19th and 20th centuries, are very modern indeed. While neither recommended specific preparation for teaching, their views are clear.

The Haldane Commission

The Royal Commission on University Education in London (the Haldane Commission) was published in 1913. It looked carefully at university education and early on concludes:

...it is essential that the regular students of the university should be able to work in intimate and constant association with their fellow students, not only of the same but of different faculties, and also in close contact with their teachers.[67]

It contrasts other places of learning such as school or technical colleges with that of the university:

...the whole organisation ought to be adapted to the attainment of the end in view. Knowledge is of course the foundation and the medium of all intellectual education, but in a university knowledge should be pursued not merely for the sake of the information to be acquired, but for its own extension and always with reference to the attainment of the truth.[68]

The Commission agrees with a Board of Education Report of 1910 which said:

We may assume that university teaching is teaching suited to adults; that it is scientific, detached, and impartial in character; that it aims not so much at filling the mind of the student with facts or theories, as to calling forth his own individuality, and stimulating him to mental effort that accustoms him to the critical study of the leading authorities with perhaps occasional references to first hand sources of information, and that it implants in his mind a standard of thoroughness, and gives him a sense of the difficulty as well as the value of truth.[69]

So far the Commission has defined the learning process and the teachers. What about the preparation for teaching? First it notes the importance of the 'personal influence' of the teacher: 'His personality is the selective power by which those who are fittest for his special work are voluntarily enlisted to his service, and his individual influence is reproduced and extended by the spirit which actuates his staff'.[70] This is an important conclusion. Teaching is about the transmission of enthusiasm for, and of love of, the subject, of handing on learning. It is about learning being caught, not taught.

However, the report is clear that if the right teachers are appointed and allowed to get on with it without interference, they can set their own syllabus and examinations. No one else needs to bother. Such a view will still find echoes of support in many parts of the university system. They say, for example, that:

> *we shall make recommendations which will dispense with the necessity of the syllabus, by ensuring the appointment of teachers who can be trusted with the charge of university education. Teachers who can be trusted with this far more important and responsible duty can also be trusted with the conduct of examinations, in so far as they are accepted as proper and necessary tests for the degrees of the University.*[71]

Life for a vice-chancellor would be so much easier in such circumstances. Appoint the right people and let them get on with it.

But are there to be no controls? The report reiterates the importance of securing for the teacher the freedom to teach as he thinks best, and if there is freedom for the teacher the learner will follow. But yes there are constraints:

> *If Faculties are to be entrusted with the powers we have set out above, and the teachers are to be freed from the restrictions imposed…it is necessary to make sure that the teachers…are worthy of the trust that will be put in them. Some test must be applied to the existing schools of the university in each Faculty in order to ascertain that they are of such standing as to justify their admission to the privileges proposed for their teachers.*[72]

Such a test is defined in Appendix II in a note from the University of London entitled: 'Regulations with regard to the conferment of the titles of University professor and Reader'. It sets out the appointment process, which includes three external assessors. The candidates should be judges on:

1. contribution to research to the advancement of science and learning
2. his powers as a teacher
3. generally his eminence in his subject or his profession.[73]

Unfortunately how his 'powers as a teacher' should be assessed is not discussed further.

By the 1940s there was increasing concern about this issue and general expressions of discontent. This is well summarised in Matheson's monograph (1981) which sets out the position to date.[74] He notes that many reports have been written, including reference to a delightful book by Fitch (1881) on the art of teaching.[75] This remarkable book is subtitled 'First Course of Lectures in the Art of Teaching addressed to members of an English University'. Fitch subsequently developed his work[76] and this contains a fascinating section on women in universities, which includes concerns about their ability to withstand the rigours of academic life!

Truscott noted how appalling things were and made some suggestions.[77] In the 1950s, a number of initiatives were taken, usually in the form of short courses. The Association of University Teachers (AUT), the Committee of Vice Chancellors and Principals (CVCP) and the National Union of Students (NUS) all became involved and interested.

First World Conference on Medical Education

In the Proceedings of the First World Conference on Medical Education, it is interesting to note that while the role, characteristics and importance of the teacher are mentioned there is only one short chapter on teaching the teachers.[78] This chapter advocates more structured assistance to aspiring teachers. It makes the point that if you believe teachers are born, not made, then there is little point in reading further. If, on the other hand, you think things could be improved, he suggests several ways forward: first by improving diction and delivery, and second by changing the content and arrangement of the teaching. He also advocates programmes for young teachers to be assessed on their presentations by experienced teachers. This was exactly how the author of this volume was shown how to do things better: by public presentations of research work to a critical audience who were as concerned about the presentation and quality of the delivery as they were about the science. It was a hard but very effective process.

This view is contradicted in several other chapters. For example, in a section on the aims of the medical curriculum one very distinguished and senior academic contrasts teaching in schools and teaching in university. Arnott writes:

> ...whereas the former consists essentially of the presentation of a limited body of data to children and adolescents, the proper task of the latter is surely to escort the student to the railhead, as it were, of knowledge and then leave him adequately equipped for further exploration. While the pedagogic facility is certainly an advantage, I maintain that it is a quite subsidiary qualification and not even essential in education at a university level.[79]

This debate continues and will be discussed again in subsequent sections.

The Hale Committee

By 1961, things had begun to move. The Hale Committee on University Teaching Methods was established by the University Grants Committee, and reported in 1964. It made some important recommendations and this occurred at the time of expansion in university education following the publication of the Robbins Report. The Hale Report interestingly covered all aspects of university teaching but excluded medicine, dentistry and veterinary science. It takes aspects of teaching, such as lectures and discussion periods, and quotes from Boswell's *Life of Johnson*:

> *Lectures were once useful; but now, when all can read, and books are so numerous, lectures are unnecessary. If your attention fails, and you miss part of a lecture, it is lost; you cannot go back as you can with a book.*[80]

There is a fascinating chapter on equipment for teaching, which begins with the importance of books and libraries. Various types of visual aids are used by staff with considerable variation among subjects taught. There is a comment on the use of 'teaching machines' which have 'no virtue apart from the programme for which it is used. It is simply a device for displaying the frames one by one in the correct sequence and so ensuring that the programme is used in the correct manner'.[81] The report makes the comment that programmed learning is no novelty and 'has been the practice of those who have given individual teaching since the days of Socrates'.[82]

Of particular interest is the chapter on 'University teaching as a matter for training and study'.[83] As part of the report, a study was done which noted that 10% of staff said that they had completed courses of training for teachers, and 17% said they had received some instruction or guidance. Interestingly, those who responded were asked whether or not they had ever checked on the efficiency of their lecturing technique, and 67% said yes. Universities were asked what provision was available, and Nottingham was the only university which had centrally organised courses. The committee had discussed the question of what training a university teacher should receive. The answer was that any proposal to make a full-time course lasting for a year, say, would receive no support at all. Any such arrangements might be a serious deterrent to recruitment. As to what should be done, they break the response into several categories. For laboratory demonstrating, this should be done 'on the job', with no further arrangements necessary. Giving a tutorial could benefit from help by an experienced practitioner, which would 'make him effective far sooner than if he were left to learn from his own mistakes'. As far as the lecture is concerned, the case for some training seemed especially strong. In addition to training there should be a method of assessing the teacher, and a number of ways are put forward. The committee suggests it is not good enough that the first a department hears about a poor teacher is by student complaints. They quote the considerable amount of work done in America, funded by the Ford Foundation, and offer one or two examples in this country.

There is one quote which is particularly relevant:

It has been remarked that University teachers who devote so much of their time to inquiry and experiment, and who are never backward, in their own subjects, in challenging accepted views for which evidence is lacking, seem nevertheless in their teaching to be often content with somewhat uncritical acceptance of traditional methods.[84]

They suggest more research is required, and propose the setting up of a body to coordinate this and to publish the results. Summer schools for teachers of particular subjects might help and the organisation might provide advisers in lecturing techniques who could visit a university, if requested, and assist. The report adds: 'However it would be a mistake to define too closely at the outset the scope and functions of such an organisation; its growth would depend on the demand for its services'.[85]

The Hale Report was an important milestone in university teaching. It began to define the problems and grasped at a solution. It would be three decades before a definitive solution would be set out and accepted.

Society for Research into Higher Education (SRHE)

In 1964, the Society for Research into Higher Education (SRHE) was formed. Numerous reports and working parties were assembled, one of the most influential being the Brynmor Jones working group on the training of university teachers, which published its report in 1972.[86] This included proposals for induction training, initial and continuing assistance, further training and specialist courses.

The CVCP then set up the Committee for the Coordination of Training of University Teachers (CCTUT) which began to work across the university sector. In an SRHE pamphlet by Greenaway, the situation in Britain's universities in 1971 was set out.[87] Most universities had short courses and it was clear that there were a number of academic staff who toured the country speaking on the subject and encouraging involvement. This review notes that the majority of universities had begun their teaching course between the early 1960s to the 1970s. There were considerable variations in the length and curriculum.

By the 1980s there was a much greater range of courses available, but these were not compulsory and some universities did not comply. Debate continued and in the midst of this the CVCP decided to review the work of the CCTUT. This was carried out under the chairmanship of Sir Harry Pitt and was circulated to members in 1980. It recommended the continuation of a central body with some enhanced activity. However, the CVCP was unable to support the report and the CCTUT was to be phased out in spite of protests. In its place a Committee on the Training of University Teachers was to be established and set up from 1981–2.

Recent developments

In the 1980s and 1990s, teacher preparation became much more of a part of university induction processes and numerous courses were set up. The Staff and Educational Development Association began a process of voluntary registration by universities of their teaching programmes. However, it was the Dearing Report in 1997 on 'Higher Education in the Learning Society' which really changed things. It advocated the establishment of an Institute of Learning and Teaching in Higher Education which would not only encourage the preparation of teachers but would accredit courses in each institution. In addition it would stimulate research, development and innovation in teaching and learning. This was set up in 1999 and by 2003 had over 14,000 members, and had accredited over 100 institutions. In 2004, it merged with several other bodies involved in teaching and learning and became the Higher Education Academy. One of the functions of the Academy, following on from the Institute of Learning and Teaching, will be to continue to elevate the status of the university teacher, including those in medicine, and to improve the quality of the student experience. For the first time, all academic staff and a wide range of academic-related staff will have the opportunity to obtain a qualification in teaching. This is a major achievement, and over the next few years it is expected that the majority of staff will take up this opportunity.

From a particularly medical perspective, the GMC produced a short but important pamphlet on *The Doctor as Teacher* in 1999. This not only set out the educational obligations of doctors but described the professional attributes of the doctor with responsibilities for clinical training/educational supervision. This is a very important list and includes:

+ maintaining a high standard of professional and personal values
+ being available and accessible to patients
+ maintaining a high standard of clinical competence
+ an ability to communicate effectively
+ a commitment to personal and professional development as a doctor

+ a commitment to professional audit and peer review

+ a commitment to team working in a multi-professional environment

+ an understanding of the multicultural society in which medicine is practised.[88]

There follows a description of the attributes of the clinical teacher which include: enthusiasm, a personal commitment to teaching and learning, sensitivity and responsiveness to educational needs, an understanding of the principles of education as applied to medicine and an understanding of the research method. In addition are some attributes which might not have been recognisable a century ago but are now increasingly important: practical teaching skills, a commitment to audit and peer review in teaching, the ability to use formative assessment and the ability to carry out a formal appraisal of the learner. There is an imperative that universities and NHS bodies should ensure that formal training in teaching skills should be provided for all new appointees. This latter comment being of especial importance.

Over the last 25 years we have come a long way in the preparation of teachers. Much still remains to be done but the foundations have been laid and the omens look good. In addition there is now increasing evidence that such preparation does indeed make a difference. Gibbs and Coffey (2004) carried out a study of two groups of university teachers.[89] The first group were involved in a training programme and the second, without such a programme acted, as a control. The results (using objective criteria) showed improvement in rating scores for the trained group, with deteriorating scores in the control group: evidence that good teaching assisted learning and improved the student experience. Similarly, a study on training the trainers by Godfrey and Welsh (2004) records a similar outcome—a conclusion with which Osler and Welch would certainly have agreed.[90] In a clinical setting Godfrey et al noted that a course for clinical teachers increased their ability in the range of teaching skills and provided evidence of sustained change.[91]

CONCLUSIONS

While this chapter began by noting that the curriculum should be led by the aims/roles of medicine and the competencies required of doctors, it is clear that the curriculum still dominates education training. From the evidence presented here the learning process must be:

+ relevant to practice and to helping patients
+ directed to specific issues and targeted
+ practice-based and delivered with regular reminders
+ effective and evidence-based, and supported by the peer group
+ easy to use and efficient in the use of time
+ cost effective.

The evidence base must be strengthened and more research is required if we are to improve the quality of care provided to patients. This could be one of the most powerful ways of improving patient care.

REFERENCES

1. Martial, The Epigrams. I xLvii. Translated by Ker C A. London: Heinemann; 1920–25.
2. Galen, Selected works. Singer P N. Oxford World Classics. Oxford: Oxford University Press; 1997; 345.
3. Bacon F. Organum novum. First book, para 90.
4. Newman G. Some notes on medical education in England. A Memorandum presented to the President of the Board. 1918, London: HMSO; 1918; 24.
5. Wilson R N. The beloved physician: Sir James MacKenzie. London: Murray; 1926; 24.
6. Perry W G. Forms of intellectual and ethical development in the college years. A scheme. New York: Holt Rhinehart and Winston; 1970; 9–10.

7. Lempp H, Seale C. The hidden curriculum in undergraduate medical education: qualitative study of medical student's perception of teaching. BMJ 2004; 329: 770–3.

8. Calman K C, Downie R S. Education and training in medicine. Med Educ 1988; 22: 488–91.

9. Bryans P, Smith R. Beyond training: reconceptualising learning at work. J of Workplace Learning 2000; 12: 228–235.

10. Jagsi R, Lehmann L S. The ethics of medical education. BMJ 2004; 329: 332–4.

11. Leinster S. Medical schools: are we paying for education or for technical training? J Roy Soc Med 2004; 97: 3–5.

12. Rees C. The problem with outcome-based curricula in medical education: insights from educational theory. Med Educ 2004; 38: 593–98.

13. Newble D, et al. Developing an outcome-focussed curriculum, Med Educ 2005; 39: 680–87.

14. Prideaux D. Clarity of outcomes in medical education: do we know if it really makes a difference? Med Educ 2004; 38: 580–1.

15. Schol S, et al. Individualised training to improve teaching competence of general practitioner trainers: a randomised controlled trial. Med Educ 2005; 39: 991–98.

16. Tauber A I. The two faces of medical education: Flexner and Osler re-visited. J Roy Soc Med 1992; 85: 598–602.

17. Dornan T. Osler, Flexner, apprenticeship and the "new medical education". J Roy Soc Med 2005; 98: 91–95.

18. Ward J P T, et al. Communication and information technology in medical education. Lancet 2001; 357: 792–96.

19. Hamilton J. Problem-based learning: from where to where? Clinical Teacher 2005; 2: 45–48.

20. Barrows H S, Tamblyn R M. Problem-based learning: an approach to medical education. New York: Springer Publishing Co; 1980.

21. Hinduja K, Samuel R, Mitchell S. Problem based learning: is anatomy a casualty? Surgeon 2005; 3: 84–87.

22. Prince K J A H, et al. Advances Health Sci Educ, 2000, 5, 105–16.

23. Prince K J A H, et al. Does problem based learning lead to deficiencies in basic science knowledge? An empirical case on anatomy. Med Ed, 2003, 37, 15–21.

24. Distlehorst L H, Dawson E, Robbs R S, Barrows H S. Problem-based learning outcomes: the glass half full. Acad Med 2005; 80: 294–99.

25. Fergusson K J. Problem based learning: let's not throw the baby out with the bath water. Med Ed 2005; 39: 352–53.

26. Dolmans D H J M, de Grave W, Wolfhagen I H A P, van der Vleuten I H A P. Problem-based learning: future challenges for educational practice and Research Med Ed 2005; 39: 732–41.

27. Iputo J E, Kwizera E. Problem-based learning improves the academic performance of medical students in South Africa. Med Educ 2005; 39: 388–93.

28. Burke J, Matthew R G, Field M, Lloyd D. Students validate problem-based learning. BMJ 2006; 332: 365.

29. Norman G. Beyond PBL. Adv Hlth Sci Educ 2004; 9: 257–60.

30. Bradley P, Bligh J. Clinical skills centres: where are we going? Med Educ 2005; 39: 649–50.

31. Simulation in clinical medicine. Med Educ 2003; 37 Suppl 1.

32. Dent J A. Adding more to the pie: the expanding activities of the clinical skills centre. J Roy Soc Med 2002; 95: 406–410.

33. Hamilton J D, Ogunbode O. Medical education in the community: a Nigerian experience. Lancet 1991; 338: 99–102.

34. Ogumbode O. Community based medical education. Single philosophy, varied cocktail. Nigeria; 2004.

35. Boaden N, Bligh J. Community based medical education: towards a shared agenda for learning. London: Arnold; 1999.

36. Tamblyn R, et al. Effect of a community oriented problem-based learning curriculum on quality of primary care delivered by graduates: historical cohort comparison study. BMJ 2005; 331: 1001–5.

37. Reforming undergraduate medical education for rural practice. Final Report. Commonwealth Department of Human Services and Health, Australia.

38. Hunter W. An anatomical description of the gravid uterus and its contents. London: J.Johnson and G. Nicol; 1794.

39. Crosby R W, Cody J. Max Brödel: the man who put art into medicine. New York: Springer Verlag; 1991.

40. O'Keefe M, Britten N. Lay participation in medical school curriculum development: whose problem is it? Med Educ 2005; 39: 651–2.

41. Wykurz G, Kelly D. Developing the role of patients as teachers: literature review. BMJ 2002; 325: 818–21.

42. Buchan J, Calman L. Skill mix and policy change in the health workforce: nurses in advanced roles. OECD Health Working Papers 17; 2005.

43. Armitage M. Advanced care practitioners—friend or foe. Lancet 2006; 367: 375–77.

44. Carlisle C, Donovan T, Mercer D, eds. Interprofessional education: an agenda for health care professionals. Salisbury UK: MA Healthcare Ltd; 2005.

45. Zwarenstein M, et al. Interprofessional education. Effects on professional practice and health. Cochrane Collaboration, Oxford. Issue 2. Chichester: John Wiley & Sons; 2005.

46. Class Ticket from the University of Glasgow. University of Glasgow Archives.

47. Schuwirth L, Cantillon P. The need for outcome measures in medical education. BMJ 2005; 331: 977–8.

48. Bolton G. Reflective practice: writing and professional development. 2nd edn. London: Sage Publications; 2005.

49. Rees C, Sheard C. Undergraduate medical students' views about a reflective portfolio assessment of their communication skills learning. Med Educ 2004; 38: 125–8.

50. Norman G. Research in clinical reasoning: past history and current trends. Med Educ 2005; 39: 418–27.

51. Kilpatrick D L. Evaluation of training. In: Craig R L, Bittel L R, eds. Training and development handbook. New York: McGraw Hill Book Company; 1967.

52. Prystowsky J B, Bordage G. An outcome research perspective on medical education: the predominance of trainee assessment and satisfaction. Med Educ 2001; 35: 331–6.

53. Segouin C. Hdges B. Educating doctors in France and Canada: are the differences based on evidence or history? Med Educ 2005; 39: 1205–1212.

54. Bligh J. Research in medical education at the start of the century. Med Educ 2002; 36: 1000–1.

55. Davies M H, Ponnamperuma GG. Medical education research at the crossroads. Lancet 2006; 367: 377–8.

56. Dauphinee W D, Dauphinee G W. The need for evidence in medical education: the development of best evidence medical education as an opportunity to inform, guide and sustain. Acad Med 2004; 79: 425–30.

57. Norman G R, et al, eds. International handbook of research in medical education. Dordrecht: Kluwer Academic Publishers; 2002.

58. Norman G R. Research in medical education: three decades of progress. BMJ 2002; 324: 1560–2.

59. Education Group for Guidelines on Evaluation. Guidelines for

evaluating papers on educational interventions. BMJ 1999; 318: 1265–67.

60. Morrision J, Prideaux D. Ethics approach for research in medical education. Med Educ 2001; 35: 1008.

61. McDougall J, Drummond M J. The development of medical teachers: an enquiry into the learning histories of 10 experienced medical teachers. Med Educ 2005 39: 1213–20.

62. Dahlgren L O, et al. To be and to have a critical friend in medical teaching. Med Educ 2006; 40: 72–78.

63. Osler W. Aequanimitas: teacher and student. New York: McGraw Hill; 1906; 27.

64. Welch W. Humane aspects of medical science. In: Papers and addresses by Willian Henry Welch. Vol. III. Medical Education. Baltimore: Johns Hopkins Press. MDCCCCXX; 6.

65. Welch, 17.

66. Welch, Advancement of Medical Education; 43.

67. Royal Commission on University Education in London. Final Report 1913 (The Haldane Commission) London: HMSO; 1913: Cmnd 6717; 26.

68. Ibid, 27.

69. Board of Education Report of 1910. Special Report of H M Inspectors on Worker's Educational Classes. App X to 3rd Report; 94.

70. The Haldane Commission, 29.

71. Ibid, 36.

72. Ibid, 56.

73. Regulations with regard to the conferment of the titles of professor and reader. University of London; 1912, Appendix II.

74. Matheson C C. Academic staff training and development in universities of the United Kingdom. A Review 1961–81. Issued and distributed by the Co-ordinating Committee for the Training of University Teachers; 1981.

75. Fitch J G. Lectures on teaching. Cambridge: Cambridge University Press; 1881.

76. Fitch J G. Educational aims and methods. Cambridge: Cambridge University Press; 1909; 414–15.

77. Truscoll B. Red brick university. London: Faber and Faber; 1943.

78. Laurence R D. Teaching the teacher to teach. In: First World Conference on Medical Education, 1953. Oxford: Oxford University Press; 1954; 539–44.

79. Arnott W M. The aims of the medical curriculum. In: First

World Conference on Medical Education, 1953. Oxford: Oxford University Press; 1954; 280.

80. University Grants Committee. Report of the Committee on University Teaching Methods. [Chairman, Sir Edward Hale.]. London: HMSO; 1964; 52.

81. Ibid, 100.

82. Ibid, 101.

83. Ibid, 103-112.

84. Ibid, 108.

85. Ibid, 112.

86. CVCP. Training of university teachers: report of the working group. (Brynmor Jones Report); 1972.

87. Greenway H. Training of university teachers. SRHE; 1971.

88. General Medical Council. The doctor as teacher. London: HMSO; 1999.

89. Gibbs G, Coffey M. The impact of training of university teachers on their teaching skills, their approach to teaching and the approach to learning of their students. Active Learning in Higher Education 2004; 5 ; 87–100.

90. Godfrey J, Dennick R, Welsh C. Training the trainers: do teaching courses develop teaching skills. Med Educ 2004; 38: 844–47.

91. Ibid.

15

Beyond learning

When questioned by a student that he had altered his views from last year, John Hunter replied: "Very likely I did. I grow wiser every year".

"Never ask me what I have said or written; but if you ask me what my present opinions are, I will tell you."[1]

John Hunter

Man, as the servant and interpreter of nature, does and understands as much as his observations on the order of nature, either with regard to things or the mind, permit him, and neither knows or is capable of more.[2]

Francis Bacon in *Organum Novum*

INTRODUCTION

*L*earning is the process of acquiring knowledge, skills and attitudes which others already know. This is a valuable activity and, indeed, is the main substance of this book. However, doctors need to go beyond such learning and discover new ideas and see things in a different light. To be interested in changing practice and to be curious about the world is a function of all doctors. Some—the research scientists—will make discovery the main task of their lives.

Others will see research and development only as a part of what they do. Each, however, has the ability and the responsibility of changing and improving health and healthcare. They need to want to do things better and improve the lot of patients and the public. This can take many forms, from detailed work on genetics, molecular biology or pharmacology to changes in the way the service is delivered, or improvements in communication with patients and the public.

One of the great lessons in the writing of this book has been how people—individual doctors or groups of doctors—have been unable to change and adapt to new knowledge and rethink what they do. The geographical journey described in Part 1 of this book shows clearly how, time after time, centres of excellence lost their pre-eminence by getting left behind. They pioneered new ways of thinking, but could not take these further and were overtaken. There is no reason to suppose things will change. Those ahead now, in whatever field, will get left behind unless there is a positive wish to learn from others and keep ahead. This emphasises the need for every doctor and every group of doctors to keep this in mind. The medical profession itself has sometimes not been as forward thinking as it might. An examination of the 50 years or so it took to set up the GMC in the 19th century is a good example of this.

How can we engender this spirit of enquiry? The educational process should encourage students and those in specialist training to think, analyse, problem solve, ask questions and keep asking them (as has been noted before, the ability to solve problems is distinct from problem-based learning). Those who have the privilege of teaching—facilitating the learning—must encourage this spirit and create a climate of questioning and curiosity. Thus, the method of learning is crucial and should not be authority based or reliant on rote learning. The rewards of learning should be based on the ability to reflect, solve problems and deal with difficult issues, as well as retaining facts. The thoughts of Sir James Mackenzie, quoted earlier in this book, on those who do well in medicine are worth further consideration (p. 426). We have come full circle and returned to the role of medicine and its aims and roots: improving health and healthcare, and the process of healing.

Some of this is about the development of wisdom, which also goes beyond learning. Wisdom is the ability to look at a problem—a complex and an uncertain one—and come to a judgement on the appropriate course of action. It is not easy and takes experience and long practice, but it is an essential part of being a doctor. It takes the doctor into theories of complexity and the management of very difficult problems, and combines the need for detailed knowledge with a broader holism about the patient and the community.[3] It is also about the unity of knowledge—the consilience that Edward O. Wilson has written about; bringing knowledge of the arts, sciences and social sciences together in solving the problem. The separation of the silos of knowledge has hindered the development of many specialties.[4]

MEDICAL MAGNETS

An integral part of the history and the geographical movement of expertise over the last 4000 years has been the concept of the 'medical magnet'. This is one of the most interesting conclusions of this book and draws attention to the fact that those who wish to learn medicine have always sought the best. Whether this is in Leiden, Edinburgh, Houston or Cape Town, it matters not. They go because of a new technique (especially in the 20th century), a new method of teaching or new knowledge. Such centres draw students from all over the world and attract staff to work there. These places and people have special characteristics—they are leaders. They have generally gone beyond learning and done something different and new. This trend is likely to continue, and while less prevalent in undergraduate programmes (most programmes are now very good) it is still much the case in specialist and research training. This implies travel of staff to other places and countries. In doing so these individuals establish long-lasting contacts and continuing research and development.

It is interesting to ask the question: 'If I wanted to be a cardiologist (or oncologist, neurologist etc.) where would I go to learn if I had the opportunity?' Perhaps even more interesting: 'Where would I go if I wanted to learn about medical education?' Of course some of the choices will be determined by one's own teachers who have provided the role model for the choice of career: the local medical magnet. Such influences are very powerful and long lasting.

Part of this movement to the best is associated with the atmosphere in such units and around such people. They feel pioneering and exciting, adventurous. The experience can last for a lifetime and create friends, colleagues and links that are kept. Clubs and visiting societies are created around them and perpetuate the fellowship. The leadership passes on and continues. One of the interesting parts of this history has been the continuity of learning and discovery across the years and the recognition that no matter who you are someone else will do it better at some point. Martin Buber in his book *I and Thou* describes this well.[5] He notes that the relationship between the teacher and the pupil changes at some point, and instead of the teacher knowing all of the answers, the pupil begins to take to lead. There is a changeover in the balance from 'I and You' to 'I and Thou'. There is little doubt that one of the most rewarding parts of being a teacher is seeing this progress and watching the pupil become the master, and outdo the work and improve the process of care. It is perhaps one of the most exciting aspects of the learning process for the teacher, when the 'pupil' takes off and goes further and faster...

The characteristics of the medical magnets

From the descriptions of medical magnets in this book, a number of characteristics can be identified which are independent of time and, indeed, of profession. These include:

1. **They developed something new and different.** They took a different path and made people think differently. This

change in direction could be related to a new discovery, technique or procedure, diagnostic test, research programme or a new way of presenting knowledge.

2. **They had considerable connections and networks.** They had contacts on a worldwide basis. They corresponded with like minds wherever they happened to be. Students moved between them and bonds grew up. They travelled widely and knew other leaders personally.

3. **They were passionate about their subject.** They told stories about it and were able to link their own areas of interest to many others. They enthused and inspired.

4. **They enjoyed teaching and passing on their learning.** They were interested in their students, taking a personal interest in their development. Students remembered them, their teaching and their kindness. When the special interest they had was in teaching, they presented this in a systematic way which was new and exciting. Cullen and Boerhaave would be good examples of this, with their integrated approach to their subject.

5. **They had many disciples and acolytes.** This is an important characteristic. Such individuals travelled across the world carrying the messages and knowledge of the master. In more recent times, travelling clubs and societies were formed to bring people together and continue to share experiences.

6. **They were associated with strong teams.** They rarely worked alone, generally having colleagues of equal distinction working with them. Indeed, it was often the team which drew students. They often had a special facility, equipment or technique which was unique and attracted people to work with them.

7. **The environment was conducive to new thinking.** They created an environment which encouraged different ways of thinking, and they took risks to achieve their goals.

In some instances, the external environment was especially favourable, as in the case of the Hunters in London where there was a real vacuum because of the weakness of Oxford and Cambridge at the time. In a similar way in the 18th century, Edinburgh welcomed a new medical school while Glasgow did not. Religious and political reasons sometimes meant that people moved, or did not move, to a particular geographical area. Oxbridge required the passing of a religious test which did not suit non-conformists, who went to Holland or Scotland. In more recent times the environment in the universities and research institutions has also been a major factor. Some of this is externally driven (funding, opportunities, etc.), and some is determined internally by institutional leaders.

8. **They were enormously hard working.** Diaries and records of the medical magnets show that they worked long hours, teaching and in the laboratories and clinics. Their passion for their subject meant that they were devoted to it and lived it 24 hours a day.

9. **They had broader interests.** In spite of the hard work they seemed to have time for broader interests outside medicine: literature, collections, music, art. They often had broader social connections which brought them into contact with the great and the good of their day. Another aspect of the networks they developed.

10. **Leadership.** This was the important characteristic. While they all had different personalities, they had qualities which marked them out as special. They were able to motivate others and effect change. They became legends and heroes; people talked about them and wanted to visit them and learn from them. They were true leaders.

It is interesting to look at this list and consider how current medical practice stands up to it. It describes an outward-looking person, who works incredibly hard, with lots of contacts, interested in people and teaching (handing on learning), working with others and presenting something new. Such individuals require wide experience and have generally worked in several places. They are leaders. It is suggested, therefore, that if places and people are to be able to attract others to them, then some or all of these characteristics need to be satisfied. This becomes an interesting checklist against which to measure one's own performance.

Such a list has consequences not only for individuals—as noted above—but also for organisations and institutions. To keep an institution refreshed requires new ideas, new blood, outside contacts and leadership. When an organisation becomes complacent, does not change, makes too many internal appointments and rests on its laurels then another institution will take over the leading place and become the magnet. This is one of the main lessons from the historical survey in this book. It requires that the head of the institution is creative, and develops an environment which encourages new thinking and is able to take risks, in spite of external pressures.

RESEARCH AS A FUNCTION OF THE DOCTOR

Throughout this volume, the importance of curiosity has been emphasised. This is characteristic of an inquiring mind and the ability to see how things might be explained and understood more fully. In the history of medical education this really began in the 15th and 16th centuries with Vesalius, Harvey, Bacon and Paracelsus challenging the conventional wisdom. The classic dialogue between John Hunter and Edward Jenner on trying out vaccination resulted in Hunter's response: 'But why think. Trie the expt'. The re-examination of the biological process by Descartes opened up new doors, and the French scientists, such as Claude Bernard in his *Introduction to Experimental Medicine*, and the great German experimentalists, Billroth and Virchow, began to set the pattern that disease could be investigated and might be understood better, and on that basis improved treatment developed. Experiments could be devised and hypotheses tested. There is also the important task of learning to evaluate data and information, of devising hypotheses and testing them and in producing original results. Such activities should be part of the learning process and done in association with those who are active in research.

Another thread which runs through this book is the value of teaching and research going hand in hand. It has been supported by many authorities, but has recently been challenged. Why is the link important? How can you justify the statement? In one sense it is answered by the question: 'What puts the higher in higher education?' The assumption is that all one needs is a good teacher, who may or may not be a good research worker. But this response concentrates on teaching, not learning. In a higher education environment, part of the function is to ensure critical thinking and questioning, and this can only be shown by those working at the coal face on real problems. Such individuals perform one of the other functions of the teacher, that of role model and one who enthuses about the subject. That is the bit that makes all the difference.

George Miller's book *Educating Medical Teachers* ends by exhorting those in power to recognise the value of teachers.[6] In a culture dominated by research, teaching may seem to have lesser value and might even be seen as having a lower status. This does not need to be so if the right assumption (learning is not just about being taught) is made.

Finally, there is the issue of research in medical education. We have already noted the scathing remark in the Todd Report of 1967, in which it made clear that the evidence base in medical education was weak and limited. It is generally under-funded and seen to be not quite as good as biomedical research. Yet its value must be considerable. In this section of the book alone—the emerging themes— there is a huge range of research issues which present themselves:

+ selection of students

+ processes of assessment

+ mechanisms of learning

+ diffusion of innovation...and many others.

Each of these topics requires significant research efforts, without which it will not be possible to know whether or not a new learning experience has been worthwhile. Research-based groups, such as the Association for the Study of Medical Education, provide a forum for the presentation of findings, discussion and learning of new methods. Many reports have called for investment and better organisation of research into medical education, and by extension research into the education of other health professionals. Yet little has happened, and the sums of money given for research are not very considerable. One of the conclusions of this book is that research into medical education is one of the most important aspects of improving the quality of the profession and of patient care.

THE ROLE OF THE RESEARCH COUNCILS AND MEDICAL CHARITIES IN MEDICAL EDUCATION

The research councils and the medical charities have played a very significant role in the education of the doctor. They have provided training fellowships, research posts and travel for young doctors over the last 80 or so years. The Medical Research Council, founded in 1913, was the first and over the years has had a substantial impact. The Wellcome Trust (1936) has been equally important in encouraging education and training in research, and particular aspects of research. These were followed by the many medical charities, Cancer Research UK (a combination of the Imperial Cancer Research Fund and the Cancer Research Campaign), the British Heart Foundation, Macmillan Cancer Relief, Leukaemia Research and many many more. The opportunities presented have been crucial in training the next and future generations of research workers and professional leaders. They have actively supported research in new and developing areas, and provide a resource without which patients would not have the up-to-date treatment and diagnostic facilities available now.

The medical research councils and charities are joined by the other research councils in the sciences, social sciences and the arts. They too play a part in improving the research base, expanding both the capacity and capability to carry out research, and improving the quality of care. There is increasing interest in the arts and health, for example: an area of research concerned more with quality of life, including in its portfolio music, art, literature, theatre, dance and architecture. The bringing together of medical science, the physical sciences, social science and the arts and humanities is an important development at the beginning of the 21st century and one of which Osler would have approved.

The research councils and medical charities listed above can be duplicated in other countries, and are given here only as examples of the great debt owed by medicine and by patients to the generosity of such bodies and the public, who give willingly to support others.

DEALING WITH NEW MEDICAL KNOWLEDGE

Part of the process of going beyond learning involves how the medical profession deals with new knowledge and innovation. Evaluating and implementing new knowledge is an important part of the role of the doctor. Whether this is in the dissemination of new ideas and concepts, new treatments or diagnostic tests, or in the changing of the delivery of the service, these are all part of the process of change and innovation, and are different from 'discovery' and research which aim at finding out new ways to do things. It is therefore assumed that the evidence is available, that the change is effective and an improvement for patients or the public. The key issues are how such innovations are evaluated and diffused through the professional practice. It is in no sense a new issue and there are innumerable examples in this book of how doctors have been slow to change and unwilling to give up strongly held views, even in the face of overwhelming evidence. This section will examine some of the reasons why and discuss the ethical issues which result from not keeping up to date.

The diffusion of innovation

When knowledge was limited and changed only slowly, there was little need to keep up to date. Most of the work of the scholars and professors was in the interpretation of the ancients and writing commentaries on their work. The big change occurred in the 16–17th centuries, when the discoveries in anatomy and physiology changed concepts of how the body worked. Harvey and Paracelsus challenged assumptions and created new paradigms of thinking, altering the understanding and classification of disease. As the science of pathology took off and was translated into better ways of treatment, so much more needed to be learned. By the 18th and 19th centuries the knowledge base had expanded considerably, and in the 20th and 21st centuries the pace of change has been even greater, with even more relevance to patient care. This needs to be thought of in what seems to be the innate conservatism of the medical profession. This is perhaps best illustrated by a quote from Molière, writing in the 17th century in *Le Malade Imaginaire*:

> *What pleases me most, and in this he is following my example, is that he holds blindly to the ancients, and has never wished to understand or listen to the so-called discoveries of the century on the circulation of the blood and other questions of the same kind.*[7]

Some background issues

There is a very significant literature in this field: for example, in the textbook *Diffusion of Innovations*, Everrett M. Rogers summarises the literature.[8] He begins by setting out the problem, getting a new idea adopted. This may require a lengthy period and the key question, relevant to all ideas which someone hopes will be adopted, is how to do it, and do it faster. The issue is well beyond medicine.

Diffusion requires communication of an idea within a social system: in this instance the medical profession or subsets of it. The communication will be directed toward reaching a mutual understanding of the value of the idea (defined very generally as a drug, technique, diagnostic procedure or change in management, etc.). Rogers' initial example is the use of lime juice to control scurvy.[9] In 1601 an English sea captain James Lancaster conducted an experiment to evaluate the effectiveness of lime juice in preventing scurvy. The results showed that it was effective. However, it was not introduced and was re-discovered by James Lind in 1747 who knew about Lancaster's results and conducted another experiment, with similar success. But it was not until 1795–98, 40 years later, that the British Navy adopted the use of lime juice. The reasons for the delay are not clear.

The characteristics of successful introduction of innovations might include the following:

+ *Relative advantage*: the innovation is better than the current method.
+ *Compatibility*: it is consistent with current values, past experiences and needs of adopters.
+ *Complexity*: the innovation needs to be understandable and usable.
+ *Trialability*: is the degree to which the innovation can be tried in a limited way.
+ *Observability*: the degree to which the innovation is observable to others. The result can be seen easily.[10]

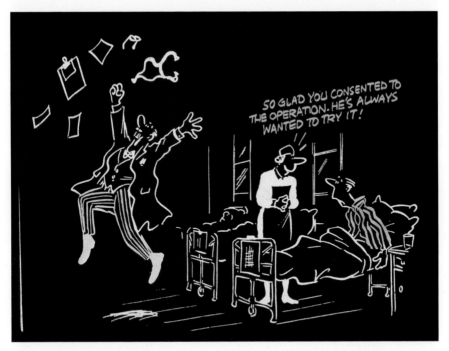

The importance of research and patient involvement. Cartoon by Bill Tidy, with permission.

The rate of adoption will vary depending on these factors.

The process of diffusion is generally described as an S-shaped cure. The process begins slowly, increases more rapidly then levels off. The first phase is where the innovators start the process. Next the early adopters become involved, and this is a key step. If such early adopters are influential people with some standing, in the next phase the majority (divided into early and late if required) will take up the innovation more readily. Finally, there are the laggards. The overall time scale for this process will of course vary.

Some examples

The literature is full of examples of ideas, procedures and treatments which have been introduced, with analysis of the process and time taken for them to be adopted. In all instances there is a delay, and this can be explained generally using the factors listed above.[11,12,13,14]

The paper by McKinlay[12] in the *Millbank Quarterly* takes a slightly different tack. It considers the life stages of a discovery from original enthusiasm, its take up by the majority and then its displacement by something better. This is considered a slow and ineffective process and could be shortened. The 'hype' surrounding some innovations makes then difficult to evaluate, and those involved find it difficult to let go. Sooner or later, however, the new innovation finds its place.

As one example of this, L. Granshaw examines the introduction of antisepsis in Britain from 1867 to 1890.[15] It has as its title a phrase used by Lister, 'Upon this principle I have based a practice'. The article begins with the problem: mortality rates in surgical wards in the mid-19th century and the development of a possible solution by Joseph Lister in the surgical wards of the Royal Infirmary of Glasgow in 1867. Lister was introduced to Pasteur's germ theory by Thomas Anderson, professor of chemistry at Glasgow, and using carbolic acid spray tested the method. He presented his findings 'On the antiseptic principle in the practice of surgery' to the Annual Meeting of the British Medical Association in 1867. His approach to the introduction was limited. He did not attempt to explain the theory and presented little in the way of results. The paper was published in both the *BMJ* and *The Lancet*. While some tried the method, there was scepticism from some powerful people, such as James Young Simpson, who noted that the idea was not original and there were other ways of achieving similar results. Lister moved to Edinburgh and London where the debate continued. The method was cumbersome and expensive, and Lister did not present many results in spite of requests to do so. He had his disciples who carried on the work but the debate shifted to spray and gauze versus cleanliness. His move to London helped in moving the debate forward at the same time as the evidence for cleanliness became clearer. Surgeons in Germany were much more positive about the method and assisted in the acceptance of the technique. By 1887 *The Lancet* at last accepted that that the use of the spray and the associated dressing had had an effect. The later history of the innovation portrayed Lister as a hero. One very interesting story is recounted by Granshaw from Hector Cameron:

> ...to the spectator, the spray and the cloud of highly irritating vapour which it emitted to envelope the operator and his assistants, was the most striking feature of the scene. As Lister entered the crowded theatre, his mobile face set and solemn as he bethought himself of the responsibilities he was about to undertake, he was followed in procession by his train of dressers, the first of whom bore aloft the sacred spray. Once the silence was broken by some ribald student whose voice was heard intoning, "let us spray."[16]

A further example of diffusion of innovation is covered in an article by Lawrence.[17] This article deals with the medical professions reaction to new technology and in particular the sphygmomanometer and the thermometer. While there was a view that science was important, the medical elite were content to play to the art. Lawrence records the words of Patrick Black, a physician of St Bartholomew's Hospital, who told his students:

> Your profession demands from you that you shall possess what is called scientific knowledge, and it is expected from your acknowledged station in society that you should not be wanting in those accomplishments which distinguish the position of gentlemen.

A classical education was important, as was maintaining an image. The most valuable knowledge was that acquired by long experience and observation, and this could be easily communicated to others orally or in writing: a good example of secret knowledge.

In spite of proponents of the science, like Clifford Allbutt, the profession remained generalist with little specialisation, and physicians tended to despise the stethoscope, the ophthalmoscope and the microscope. *The Lancet* noted in 1860 that 'it may be doubted whether these instruments, though very ingenious, will ever prove actually useful in practice'.[18] Another quote in Lawrence states: 'Physicians should eschew instrumental aids and educate the "finger"'.[19] London medicine was filled with gentlemen and science had a hard time gaining a foothold.

Some more recent examples

The examples above refer to topics which were active some years ago. There are many others including: vaccination, serum therapy for diphtheria, X-ray technology in obstetrics, sanatorium treatment, the use of aspirin in chest pain and the introduction of many new and effective drugs. In the past 15 years, new mechanisms have been developed for changing practice, including the use of guidelines, national service frameworks and evidence-based clinical procedures. Advice issued from organisations such as the National Institute for Clinical Excellence (NICE) have provided a way in which such guidance can be assessed in practice, along with the mechanisms available to achieve more rapid implementation. The guidance (or evidence) has generally been gathered using a variety of methods (e.g. clinical trials) and assessed by the relevant specialist group. The evidence or guidance is generally well publicised. If recommended, the evidence is thus clear, readily available and it is backed by colleagues with influence. The last few years have therefore seen a series of publications monitoring whether or not the guidelines have been implemented. In an editorial, Fiona Godlee analyses some of the issues and concludes that while things are complex the topic is one which needs to be tackled.[20] Books have followed, such as *Getting Research into Practice* and *Innovations in Health and Medicine. Diffusion and resistance in the 20th century*, as well as publications such as *Clinical Evidence* published regularly by the *BMJ* and American College of Physicians since 1999.[21,22] The following are some examples of the results of such investigations:

Closing the gap between research and practice; an overview of systematic reviews of interventions to promote the implementation of research findings.[23] This article was part of a series which looked at the gap between research and practice. The literature was searched for reviews of interventions to improve professional performance, and 18 met the criteria and covered a wide range of interventions. Following the analysis the authors listed the issues which affected the outcome.

Interventions to promote behavioural change among health professionals:

1. Consistently effective interventions

    + Educational outreach visits

    + Reminders (manual or computerised)

    + Multifaceted interventions

    + Interactive educational meetings

2. Interventions of variable quality

    + Audit and feedback

    + The use of local opinion

    + Local consensus processes

    + Patient-mediated interventions

3. Interventions that had little or no effect

    + Educational materials—distribution of recommendations

    + Didactic educational meetings.

These should come as no surprise to those who have followed the educational history in this book: involvement, interaction, local consensus, etc. The authors note: 'It is striking how little is known about the effectiveness and cost effectiveness of interventions that aim to change the practice or delivery of health care'.

The case for knowledge translation: shortening the journey from evidence to effect.[24] This paper also covers the literature on the effectiveness of education. The most relevant strategies are those which are active, multiple, based on an assessment of need and aimed at overcoming barriers to change. These strategies may be limited for a variety of reasons. The authors suggest a new model: that of knowledge translation. This focuses on the setting within the practice, the targets (all participants in the health care practice including patients), the use of evidence-based research and a more holistic view linking the practitioner–learner to the healthcare system.

Re-inventing continuing medical education.[25] This paper again notes the difficulties with CME and presents evidence for practice-based learning with practice improvement strategies and then re-certification.

The assessment of NICE guidelines on two surgical procedures.[26] This article considers the effect of NICE guidelines on two surgical procedures: wisdom tooth extraction and primary total hip replacement. The analysis showed that the NICE guidance was not the primary reason for the downward trend in extractions, and that for total hip replacements there was no significant change in behaviour away from the non-cemented hip prosthesis. The conclusion was that the guidance had little effect.

What is the evidence that NICE guidance has been implemented? Results from a national evaluation using time series analysis, audit of patients' notes, and interviews.[27] This is a very large study and uses a variety of topics, such as the control of obesity, taxanes for cancer, extraction of wisdom teeth, and drugs for Alzheimer's disease. The conclusion was:

> ...that the implementation of NICE guidance has been variable. Guidance seems more likely to be adopted when there is strong professional support, a stable and convincing evidence base, and no increased or unfunded costs, in organisations that have established good systems for tracking guidance implementation and where the professionals involved are not isolated. Guidance needs to be clear and reflect the clinical context.

Again the implications are clear. So does an effective educational programme help? This was answered in a paper entitled: *What is the evidence that postgraduate teaching in evidence based medicine changes anything? A systematic review.* Twenty three studies were evaluated and there is a clear conclusion: 'Teaching of evidenced based medicine should be moved from classrooms to clinical practice to achieve improvements in substantial outcomes'.[28]

What does all this mean? The results above represent a brief review of the work in this area; however, the results are typical. They indicate that changing practice is complex and that to do so requires considerable thought. Like many educational areas, it is simply assumed that teaching is all that is needed. A good lecture will do the trick, especially if it is by a distinguished visiting professor. So much for the work of the last 4000 years. What does change practice? How can it best be achieved? These are still questions which haunt the educationalist. Learning is more than just listening and reading. It is about changing behaviour and acting differently. The need for research is greater than ever.

One way of thinking about this, based on the work noted above, is to make the assumption that diffusion of innovation depends on a process of learning. In this instance, learning is defined as the process by which an individual changes behaviour in response to new knowledge, skills or attitudes. Such a statement does not define the content or the method of learning. On the basis of the work described above, this learning should be:

+ practice-based
+ inclusive of all members of the team
+ associated with improved practice delivery
+ active and involve the individual
+ based on a strong evidence base
+ relevant to clinical care.

ETHICAL ISSUES OF NOT KEEPING UP TO DATE

This is an issue which follows from the discussion above. It is an ethical responsibility to keep up to date, hence the importance of regular peer review and revalidation. Patients need to be assured that when they are seen by a doctor, the most up-to-date methods and treatments are being deployed. Or if these methods and treatments are outside the knowledge and skills of that doctor, the patients should be referred elsewhere. This is not just a platitude, but a fundamental part of being a doctor.

CONCLUSIONS

Beyond learning takes the medical practitioner into a different way of thinking. Not only must they continue to learn from others, they must also ensure that they remain curious and open to fresh views. They must continue to pursue new concepts and improve patient care. There is an aboriginal saying which encapsulates this:

There are no paths, paths are made by walking.

Doctors need to continue to search for new 'paths' to find better ways of healing and delivering care.

REFERENCES

1. Moore W. The knife man. London: Bantam Press; 2005; 245.
2. Bacon F. Organum novum. First book, para 1.
3. Downie R S, Macnaughton J. Clinical judgement: evidence in practice. Oxford: Oxford University Press; 2000.
4. Wilson E O. Consilience: the unity of knowledge. London: Abacus; 1998.
5. Buber M. I and thou. Edinburgh: SCM Press; 1958.
6. Miller G E. Educating medical teachers. Cambridge, Mass: Harvard University Press; 1980.

7. Molière. Le Malade Imaginaire.

8. Rogers E M. Diffusion of innovations. 4th ed. New York: Free Press; 1995.

9. Ibid, 7–8.

10. Ibid, 15–16.

11. Fenell M M, Warnecke R B. Diffusion of Medical Innovations: an applied network analysis. New York: Plenum; 1988.

12. McKinlay J B. From Promising report to standard procedure: seven stages in the career of a medical innovation. Millbank Fund Quarterly 1981; 59: 374–411.

13. Coleman J S, et al. Medical innovations: a diffusion study. In: Pickstone J V. Medical Innovations in Historical Perspective. New York: St Martin's Press; 1992.

14. Gabbay J, Walley T. Introducing new health interventions. BMJ 2006; 332:64–65.

15. Granshaw L. Upon this principle I have based a practice. In: Pickstone J V. Medical Innovations in Historical Perspective. New York: St Martin's Press; 1992.

16. Ibid, 29.

17. Lawrence C. Incommunicable knowledge: science, technology and the clinical art in Britain 1850–1914. J Contemporary History 1985; 20: 503–20.

18. Lancet 1860; (i): 435.

19. Lawrence S C. Charitable knowledge: hospital pupils and practitioners in eighteenth century London. Cambridge: Cambridge University Press; 1966; 516.

20. Godlee F. Getting evidence into practice. BMJ 1998; 317: 6.

21. Clifford C, Clark J. Getting Research into Practice Edinburgh: Churchill Livingstone; 2004.

22. Stanton J, ed. Innovations in Health and Medicine. Diffusion and resistance in the 20th century. London: Routledge; 2002.

23. Bero L A, et al. Closing the gap between research and practice; an overview of systematic reviews of interventions to promote the implementation of research findings. BMJ 1998; 317: 465–8.

24. Davies D, et al. The case for knowledge translation: shortening the journey from evidence to effect. BMJ 2003; 327: 33–35.

25. Clancy C. Re-inventing continuing medical education. BMJ 2004; 328: E291.

26. Ryan J, Piercy J, James P. The assessment of NICE guidelines on two surgical procedures. Lancet 2004: 363: 1525–26.

27. Sheldon T A, et al. What is the evidence that NICE guidance has

been implemented? Results from a national evaluation using time series analysis, audit of patients' notes, and interviews. BMJ 2004; 329: 999–1004.

28. Coomarasamy A, Khan K S. What is the evidence that post-graduate teaching in evidenced based medicine changes anything? A systematic review. BMJ 2004; 329: 1017–9.

PART 3
The future

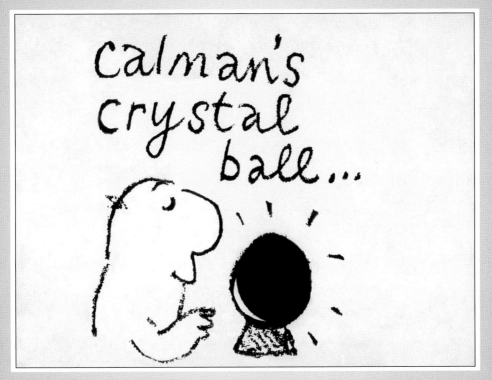

The future of medical education, bright and confident. © S.&C. Calman.
Reproduced with permission.

16

Conclusions

Oh wad some pow'r the giftie gie us to see oursels as others see us.[1]

Robert Burns

The fault dear Brutus is not in our stars but in ourselves that we are underlings.[2]

William Shakespeare

Human progress is neither automatic or inevitable...Every step towards the goal of social justice requires sacrifice, suffering and struggle and the passionate concerns of dedicated individuals. This is no time for complacency. It is a time for vigorous and positive action.[3]

Martin Luther King

INTRODUCTION

The three quotations which head this final chapter have been chosen with care. They illustrate some of the major issues in medical education. First, the medical profession needs to see itself dispassionately and from the outside, and recognise that others may not be as happy with medical education, and hence medical practice, as is the profession.

Second, it is likely that the problems and their solutions lie within the profession and not in outside forces. Of course, the environment will change, and there will be changes in the organisation of practice, which the profession may not like. But the profession can still continue to provide a service to patients and the public with compassion and care. The solutions lie within the profession, hence the need for leadership at all levels. The profession should set the agenda, not be led by it.

The final quotation gives the answer. The profession must take the lead and show that it can continue to improve care and provide a service to patients and the public. This is what the section on 'Aims of medicine' (p. 345) was all about. It is not a time to be complacent—perhaps it never was—but this is certainly the time for action.

The profession is often viewed from the outside as conservative and unable to change. Numerous examples have been noted in this book—from the past and the present—in which opportunities have been missed or delayed. In such circumstances, the profession is seen to react to events rather than leading and creating opportunities. This is perhaps the first and most important lesson from this book. The profession has to change and to lead the process of change.

This book has taken a particular view of the history of medical education, that of a profession passionately concerned about standards, quality, care and compassion. Not everyone will agree with this approach, or the conclusion. There might have been many other ways of tackling the issues raised in this book. In spite of all of the changes over the centuries, medicine remains a great profession. The efficiency of the process of medical education (numbers entering compared to numbers gaining awards) is very high. We do it well, but could do better. Thousands and thousands of graduates and specialists reach high standards each year, able to provide assistance to the process of healing to millions of people, day in and day out. Their actions are related to the overall aim of medicine, improving health, healthcare and quality of life.

If we return to the beginning of this book we imagined a group of medical students and young doctors together with patients asking questions about their future and the future of medicine. Have their questions been answered? To some extent they have. The educational process has been described, and is now better than it has ever been. There is a much greater interest in learning and in the outcome of the process itself (what it is for) rather than in the mechanisms and minutiae of curriculum development. There is much activity at present in this area, and this must be a good thing if we are to take the second of the big messages of this book to heart—the questioning of conventional wisdom and challenging the norm. The fact that the current evidence base remains weak in many aspects of medical education is a major problem; more needs to be done.

But to return to our medical students on their first day of term. What do they need to set them off on their journey? What do they need to explore the world of learning medicine and begin their adventure?

+ A wish to be a doctor, and be selected for entry to a medical school—the selection process.

+ An objective and a direction of travel—a goal to aim for, a compass to act as a lodestone to refer to. This sets the goals, values and beliefs to return to each time.

+ A map, background information and a guide book—these are the learning resources available and include everything from books to people.

+ A guide, mentor, master, teacher—to give advice, interpret and support, to provide correction where appropriate and to inspire, enthuse, rebuke and be a role model. The need for such guides will vary depending on where the doctor is on the journey, but they are always necessary.

+ A good pair of boots to get started, and real experience—this is not an armchair job, practical experience of seeing and doing is necessary.

+ A record of progress towards objectives—a diary or journal to log the stops on the way, reflections and an analysis of progress.

+ An overall progress report by other travellers.

Such a list presents medicine as an adventure, as a journey of exploration and discovery. It is not a boring or repetitive journey, though there will be times when progress seems slow and difficult. However, it is the objective—the aim—which provides the energy to keep going.

History has shown how the educational process has progressed and been able to deal with enormous changes in knowledge and skills, and the changing role of medicine in society. There have been significant shifts in attitudes, values and beliefs, and a changing relationship with patients and the public. These changes are likely to continue and the pace will quicken.

The learning environment has also changed enormously over the centuries. While some key aspects endure (lectures, small-group teaching and the use of the book), new methods have been added: laboratory work, skills labs, problem-based learning, special study modules and simulated patients. New methods of assessment have also developed and again are likely to continue to change.

In the early days of medical education, the emphasis was on the undergraduate part of the course, now it encompasses specialist education and continuing professional development. The continuity between the phases is recognised and the transition between them more appropriately managed. There is a greater interest now in the role and aims of medicine, and the current interest in the concept of a profession and a professional is an important return to the roots of medicine. Defining the characteristics and qualities, and identifying the competences, allows better selection, and the determination of a curriculum (at all levels) which meets the needs of patients and the public is now much more of a reality.

The next few decades are likely to see the pace of change accelerating, partly related to changes in knowledge. In particular, however, the relationship with patients and the public will be re-assessed. There will be much more of a partnership and increased involvement. There will be greater emphasis on revalidation (or whatever it will be called) to assure the public of the quality of the learning and of the competence of doctors. Doctors should lead this debate and see it as an opportunity, not a threat.

As we move further into the 21st century, there are a number of factors which are likely to determine the way forward. Predicting the future is not part of the remit of this book, but the following topics will possibly shape the direction of medical practice and education.

THE CONTEXT

Reference has already been made to the potential increase in knowledge and skills which will be required of doctors. Somehow this will need to be encompassed in learning programmes without recourse to filling every minute of the curriculum, the bane of the medical student and postgraduate's life. This will mean more careful planning and, at the same time, freeing up the learner to pursue special interests and aptitudes. The pace will increase and new discoveries may totally alter the knowledge and skills required of the doctor. The content of the curriculum may be radically different from the present. Educational programmes must reflect this.

The second contextual issue is that of the health service which, if past experience is anything to go on, will continue to change and be reorganised. This may affect the ability to deliver effective learning; educators will need to be one step ahead of the game. This not peculiar to the UK but is likely to be a worldwide phenomenon as politicians try to deliver an increasingly effective service with improved efficiency. The educational process should not be determined by such changes but will need to use them to best effect.

In a similar way, the social context within which medicine is practised is likely to alter. Changes in social policy and demography—and expectations—will impact on the kind of service patients and the public will require. Expectations will rise and, with this, requirements for more information and support. Greater public and patient involvement will be the norm, and—as we have discussed—this should be welcomed and encouraged. After all, it is their body, their health and quality of life, and they have a right to be part of the process.

In addition to demographics, changes in the determinants and distribution of disease will feature in the future. New diseases and patterns of disease will appear and old ones will change their characteristics. Lessons from the past mean that educators need to reflect these changes by modifying the curriculum to suit. How medicine responds to these new challenges will be determined partly by our ability to better understand disease and partly by the development of new interventions to improve care. The international dimension of health and disease will become more prominent as new diseases develop and populations move around the globe. As the population ages, chronic diseases and the processes of ageing will become more prominent.

The last 100 years has seen considerable expansion in the role of the specialist. This brings benefits and some disadvantages. It is possible that there will remain the need for some who are 'generalists' and can see clinical problems with a broad vision.

LEARNING MEDICINE

Driven by these contextual factors, the processes, methods and outcomes of learning are likely to change. Perhaps the first of these changes will be the need for greater preparation of teachers for the task. As we have discussed, preparation for teaching is a relatively recent phenomenon. It is just assumed that doctors will be good at it. Yet there is much to be learned and appreciated about education and learning. New educational methods (in learning and assessment) will need to be recognised and prepared for in addition to updating the medical skills and knowledge base.

It is hoped that there will be more emphasis on developing the evidence base for medical education. This is progressing but much more needs to be done. There is a need for investment in this area and the provision of a much needed research base in order that the learning process can be improved. Much can be learned from other disciplines (education, anthropology, philosophy, social sciences) and from experience in medical education around the world. The role of journals, books, seminars and meetings in this process is important if knowledge is to be shared. The expertise available is limited, and the establishment of centres for research and development on medical education should be part of this. As a subset, there needs to be a greater understanding of how new knowledge is disseminated and introduced into practice. This needs to be a priority for research. Why don't doctors take up new ideas in clinical practice as rapidly as they might? How can they get better at keeping up to date? These are not questions peculiar to medicine but to all professions. Curiosity and a wish to do better are part of the role of being a doctor. This leads to a further point: the need for a stronger evidence base and for the profession to learn from such a base more effectively.

The potential conflict between research and teaching is often raised as a reason for downgrading the status of the teacher. How is it possible to do both well—after all, research brings in more money and prestige? Yet this is a false antithesis. Teaching and research can and should go hand in hand. As has been noted, the question can be posed in another way. What is it that puts the higher in higher education? It is the learning which should proceed in an environment of research, experiment and scholarship. Teaching itself is not enough without the atmosphere of inquiry and discovery. Being close to where knowledge is being developed is at the heart of learning medicine. This is also one of the reasons that learning medicine should continue in a university environment. As the knowledge base expands and the practice of medicine requires input from across the spectrum, from the big sciences to the arts and humanities, so there is a need to remain close to such subjects, and the best place to do this is in a university. Interdisciplinarity will be the future and needs to be reflected in the learning environment.

This relationship with other subjects will also need to be reflected in the ways in which students and postgraduates interact with other health and social care professionals during learning. At present, a number of methods are employed to encourage and support such learning and it is envisaged that these will increase and be modified as the results of research are published and disseminated. Such learning will reflect the changing roles of the various professions. In addition, there will be changes in the healthcare organisation of the country or region, and the impact of these changes on the process of education will need to be taken into account.

As well as learning the scientific basis of medicine, the doctor of the future is likely to have a greater interest in social sciences, the arts and humanities. Ethical issues will remain important as better methods of helping doctors to think through their own ideas, values and beliefs become available. The role of the arts and humanities is likely to grow with a greater emphasis on issues such as quality of life, care and compassion, and as the aim of medicine is discussed and debated. The holistic view of health is part of this thinking. The rise of interest in professionalism will add to this.

In educational terms, many questions remain. How can we better select those who are to become doctors and those who will be specialists? In no sense are these new issues but the pressure now is to get better at selection and thus allow greater public reassurance and better care. In addition it is likely that new methods of education will be introduced, including new types of assessment which should strengthen this outcome.

There will be a continuing debate on the role of books and developments in IT. The potential for learning is huge using the developing technologies and specialities, such as rural medicine, and health can flourish and grow using such methods. The ability to transmit data and images, carry out live conversations and consultations by digital technology is likely to have an immense impact on patient care. In the same way, contact with a master (the apprenticeship process) will remain an important part of learning and the passing on of wisdom and values. It is in such ways that secret or tacit knowledge is passed on. Medicine is likely to remain an inexact science for some time. It is thus essential to ensure that doctors are able to deal with uncertainty and unexpected and new developments as they occur.

On a personal note, the most powerful learning experience for the author of this book was in setting up a series of support groups for cancer patients (Tak Tent Groups after the old Scots phrase for take care). As a high quality oncology unit (or so we thought), it was salutary to meet patients in an informal setting, get to know them and realise that their experience was worth much more than mine. They had so much to give if they were allowed to contribute and be involved. They taught me what it was like to suffer from cancer and how I could help them and others in a more effective way. I have always been grateful for that privilege.

THE MEDICAL PROFESSION

It has already been noted that the profession itself should lead the debate about its future. Much will change and the profession needs to be flexible and able to respond rapidly and effectively. Over the years it is clear that the profession has not acted with a single voice, and power struggles have been characteristic of the response. Perhaps now is the time to have a single 'academy' which brings together all aspects of the profession of medicine. Individual societies (local, national and international) and specialist groups are an essential part of this, providing input from the front line and immediate contact with patients and the public. But there is a bigger goal than the interests of individual groups, that of creating a profession dedicated to healing. One major reason for this is that the boundaries between related professional groups and medicine will continue to change, and medicine will have to re-define itself on a regular basis. Hence, the need for leadership and taking the initiative on the future of medicine, its scope and regulation.

There is also a significant debate to be had on the detailed structure of education and medical practice. For example, there is an increasing tendency to specialise in particular fields of clinical practice. This has a positive benefit for patients in that they will have access to up-to-date specialist care. There is also a downside, that of being too specialised, as doctors learn more and more about less and less. This emphasises the need for a generalist, the wise doctor (physician, surgeon, gynaecologist, etc.) who can see the whole picture, the whole patient. As some medical tasks are taken over by other professional groups, so we will need such people. Medicine has always been blessed by such generalists, men and women to whom the difficult problems are referred not for specialist care but for diagnostic skills. Such generalists have three functions:

understanding disease and illness

understanding people

understanding the concept of 'diagnosis'.

Of course, specialists have the same skills but generally in a narrower area. In the future, just as the generalist will need to keep up to date with specialist practice, the specialist will need to be familiar with subjects across the medical field. Post-graduate training, CPD programmes and the process of revalidation will need to reflect such requirements.

Part of this requires that the profession is clear about what it means by competence. The definition of competence developed in this book —the application in practice of knowledge, skills and attitudes to real problems in real time—needs further thought and reflection by each of the specialty groups. This includes the ability to deal with the unexpected, to remain calm and in control during periods of high activity and stress, such as in dealing with emergencies. Defining competence is a fundamental task and one which each speciality group (including generalists) needs to undertake for itself. There is an international dimension to this as there is to other aspects of clinical and public health practice.

This also relates to how medicine is regulated. The current debate (2005) on the role of the GMC in the UK is an important one. Difficulties in the recent past have meant that medicine is now scrutinised as never before. This can be seen as a threat or as an opportunity to show how the safety of patients and the quality of care provided leads the agenda for change. The next few years will be crucial to the profession of medicine. Much of this will require that doctors are convinced that change is essential and urgently needed. The saying 'mural dyslexia' (the inability to see the writing on the wall) may be relevant here. Current debates on professionalism are to be encouraged.

Finally, in this section there is the need to discuss some related issues. First, the dichotomy between the clinician and the medical scientist; second, medicine as an art or a science. We need both clinicians and research scientists working to improve care for patients and provide better public health. There is a continuum between the two ends of the spectrum in both cases, and it may vary with time for each doctor. The classic difference was noted in the contrast between Sydenham, the clinician, and Boyle, the clinical scientist. Both were necessary to change medical practice, and indeed both were good friends.

Medicine is also both an art and a science. This is neatly summarised by Weatherall:

The principal problem for those who educate our doctors of the future is how, on the one hand, to encourage a life long attitude of critical scientific thinking to the management of illness and, on the other, to recognise that moment when the scientific approach, because of ignorance, has reached its limit and must be replaced by sympathetic empiricism. Because of the dichotomy between the self-confidence required at the bedside and the self-critical uncertainty essential in the research laboratory, it may always be difficult to achieve this balance. Can one person ever combine the two qualities? Possibly not but this is the goal to which medicine must aspire.[4]

Judgements remain difficult as Hippocrates noted some time ago, and until the science has caught up with uncertainty and all patients behave in the same way, there will be a role for the art of medicine. Ethical issues will remain of crucial importance as will experience, wisdom and judgement. Sometimes, of course, the 'art' can be seen as an excuse for sloppy thinking and a lack of awareness of the evidence available. Most times it is a proper response to uncertainty and the choices of patients.

THE ROLE OF MEDICINE

All of the discussion above is predicated on a clear understanding of the role of medicine, its aims and how such aims can be put into practice. The outcome of medical education has such potential benefits for patients and the community; if we can continue to improve it, it will be people who will reap the harvest. Current debates about boundaries between the various health care and social care professions simply sharpen the need to be clear about the purpose of medicine. This topic has been dealt with at length in a previous chapter, but the aims and characteristics might be conveniently summarised now:

+ Assisting in healing and all that this implies.
+ An interest in people.
+ A recognition of the needs of patients and the public.

+ An understanding of disease and illness.

+ A system of professional governance to support these aims.

The history of medical education provides a rich seam to mine, full of examples of best and worst practice, and gives hope for the future. There is more to be done and learned from the past. Medicine remains an adventure, an exciting and wonderful profession within which there are places for different approaches and styles. Above all, the profession needs to be clear about its role, defined in this book as the assistance in healing of body, mind and spirit. Doctors and the profession need to continue to learn for the benefit of patients and the community.

And finally, every doctor also needs:

+ A sense of purpose and excitement to know where we are going.

+ A sense of confidence without arrogance. Humility is a great virtue.

+ A sense of competence—but always willing to learn.

+ A sense of courtesy and respect for the feelings of others.

+ A sense of commitment to maintaining standards in personal and professional life.

+ A sense of contentment with interest outside work.

+ A sense of humour to keep us going when things get tough.

The *Regimen Sanitatis Salerni* translated by Sir John Harrington in 1607 has already been referred to in an earlier chapter. Its last paragraph is a splendid way of ending this book:

> *And here I cease to write, but will not cease*
> *To wish you live in health and die in peace*
> *And ye our physic rules that friendly read*
> *God grant that physic you will never need.*[5]

REFERENCES

1. Burns, R. To a mouse. 1786.
2. Shakespeare W. Julius Caesar. Act 1, scene 2.
3. King M L. Strive toward freedom: the Montgomery story. London: Victor Gollancz Ltd; 1959; 187
4. Weatherall D J. Science and the quiet art. Oxford: Oxford University Press; 1995.
5. Regimen Sanitatis Salerni. Translated by Sir John Harrington in 1607. Salerno: Ente Provinciale per il Turismo; 1966.

Further reading

History of medicine and medical education

Barzansky B, Gevitz, N, eds. Beyond Flexner: medical education in the twentieth century. New York: Greenwood Press; 1992.

Bernard C. Experimental medicine. Translated by Greene H C, Henderson L J. New York: Macmillan Company; 1927.

Billroth T. The medical sciences in the German universities. Translation and introduction by William Welch. New York: Macmillan and Co.; 1924.

Bonner TN. Becoming a physician. Oxford: Oxford University Press; 1995.

Buchan W. Domestic medicine. Edinburgh; 1824.

Burnham J C. How the idea of profession changed the writing of medical history. Medical History, Suppl.18. London: Wellcome Institute for the History of Medicine; 1998.

Castiglione A. Histoire de la Médecine. Paris: Payot; 1931.

Davies N. Europe: a history. Oxford: Oxford University Press; 1996.

Edelstein L. In: Temkin O, Temkin C, eds. L. Ancient Medicine, Selected Papers of Ludwig Edelstein. Baltimore: John Hopkins Press; 1967.

The Flexner Report on Medical education in the United States and Canada. 1910. Carnegie Foundation for the Advancement of Learning.

Gairdner W T. The physician as a naturalist. Glasgow: James Maclehose; 1889.

Garrison F H. An introduction to the history of medicine. 4th edn. Philadelphia and London: W B Saunders Company; 1929.

Gribbin J. Science: a history, 1543–2001. London: Allen Lane, The Penguin Press; 2002.

Guthrie D. History of medicine. Edinburgh: Thomas Nelson; 1958.

Guthrie D. Extramural medical education in Edinburgh, and the School of Medicine of the Royal Colleges. Edinburgh E S Livingstone; 1965.

Kuhn T S. The structure of scientific revolutions. 3rd edn. Chicago; University of Chicago Press; 1996.

Morton L T, ed. Garrison and Morton's medical bibliography. 2nd edn. London: Andre Deutsch; 1965.

Newman C. The evolution of medical education in the nineteenth century. Oxford: Oxford University Press; 1957.

Newman G. Some notes on medical education in England. A memorandum presented to the president of the board. London: HMSO; 1918.

Nutton V, Porter R. eds. The history of medical education in Britain. Amsterdam–Atlanta GA: Clio Medica. Rodopi; 1995.

O'Malley C D, ed. The history of medical education. Los Angeles: University of California Press; 1970.

Osler W. Aequanimitas: with other addresses to medical students, nurses and practitioners of medicine. London: H.K.Lewis; 1904.

Porter R. The greatest benefit to mankind. London: Fontana Press; 1999.

Poynter F N L, ed. The evolution of medical education in Britain. London: Pitman Medical Publishing Co; 1966.

Puschmann T. A history of medical education. Translated and edited by Hare E H, Lewis H.K. London; 1891.

Report of the Inter-departmental Committee on Medical Schools. (Goodenough Report) 1944. HMSO.

Weatherall D J. Science and the quiet art: medical research and patient care. Oxford: Oxford University Press; 1995.

General education

Ayer A J. The problem of knowledge. Harmondsworth: Penguin Books; 1956.

Bacon F. The advancement of learning. 1605.

Buber M. I and Thou. Translated by Smith R G. 2nd edn. Edinburgh: T and T Clark Ltd; 1958.

Dent H C. The training of teachers in England and Wales. London: Hodder and Stoughton; 1977.

Edmonds D, Eidinow J. Wittgenstein's poker. London: Faber and Faber; 2005.

Faraday M, Bragg L. Advice to lecturers: an anthology. Royal Institution; 1974.

Fitch J G. Lectures on teaching delivered in the University of Cambridge during the Lent Term, 1880. Cambridge: Cambridge University Press; 1881.

Jarvis P, Holford J, Griffin C. The theory and practice of learning. London: Kogan Page; 1998.

Locke J. Some thoughts concerning education. 1693.

Cardinal Newman. The idea of a university.

Palmer J, ed. Fifty major thinkers in education: from Confucius to Dewey. London: Routledge; 2001.

Palmer J A, ed. Fifty modern thinkers on education: from Piaget to the present. London: Routledge; 2001.

Stewart G. The story of Scottish education. London: Pitman and Sons; 1927.

Medical education

Barrows H S, Tamblyn H S, eds. Problem based learning. An approach to medical education. New York: Springer Publishing Company; 1980.

Carlisle C, Donovan T, Mercer D, eds. Interprofessional education: an agenda for health care professionals. Dinton, Wiltshire: Quay Books; 2005.

Committee of Enquiry into Competence to Practise. Competence to practise: report of a committee of enquiry set up for the medical profession in the United Kingdom (Alment Report). London; 1976.

Committee of Inquiry into the Regulation of the Medical Profession. Report of the Committee of Inquiry into the Regulation of the Medical Profession. (The Merrison Report). London: HMSO; 1976.

Dent J A, Harden R M, ed. A practical guide for medical teachers. 2nd edn. Edinburgh: Churchill Livingstone; 2005.

General Medical Council. Recommendations on education and examination. London: Spottiswood and Co; 1881.

Green J S, Grosswald S J, Suter E, Walthall D B, eds. Continuing education for the health professions. San Francisco: Jossey-Bass Publishers; 1984.

Guilbert J J. Educational handbook for health personnel. Geneva: WHO offset Publication No 35; 1977.

Guthrie D. Extramural medical education in Edinburgh and the School of the Medical Royal Colleges. Edinburgh: E and S Livingstone; 1965.

Henry R, Byrne K, Engel C, eds. Imperatives in medical education: the Newcastle approach. Newcastle, Australia: Faculty of Medicine and Health Sciences, University of Newcastle; 1997.

McGaghie W C, Miller G E, Sajid A W, Telder T V. Competency-based curriculum development in medical education: an introduction. WHO; Geneva; 1978.

Miller G E. Educating medical teachers. Cambridge, Mass: Harvard University Press; 1980.

Peyton J W R, ed. Teaching and learning in medical practice. Manticore Europe Ltd; 1998.

Pickering G. Quest for excellence in medical education. Nuffield Provincial Hospitals Trust. Oxford: Oxford University Press; 1978.

Physicians for the twenty-first century. Report of the Project Panel on the General Professional Education of the Physician and College Preparation for Medicine. Journal of Medical Education. 59; 1984 (whole volume).

Royal Commission on Medical Education 1965–68. (Todd Report). London: HMSO; 1969.

Sweet J, Huttly S, Taylor I, eds. Medical, dental and veterinary education. London: Kogan Page; 2003

Turner T B. Fundamentals of medical education. Springfield, Indiana: Charles C Thomas; 1963.

Walker R M. Medical education in Britain. London: Nuffield Provincial Hospitals Trust; 1965.

Welch W H. Papers and Addresses. Volume III Medical Education. MDCCCCXX. Baltimore: Johns Hopkins Press.

Wilson R M. The beloved physician. Sir James Mackenzie. London: John Murray; 1926.

Chinese medicine

Confucius. The Analects. London: Penguin Classics; 1979.

Cotterell A. China: a history. London: Pimlico Books; 1990.

Hsu E. The transmission of Chinese medicine. Cambridge: Cambridge University Press; 1999.

Huard P, Wong M. Chinese medicine. London: World University Press, Weidenfeld and Nicolson; 1968.

Lao Tzu. Tao Te Ching. London: Penguin Classics; 1963.

Maciocia G. The foundations of Chinese medicine. Edinburgh: Churchill Livingstone; 1989.

Morse W R. Chinese medicine. New York: Clio Medica. AMS Press; 1978. [Reprint of 1938 edition.]

Veith I. The Yellow Emperor's Classic of Internal Medicine. Los Angeles: University of California Press; 1972.

Wong K C, Wu L–T. History of Chinese medicine. China: The Tientsin Press Ltd; 1932.

Egyptian medicine

Ghalioungui P. The house of life: per ankh: magic and medical science in Ancient Egypt. Amsterdam: B M Israel; 1972.

Hurry J B. Imhotep: the Vizier and Physician of King Zoser and afterwards, the Egyptian god of medicine. Oxford: Oxford University Press; 1926.

Mahfouz N B. The history of medical education in Egypt. Cairo Government Press; 1935.

Nunn J F. Ancient Egyptian medicine. London: British Museum Press; 1997.

Greek medicine

Anonymus Londonensis. Translated by Jones W H S. Cambridge: Cambridge University Press; 1947.

Hippocratic writings. Translated by Chadwick J, Mann W N. London: Penguin Books; 1978.

Hippocrates. Translated by Jones W H S, Withington W H S. LCL 4 vols. London: Heinemann; 1923–31.

Roman medicine

Allbutt T C. Greek medicine in Rome. London: Macmillan and Co; 1921.

Galen. Selected Works. Translated by Singer P N. Oxford: Oxford University Press; 1997.

Jackson R. Doctors and diseases in the Roman Empire. London: British Museum Publications; 1988.

Nutton V. The perils of patriotism: Pliny and Roman medicine. In: French R, Greenaway F, eds. Science in the early Roman Empire: Pliny the elder: his sources and influence. London: Croom Helm; 1986.

Arabian medicine

Browne E G. Arabian medicine: the Fitzpatrick lectures 1919–20. Royal College of Physicians. Cambridge: Cambridge University Press; 1962.

Gruner O C. A treatise on the Cannon of Medicine of Avicenna. Incorporating a translation of the First Book. London: Luzac & Co; 1930.

Jumay I. Treatise to Salah ad-din on the revival of the art of medicine. Translated by Fahndrich H. Wiesbaden: Deutsche Morgenlandische Gesellschaft; 1983.

Maimonides. The Book of Knowledge. Translated Russell H M, Weinberg J. Royal College of Physicians of Edinburgh; 1981.

Middle Ages

Bannerman J. The Beatons: a medical kindred in the classical Gaelic tradition. Edinburgh: John Donald Publishers Ltd; 1998.

Bayon H P. The masters of Salerno and the origins of professional medical practice. In: Underwood E A, ed. Science medicine and history: essays on the evolution of scientific thought and medical practice. In honour of Charles Singer. Oxford: Oxford University Press; 1953.

Clay R M. The medieval hospitals of England. London: Methuen and Co; 1909.

Harrington J. The School of Salernum: Regimen Sanitatis Salerni. The English Version. Salerno: Ente Provinciale per il Turismo; 1966.

Kristeller P O. The School of Salerno: its development and contribution to the history of learning. Bulletin of the History of Medicine. XVII; 1945.

Lawn B. The Prose Salernitan Questions. Oxford: Oxford University Press; 1979.

Parente P P. The Regimen of Health by the medical school of Salerno. New York: Vantage Press; 1967.

Riesman D. The story of medicine in the middle ages. New York: Paul B. Hoeber; 1936.

Rossetti L The University of Padua: an outline of its history. Trieste: Edizioni Lint; 1987.

Schlesssner M R. Manuscript sources of medieval medicine: a book of essays. New York: Garland Publishing; 1995.

Siraisi N G. Medieval and early renaissance medicine. An introduction to knowledge and practice. Chicago: University of Chicago Press; 1990.

Talbot C H. Medicine in medieval England. London: Oldbourne Books; 1967.

The sixteenth century

Bacon F. The essays. John Pitcher, ed. Harmondsworth, England: Penguin Books; 1985.

Bacon F. The advancement of learning. Chicago: Encyclopaedia Britannica, Inc; 1952.

Calder A. Molière: the theory and practice of comedy. London: The Athlone Press; 1993.

Durling R J. An early manual for the medical student and newly-fledged practitioner. Martin Stainpeis' Liber de modo studendi seu legendi in medicina. Vienna 1520. Amsterdam: Clio Medica; 1970.

Gillies H C. Regimen Sanitatis: a Gaelic manuscript from the 16th Century. Glasgow: Alex MacLaren; 1911.

Grell O P, Cunningham, A, eds. Medicine and the reformation. London: Routledge; 1993.

Joseph H. Shakespeare's son-in-law. John Hall: man and physician. 1976. Privately printed.

Lowe P. The Whole Course of Chirurgerie. 1597. Facsimile Edition. Classics of Medicine Library; 1981.

Marland H, Pelling M, eds. The task of healing: medicine, religion and gender in England and the Netherlands, 1450–1800. Rotterdam: Erasmus Publishing; 1996.

More T. Utopia. Wordsworth Classics.

Pelling M, Webster C. In: Webster C, ed. Health, medicine and mortality in the sixteenth century. Cambridge: Cambridge University Press; 1979.

Siraisi N. Avicenna in Renaissance Italy: The Canon and medical teaching in Italian universities after 1500. New Jersey: Princeton University Press; 1987.

Simpson R R. Shakespeare and medicine. Edinburgh: E and S Livingstone; 1959.

The seventeenth century

Brockliss L, Jones C. The medical world of early modern France. Oxford: Clarendon Press; 1997.

Bylebyl J J, ed. William Harvey and his age: the professional and social context of the discovery of the circulation. Baltimore: Johns Hopkins University Press; 1979.

Descartes R. Discourse on method. Harmondsworth, England: Penguin Books; 1968.

Dewhurst K. Dr Thomas Sydenham (1624–1689): his life and original writings. London: The Wellcome Historical Medical Library; 1966.

French R, Wear A, eds. The medical revolution of the seventeenth century. Cambridge: Cambridge University Press; 1989.

Kaplan B B. Divulging of useful truths in Physick: the medical agenda of Robert Boyle. Baltimore: Johns Hopkins University Press; 1993.

Sydenham T. The works of Thomas Sydenham: with a life of the author by R G Latham London: The Sydenham Society; 1848.

The eighteenth century

Allen E, Turk J L, Murley R, eds. The Case Books of John Hunter FRS. London: Royal Society of Medicine; 1993.

Broadie A, ed. The Scottish enlightenment: an anthology. Edinburgh: Cannogate Classics; 1997.

Bynum W F, Porter R, eds. William Hunter and the 18th century medical world. Cambridge: Cambridge University Press; 1985.

Cunningham A, French R, eds. The medical enlightenment of the eighteenth century. Cambridge: Cambridge University Press; 1990.

Dobson J. John Hunter. Edinburgh: E and S Livingstone; 1969.

Doig A, Fergusson J P S, Milne I A, Passmore R, eds. William Cullen and the eighteenth century medical world. Edinburgh: Edinburgh University Press; 1993.

Finch E. The influence of the Hunters on medical education. Annals Roy Coll Surgeons of England 1957; 20: 205–248.

Gloyne S R. John Hunter. Edinburgh: E and S Livingstone; 1950.

Gray E A. Portrait of a surgeon. London: Robert Hale Ltd; 1952.

Houston J. Memoirs of the life and travels of James Houston, M.D. from the year 1690 to this present year 1747. Collected and written by his own hand. London; 1747.

Hunter W. An anatomical description of the gravid uterus and its contents. London: J Johnson and G Nicol; 1794.

Hunter W. Medical Commentaries. Containing a plain and direct answer to Professor Munro Junior. Interspersed with remarks on the structure functions and diseases of several parts of the human body. London: A Hamilton; 1762–4.

Hunter W. Two introductory Lectures, delivered by Dr William Hunter, to his last course of anatomical lectures at his theatre in Windmill Street: as they were left corrected for the press by himself. To which are added, some papers relating to Dr Hunter's intended plan, for establishing a museum in London, for the improvement of anatomy, surgery and physic. London; 1784.

Johnstone J. A guide for gentlemen studying medicine at the University of Edinburgh. London: Robinson; 1792.

Kaufman M H. Medical Teaching in Edinburgh during the 18th and 19th centuries. Edinburgh: Royal College of Surgeons; 2003.

Kemp M, ed. William Hunter at the Royal Academy of Arts. Glasgow: University of Glasgow Press; 1975.

King-Hele D. Erasmus Darwin: a life of unequalled achievement. London: DLM Publishing; 2000.

Knoeff R. Herman Boerhaave (1668–1738): Calvinist chemist and physician. Amsterdam: Koninklijke Nederlandse Akademie van Wetenschappen; 2002.

Lawrence S C. Charitable knowledge: hospital pupils and practitioners in eighteenth century. London: Cambridge University Press; 1966.

Lindeboom G A. Herman Boerhaave, the man and his work. London: Methuen; 1968.

Moore W. The knife man: the extraordinary life and times of John Hunter, father of modern surgery. London: Bantam Press; 2005.

Rosser L. Medical education in the age of improvement: Edinburgh students and apprentices 1760–1826. Edinburgh: Edinburgh University Press; 1991.

Smollett T. The adventures of Roderick Random. Oxford World Classics; 1979.

Underwood E A. Boerhaave's men: at Leyden and after. Edinburgh: Edinburgh University Press; 1977.

The nineteenth century

Bartrip P W J. Mirror of medicine: a history of the BMJ. Oxford: Clarendon; 1990.

Bell E M. Storming the citadel: the rise of the woman doctor. London: Constable and Co Ltd.; 1953.

Bernard C. An Introduction to the study of Experimental Medicine. Translated by Greene H C with an introduction by L J Henderson. New York: The Macmillan Co; 1927.

Billroth T. The Medical Sciences in the German Universities: with an Introduction by W.H. Welch. New York: Macmillan Company; 1924.

Bynum W F. The science and practice of medicine in the nineteenth century. Cambridge: Cambridge University Press; 1994.

Bynmu W F, Lock S, Porter R, eds. Medical journals and medical knowledge. London: Routledge; 1992.

Chadwick E. Report on the sanitary condition of the labouring population of Great Britain. 1842.

Evans R J. Death in Hamburg: society and politics in the cholera years. London: Penguin Books; 1990.

French R, Wear A. British medicine in an age of Reform. London: Routledge; 1991.

Guthrie D. Extramural medical education in Edinburgh, and the School of Medicine of the Royal Colleges. Edinburgh: E and S Livingstone Ltd.; 1965.

Ibsen H. An enemy of the people. Oxford: The World's Classics, Oxford University Press.

Keele K D. The evolution of clinical methods in medicine: being the FitzPatrick Lectures at the Royal College of Physicians 1960–1. London: Pitman Medical Publishing; 1963.

Manson-Bahr P. History of the School of Tropical Medicine in London (1899–1949). London: H.K. Lewis; 1956.

Newman C. The evolution of medical education in the 19th century. London: Oxford University Press; 1957.

Osler W. Aequanimitas and other addresses. London: H K Lewis; 1904.

Peterson M J. The medical profession in mid-Victorian London. Berkeley: University of California Press; 1978.

Roberts S. Sophia Jex-Blake: a woman pioneer in nineteenth century medical reform. London: Routledge; 1993.

Romano T M. Making medicine scientific: John Burdon Sanderson and the culture of Victorian science. Baltimore: Johns Hopkins University Press; 2002.

Simon J. English sanitary institutions. 2nd edn. London: John Murray; 1897.

Sprigge S S. The life and times of Thomas Wakley. 1879. New York: R.E.Krieger Publishing Co; 1974 reprint.

Travers G (Margaret Todd). Mona Maclean: medical student: a novel. London and Glasgow: Collins; 1892.

Welch W H. Papers and addresses by William Henry Welch. Volume III, Medical Education. Baltimore: Johns Hopkins Press; MDCCCCXX.

Wilson R M. The beloved physician: Sir James Mackenzie. London: John Murray; 1926.

Walker M E M. Pioneers of public health: the story of some benefactors of the human race. Edinburgh: Oliver and Boyd; 1930.

American medical education

Barzansky B, Gevitz, N, eds. Beyond Flexner. Medical education in the twentieth century. New York: Greenwood Press; 1992.

Bowles M D, Dawson V P. With one voice: the Association of American Medical Colleges 1876–2002. Washington: AAMC; 2002.

Brock W R. Scotus Americanus: a survey of the sources for links between Scotland and America in the eighteenth century. Edinburgh: Edinburgh University Press; 1982.

Field J. Medical education in the United States: late nineteenth and twentieth centuries. In: O'Malley C D. The history of medical education. Berkeley: University of California Press; 1970.

Flexner A. I remember. An autobiography. Simon and Schuster: New York; 1940.

Flexner A. Medical education in the United States and Canada (The Flexner Report). New York: Carnegie Foundation for the Advancement of Learning; 1910.

Flexner A. Medical education: a comparative study. New York: Macmillan Company; 1925.

Fishbein M. A history of the American Medical Association. Philadelphia: Sanders; 1947.

Hodges B. The many and conflicting histories of medical education in Canada and the USA: an introduction to the paradigm wars. Medical Education 2005; 39: 613–21.

Jonas S. Medical mystery: the training of doctors in the United States. New York: W.W. Norton and Co; 1978.

Kaufman M. American medical education. Westport, Conn.: Greenwood Press; 1976.

Ludmerer K M. Learning to heal: the development of American medical education. New York: Basic Books; 1985.

Medical Education. Final Report on the Commission on Medical Education. New York: American Association of Medical Colleges; New York.

Miller G E. Educating medical teachers. Cambridge, Mass.: Harvard University Press; 1980.

Morgan J. A discourse upon the institution of medical schools in America. With a preface containing, amongst other things, the Author's apology for attempting to introduce the regular mode of practising physic in Philadelphia. Philadelphia; 1765.

Norwood W F N. Medical education in the United States before 1900. In: O'Malley C D. The history of medical education. Berkeley: University of California Press; 1970.

Norwood W F N. Medical Education in the United States before the civil war. Philadelphia: University of Pennsylvania; 1944.

Shryock R H. Medicine in America; historical essays. Baltimore: Johns Hopkins Press; 1966.

Shryock R H. The development of modern medicine. New York: 1947.

Welch W H. Papers and addresses by William Henry Welch. Volume III, Medical Education. Baltimore: Johns Hopkins Press; MDCCCCXX.

Welche W H. Medical Education in the United States. Harvey Lectures, 1915–16. 11: 366–82.

The twentieth century

Aird I. The making of a surgeon. London: Butterworths; 1961.

Barzansky B, Gevitz N, eds. Beyond Flexner: medical education in the twentieth century. New York: Greenwood Press; 1992.

British Medical Association. Secret remedies; what they cost and what they contain. London: British Medical Association; 1909.

The Christchurch Conference on Postgraduate Medical Education. BMJ 1962; 1: 466–7.

Commission on Medical Education. Final Report on the Commission on Medical Education. New York: Office of the Director of Study, American Medical Colleges; 1932.

Committee on Higher Education. Higher Education: Report of the Committee appointed by the Prime Minister under the chairmanship of Lord Robbins, 1961-1963. London: HMSO; 1963.

Department of Health and Social Security. Report of the Working Party on the Responsibilities of the Consultant Grade. (The Godber Report) London: HMSO; 1969.

Dubos R. The mirage of health. New York: Doubleday Anchor Books; 1959.

Edinburgh Pathological Club. An Inquiry into the Medical Curriculum. Edinburgh: W.Green and Sons; 1919.

Freidson E. The profession of medicine. New York: Dodd, Mead and Company; 1975.

General Medical Council. Recommendations as to the medical curriculum. London: HMSO; 1947.

General Medical Council. Recommendations as to the medical curriculum. London: HMSO; 1957.

Hastings Center. The Goals of Medicine. Setting New Priorities. The Hastings Center Report; 1996.

Illich I D. Medical nemesis: the expropriation of health. London: Calder and Boyars; 1975.

Inter-Departmental Committee on Medical Schools. Report of the Inter-Departmental Committee on Medical Schools (Goodenough Report). London: HMSO; 1944.

Kennedy I. The unmasking of medicine. London: Allen & Unwin; 1981.

McKeown T. The role of medicine. Oxford: Basil Blackwell; 1979.

Newman G. Notes on medical education in England. A memorandum address to the President of the Board of Education. London: HMSO; 1918, Cmmd 9124.

The Royal College of Physicians of London. Revision of the Medical Curriculum. Lancet 1956; (i): 437–9.

Royal College of General Practitioners. Forty Years on. The story of the first forty years of the Royal College of General Practitioners. RCGP; 1992.

Royal Commission on Medical Education. London: HMSO; 1968.

Social Services Committee. Fourth Report from the Social Services Committee. Medical Education, With special reference to the number of doctors and the career structure in hospitals. (the Short Report). London: HMSO; 1981.

Wear D, Bickel J, eds. Educating for professionalism: creating a culture of humanism in medical education. Iowa City: University of Iowa Press; 2000.

Miller H G. Medicine and Society. London: Oxford University Press; 1973.

Roles, values, boundaries of the profession

Alberti G. Professionalism—time for a new look. Clinical Medicine 2003; 3: 91.

AMA. Professing medicine: strengthening the ethics of professionalism of tomorrow's physicians. American Medical Association; 2002.

Association of American Medical Colleges. Physicians for the 21st century. Report of the project panel on the general professional education of the physician and college preparation for medicine. J Med Educ Suppl, November 1984, Part 2.

Barrows H S, Tamblyn R M. Problem-based learning: an approach to medical education. New York: Springer Publishing Co; 1980.

Becker H S, et al. Boys in white: student culture in medical school. Chicago: University of Chicago Press; 1961.

Calman K C. Quality: a view from the centre. Quality in Health Care 1992; 1: 28–32.

Calman K C. Quality of life in cancer patients—an hypothesis. J Med Ethics 1984; 10: 124–127.

Calman K C. The potential for health. Oxford University Press; 1998.

Calman K C. The profession of medicine. BMJ 1994; 309: 1140–3.

Cogan M I. Toward a definition of profession. Harvard Educational Review 1953; XXIII: 33–50.

Couleham J. Today's professionalism: engaging the mind but not the heart. Acad Med 2005; 80: 892–98.

Francis C K. Professionalism and the medical student. Lancet 2004; 364: 1647–8.

Freidson E. Profession of medicine: a study of the sociology of applied knowledge. New York: Dodd, Mead and Company; 1970.

Hastings Center. The Goals of Medicine. Setting New Priorities. The Hastings Center Report; 1996.

Huddle T S. Teaching professionalism: is medical morality a competency? Acad Med 2005; 80: 885–91.

Hunter D, Bomford R R. Hutchison's Clinical Methods. 13th edn. London: Cassell; 1956.

Irvine D. The doctor's tale: professionalism and public trust. Oxford: Radcliffe Medical Press; 2003.

Irvine D. The performance of doctors. I: professionalism and self regulation in a changing world. BMJ 1997; 314: 1540–2.

Irvine D. The performance of doctors. II: maintaining good practice, protecting patients from poor performance. BMJ 1997; 314: 1613–5.

Medical professionalism in the new millennium: a physicians' charter. Lancet 2002; 359: 520–22.

Sritharan K, et al. Medical Oaths and declarations. BMJ 2001; 323: 1440–1.

Tallis R. Hippocratic Oaths: medicine and its discontents. London: Atlantic Books; 2004.

Veloski J J, Fields S K, Boex J R, Blank L L. Measuring professionalism: a review of studies with instruments reported in the literature between 1982 and 2002. Acad Med 2005; 80: 366–70.

Watkinson P. On professionalism. Clinical Medicine 2004; 4: 201–2.

White G E. Setting and maintaining professional role boundaries: an educational strategy. Medical Education 2004; 38: 903–910.

Beyond learning

Kuhn T S. The structure of scientific revolutions. 3rd edn. Chicago: University of Chicago Press; 1996.

Pickstone J, ed. Medical innovations in historical perspective. London: Macmillan; 1992.

McKinlay J B. From promising report to standard procedure: seven stages in the career of a medical innovation. Millbank Memorial Fund Quarterly 1981; 59: 374–411.

Stanton J, ed. Innovations in health and medicine: diffusion and resistance in the 20th Century. London: Routledge; 2002.

Preparation for teaching

Carlisle C, Donovan T, Mercer D, eds. Interprofessional education. An agenda for healthcare professionals. Salisbury, England: Quay Books; 2005.

General Medical Council. The doctor as teacher. London: HMSO; 1999.

Gibbs G, Coffey M. The impact of training of university teachers on their teaching skills, their approach to teaching and the approach to learning of their students. Active Learning in Higher Education 2004; 5: 87–100.

Godfrey J, Welsh C. Training the trainers: do teaching courses develop teaching skills? Med Educ 2004; 38: 844–47.

Greenaway H. The Training of University Teachers. Society for Research in Higher Education, Pamphlet 1; 1971.

Highet G. The art of teaching. London: Methuen and Co; 1963.

Matheson C C. Academic staff training and development in universities of the United Kingdom. A Review 1961–81. Issues and distributed by the Co-ordinating Committee for the Training of University Teachers; 1981.

The National Committee of Inquiry into Higher Education Higher Education in the learning society (The Dearing Report); 1997

Royal Commission on University Education in London. Final Report 1913 (The Haldane Commission) London: HMSO; 1913: Cmnd 6717; 26.

University Grants Committee. Report of the Committee on University Teaching Methods. [Chairman, Sir Edward Hale.] London: HMSO; 1964; 52.

Ethics, arts and humanities

Bayntun C. A medical student's experience of being taught medical ethics. Bull Med Ethics 2004; 201: 13–18.

Calman K C. A study of storytelling, humour and learning in medicine. London: Stationery Office; 2000.

Calman K C, Downie R S, Duthie M, Sweeney B. Literature and medicine: a short course for medical students. Med Educ 1988; 22: 265–9.

Downie R S, Macnaughton J. Clinical judgement: evidence in practice. Oxford: Oxford University Press; 2000.

Elster J, von Troil H, eds. How best to teach medical ethics. Report from a Workshop March 2003, Nordic Committee on Bioethics and NorFA, TemaNord. 2004: 519.

Evans M, Louhiala P, Puustinen R. Philosophy for medicine: applications in a clinical context. Oxford: Radcliffe Medical Press Limited; 2004.

Goldie J. Review of ethics curricula in undergraduate medical education. Med Educ 2000; 34:108-119.

Goldie J, Schwartz L, McConnachie A, Morrison J. The impact of a modern curriculum on students' proposed behaviour on meeting moral dilemmas. Med Educ 2004; 38: 942–9.

Gross M L. Medical ethics education: to what ends? J Eval Clin Pract 2001: 7: 387–97.

Jones A H. Carson R A. Medical humanities at the University of Texas Medical Branch at Galveston. Acad Med 2003; 78: 1006–9.

Lancaster T, Hart R, Gardner S. Literature and medicine: evaluating a special study module using the nominal group technique. Med Educ 2002; 36: 1071–1076.

Lehmann L S, Kasoff P, Federman D D. A survey of medical ethics education at US and Canadian medical schools. Acad Med 2004; 79: 682–9.

Louhiala P. Philosophy for medical students—why, what, and how. Med Humanities 2003; 29: 87–8.

Macnaughton J, White M, Stacey R. Research in the benefits of art and health. Health Education. (In Press)

Roff S, Preece P. Helping medical students to find their moral compasses: ethics teaching for second and third year undergraduates. J Med Ethics 2004; 30: 487–9.

Shapiro J, Duke A, Boker J, Ahearn C S. Just a spoonful of humanities makes the medicine go down: introducing literature into a family medicine clerkship. Med Educ 2005; 39: 605–612.

Singer P. Strengthening the role of ethics in medical education. Canad Med Assoc J 2003; 168: 854–5.

Smith S, Fryer-Edwards K, Diekema D S, Braddock C H. Finding effective strategies for teaching ethics: a comparison trial of two interventions. Acad Med 2004; 79: 265–71.

Vernon B. Teaching about ethical issues: getting down to the basics of medical practice. Clinical Teacher 2005; 2: 66–8.

Watkins P. The healing environment. Clin Med 2005; 5: 197–8.

Wayne D B, Muir J C, DaRosa D A. Developing an ethics curriculum for an internal medicine residency program: use of needs assessment. Teach Learn Med 2004; 16: 197–201.

Whong-Barr M. Clinical ethics teaching in Britain: a history of the London Medical Group. New Rev Bioeth 2003; 1: 73–84.

Index

Note: Page numbers in *italics* refer to pictures, cartoons or boxes.

E